Cultivating Compassion

Pip Hardy • Tony Sumner
Editors

Cultivating Compassion

How Digital Storytelling is Transforming Healthcare

Second Edition

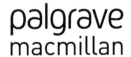

palgrave
macmillan

Editors
Pip Hardy
Patient Voices, Pilgrim Projects
Landbeach, Cambridgeshire, UK

Tony Sumner
Patient Voices, Pilgrim Projects
Landbeach, Cambridgeshire, UK

ISBN 978-3-319-64145-4   ISBN 978-3-319-64146-1   (eBook)
https://doi.org/10.1007/978-3-319-64146-1

Library of Congress Control Number: 2017953880

Cover illustration: Maciej Bledowski / Alamy Stock Photo

Printed on acid-free paper

This Palgrave Macmillan imprint is published by Springer Nature
The registered company is Springer International Publishing AG
The registered company address is: Gewerbestrasse 11, 6330 Cham, Switzerland

Foreword to the First Edition

Humans have probably been telling stories from the moment they invented language. Narrative accounts of people's experiences—factual or invented—have been a central focus of social interaction throughout history, the main means by which our ancestors shared information about the world. Stories are still a central focus of our learning. They create powerful images that help us understand and interpret events. Using stories we can describe events vividly, see them from alternative viewpoints, engage our emotions and our brains, challenge assumptions and aid creative reflection.

This is a book of stories about stories. Each chapter is written by someone who has personal experience of using digital stories to stimulate learning or improve healthcare. They describe how the stories have been used to help trainees understand and come to terms with the challenges of their new roles, how they have helped newly qualified clinicians cope with emotional traumas encountered during their work and how hospital boards have used the stories to recapture their focus on the needs of service users. Here we can learn what it's like to feature in a digital story and how to make them. Like all the best storytellers, the stories about stories are narrated in a direct and compelling manner, with detailed accounts of listeners' reactions and the circumstances in which they viewed them.

Modern healthcare is highly technical. It relies on biomedical science, sophisticated equipment, information technology, data and statistics, complex organisational systems, protocols and project management. This wealth of technologies sometimes threatens to overwhelm us, squeezing out the more personal aspects of healthcare and its essential qualities—caring, compassion and empathy. Digital stories provide a way to redress the balance. They are a powerful means of giving voice to the experiences and concerns of patients and service users, helping to ensure that those working in this complex system maintain their focus on the people they are there to help.

The reader will find here a wealth of practical ideas on how personal narratives can be used as a tool for teaching, learning and quality improvement. It reminds us that compassion must be at the heart of healthcare, and this can be achieved only when those who work in the system listen to and learn from patients' experiences. The book is a fitting celebration of the remarkable ten-year history of the Patient Voices Programme and its crucial contribution to putting the personal back into healthcare.

21 October 2013   Angela Coulter

Foreword to the Second Edition

More than a decade has passed since I first met Pip Hardy and Tony Sumner. During that time their work has evolved in ways I could not possibly imagine. In reviewing this newest edition of this collection of essays, I am struck by several things.

First, I am awed by the sheer volume of insights about the use of Digital Storytelling in the healthcare context and, by analogy, the use of Digital Storytelling as a tool in human services in general. As a story facilitator and creative writing, media and performing arts educator for more than 30 years, I have collected a significant library of books on story and storytelling in the fields of business, education, social services and health. This book is the single most complete summary of the application of story-based communication in any profession I have read.

Second, I am impressed by how completely Pip, Tony and the other collaborating writers have integrated their goals and aspirations for the methods of the Digital Storytelling workshop, this marvellous tool we as facilitators take for granted, with the goals and aspirations of the healthcare entities and institutions that have engaged them. At all points you are made aware of the deep respect that Pip, Tony and company have for the challenges of healthcare professionals, and that these same professionals seem to have for Pip, Tony and their collaborators.

Third, the book reminds me that healthcare provision is an endlessly complex issue. (*Who Knew?* as our unfortunate new US President quipped). For a society to commit to equitable lifelong health services support, the contradicting tensions are enormous, most evidently, the seeming tension between cost and compassion. This book adds weight to the argument that when we take care of people ahead of their crisis (as patients, as caregivers), when we stop and hold each other's stories with dignity and respect, we do in fact create the conditions for more efficient and cost-effective implementation.

Finally, this book is about the experience of being a patient, a carer or a health professional—all people. The most valuable component of Pip and Tony's efforts is how they serve as advocates for the voices of both those who receive and those who deliver healthcare. Big processes, big data, leaves so many, many people invisible; their needs, hopes and traumas, large and small, reduced to small ticks on an accounting sheet. This book reminds us again that every story matters, every story informs. While the great chaos of our mass communication society might privilege and surface certain stories over others, down on the ground, when a nurse or doctor greets their next patient, for that moment, no other stories matter. Two people being present, looking for a way to help or be helped, if not with a solution, then with kindness and understanding.

So as you wander this book's pages, consider yourself fortunate to have so much considered reflection on the way story, and specifically Digital Storytelling, works in our communication processes in one place.

As they delineate and explicate all these unique and wonderful projects, also be reminded that the starting point for all this work is love.

Pip and Tony love what they do.

And they bring love into every aspect of their doing it.

I hope you enjoy it as much as I have.

May 2017   Joe Lambert

Patient Voices: In Celebration

At that first digital story workshop ten years ago, the greeting said it all.

'Hello Monica, how are you?' said Pip, *not* followed by 'How's John?' For I was there about me.

It was the first time that I realised that I had losses too, for I was invited to tell MY story. Up to then it was—as it should be—about how ill my husband, John, was, how he had lost his ability to speak, to read, to eat, to move because of the stroke.

That was the first time that I, as his carer, was given my own platform.

Soon I came to feel the openness and objectivity of that platform, where pain is allowed to reveal its own prose and poetry, feeding on the experiences of others whose pain shadowed mine, yet enriched mine, showing me new ways of being.

There we all were, so different from each other. We started off in faltering, hushed tones, but soon our voices became bolder as we allowed the harshness of our daily lives to break through surfaces of politeness and reserve. That first hour was intense. I tried to find words for emotions which had not been written with, or for, words.

But when the words started to flow, they strung themselves together in a magical way, forming patterns of expression which I did not know existed within me. And pictures started to appear too. With gentle encouragement resting in long silences, the pictures emerged from somewhere within the clouds of my loss and bewilderment, giving meaning to faltering words which became sentences, paragraphs, chapters and then a story.

My story, as I saw it, for the first time being recorded for others also to see.

Not an easy task, for I have this fear of being seen as an 'angel'. It makes my senses go weird when people say, 'I don't think I'd be able to do what you're doing. You're an angel'.

I remember talking about that on that first morning. I told the group about how, returning from a regular early morning swim, my grocer-friend was, as he does each day, putting out his fruit and vegetables on the pavement, and as I passed, he called me over.

'Does John know that you're having an affair?' he asked.

I gasped. I could not believe that he had been watching me coming back from my swim three times a week, which I rushed to do while the home-help gave John his morning bath—he watched me return, not having seen me leave, believing I'd spent the night out!

And there I was on that first morning, able to talk about this. For the first time I could speak about how confused I was by this contradiction within me. For yes, I realised, I do not want to be seen as anything other than a dutiful wife, looking after her man till death us part. Yet I don't want to be seen as an angel.

How relieved I felt that morning when I could talk, and laugh, about this angel business. We talked, said things like they needed to be said, and our stories started to form their own shapes.

Talking about my journey, my understanding, my bewilderment, my anger, helped me to realise that all is well, for the strengths which I did not know I had in me slowly started to reveal themselves. I saw them through the reactions of those around me, whose stories mingled with mine in mutual tenacity and courage. Our tears, our laughter brought us together in an amazing commonality and showed us that pain does not respect education, money or class.

I spoke openly with everyone in the room about all sorts of intimate things, and they understood. Nobody judged. Nobody opinionated. Though I feared criticism, it never came. So I spoke, wrote, captured images and pictures, and, with the Pilgrims' help and careful editing, pulled the different threads into understandable digital stories.

Thank you Pilgrims, not only for the platform you make available through your workshops, but also for the skills which each of us walk away with after a day of speaking our shyness and whispering our private fears to sympathetic others. Thank you for opening up to us the opportunity to place our experiences under the microscope of realisation, acceptance and reality.

Thank you for teaching us a skill which we would otherwise not even have dreamt existed: learning to record our stories digitally for others, including the medical, health and social care professionals, to learn from. And thank you for recording their stories too, for it gives us an equal insight into their world, to learn from their stories so as to show us that we are all on the same side.

You have helped so many of us start that special process of healing which comes from honesty and acceptance, a path upon which our next generations can build and improve.

And thank you for facilitating the lasting friendships which we have come away with.

To the readers of this book I say, if you are thinking of making your story—or making it possible for others to make their stories—you are in for a surprise, for you are going to receive that special gift of freedom which can come only from acceptance and revelation. Do not be afraid to liberate yourself—and others.

Listen. Learn. Understand. Share YOUR story—your stories—and the stories of those for whom you care and with whom you work. Only then can others gain from your insights and experiences.

25 October 2013   Monica Clarke

Monica's stories can be seen at: www.patientvoices.org.uk/mclarke.htm

Preface

It was a dark and stormy November night, not many years into the new millennium. We were enjoying dinner with old friends. As the evening drew to a close, and our friends were heading for the door, Brendan turned and said 'Oh, there's something I've been meaning to show you. Have you ever heard of a digital story?' We had not.

He switched on his laptop, turned up the volume and played a very short video. But it was no ordinary video. It lasted less than two minutes, consisted of a series of still pictures, the voice of the narrator, a bit of piano music in the background and no video footage. It was a story told by a mother about her daughter—and the joy and pain of watching her grow up. Her voice cracked with emotion.

It was one of those 'Ah ha' moments.

As we wiped our eyes, we realised that this could be the solution to the dilemma of how we could, creatively and effectively, bring the voice of the patient into e-learning materials that were designed to contribute to the development of effective, safe, humane and reflective healthcare practitioners.

The digital story that we had just seen—told with unquestionable authenticity and undeniable poignancy—conveyed something that really mattered to the storyteller. We walked in the mother's shoes for those moments, and we learned a great deal about her in a very short space of time. In less than two minutes, it raised lots of questions, inviting the viewer to question assumptions and consider and re-consider values.

This short multimedia form, at that time used almost exclusively in community history and community development, seemed to us to provide the perfect vehicle for conveying 'the patient voice' and utilising these powerful personal stories to promote reflection, prompt discussion and debate, highlight opportunities for learning and improvement, encourage the cultivation of empathy and compassion, and remind all those engaged in the business of healthcare of our shared humanity. We knew that stories like the one we had just seen could transform the learning materials we were designing, by giving people a different kind of learning opportunity: one that engaged hearts as well as minds, one that prompted deep reflection and exploration of values.

A few days later we showed that first digital story to our colleague Paul Stanton, the then head of Board Development at the Modernisation Agency's Clinical Governance Support Team. We had been working closely with him on a large research and development project about clinical governance for primary care trust board teams; he was also one of the expert advisers on the Royal College of Nursing's Clinical Governance e-learning modules.

As *he* wiped *his* eyes, he commented: 'I know what you're thinking'.

And so, in 2003, we, the editors of this book, embarked on a quest or, perhaps, in retrospect, a pilgrimage. We wanted patients everywhere to be treated with justice, dignity, humanity, respect and compassion. We wanted the same for all the people who deliver healthcare.

Actually, our goal was nothing less than a transformation in healthcare which, we believed, could come about if people—healthcare providers, managers, decision-makers, policymakers—would take the opportunity to listen to and learn from the stories of the people they served. We believed that there was a new and important kind of knowledge contained in these stories that was every bit as important as knowing how to take a temperature, measure blood pressure or insert a catheter. While Evidence-Based Healthcare was intended to establish the standard for high-quality, safe and effective clinical care, we wanted to offer the Evidence of Experience to weight the scales a little more towards the person and a little less to the disease. We wanted to offer all those who design and deliver healthcare an opportunity to walk in someone else's shoes for just a few moments—to gain some insight into their experience—and then to reflect on their own practice, their own values.

Quests are rarely easy, and ours has been no exception.

Our journey has, quite literally, taken us around the world. We have been to interesting places, met extraordinary people, faced many challenges and learned many new things. We have taken wrong turns, headed up blind alleys, stumbled and picked ourselves up again. We have definitely encountered some dragons, but with our particular blend of stubbornness and idealism, we have carried on, frequently reminded that the journey is often more important than the destination.

Along the way, we have facilitated nearly 200 projects and workshops, met well over 1000 storytellers and recorded their stories, conducted research into the uses and impact of the stories, produced several publications, contributed chapters to books on digital storytelling and presented our work at dozens of conferences around the world.

As a means of educating clinicians through involving patients, carers and service users, the Patient Voices approach to digital storytelling has gained recognition throughout the international healthcare community as well as the international digital storytelling community.

The first edition of this book was published in 2014 to mark an important milestone: the celebration of ten years of the Patient Voices Programme. Now, three years on, we still haven't reached the end of our journey, and there is still more to say.

But by now, you may be asking yourself: What are Patient Voices? Who are Patient Voices? What are digital stories? How do they work? What happens in the workshops? Who actually creates the stories? What happens to them? Who benefits from the stories? Can you quantify the benefit? Why should providers and commissioners of healthcare services be interested in digital stories? Can you teach compassion and empathy? Is digital storytelling a therapy? How could I use Patient Voices digital stories in my work/with my team? Can the stories be used in education? Can they be used in research? These are some of the questions that arise when introducing Patient Voices and which this book will try to answer.

About This Book

It is a common literary device for a group of friends, colleagues, travellers or, as in Chaucer's *Canterbury Tales*, fellow pilgrims, to share their individual stories while on a communal journey. We've invited our colleagues to share with you their stories of their part of the Patient Voices journey. So, this book is written in the spirit of co-production and collaboration and in recognition that the Patient Voices Programme would not exist if it were not for all those with whom we have partnered on Patient Voices projects and workshops.

Every one of the chapters is written by someone who has commissioned or participated in at least one Patient Voices Reflective Digital Storytelling workshop as part of a larger project. When authors refer to digital storytelling, they are referring to Patient Voices. When we refer to digital storytelling, we are referring to what has become known as the 'classical' digital storytelling form, developed in the mid-1990s by Joe Lambert and StoryCenter (www.storycenter.org).

Most of the authors, whether health professional, educator or service user, made their own digital stories before advocating and facilitating their further use with other health professionals or service users. They are thus able to speak from their own personal experience while also addressing fundamental theoretical, therapeutic or practical benefits and legitimate questions and concerns about the use of digital stories and digital storytelling in healthcare.

In the chapters that follow, you will read many stories of transformation, both personal and professional. People who once thought of themselves as patients have discovered their strengths, their courage and their resilience, while people who think of themselves as clinicians have become aware of their vulnerabilities—and the courage that enables them to share their stories.

Like many of our storytellers, we have also been transformed by this work that affords us the extraordinary privilege of hearing about what matters most to people. The Patient Voices Programme has become a way of life for us, a vocation, a commitment, a call to action, an opportunity to relieve suffering through a willingness to walk alongside storytellers, to listen to and accept their stories and, through the alchemical process of digital storytelling, to see storytellers grow in confidence, gain insight and come to accept themselves and their stories with new respect and, sometimes, even love.

We hope you will enjoy reading about this work as much as we have enjoyed doing it.

Cambridge   Pip Hardy
May 2017   Tony Sumner

Acknowledgements

To all the people who have given generously of their time, expertise and experiences to contribute to this book: we are more grateful than we can say. Without you there would be no book.

To all those people (and their organisations) who have sponsored workshops: thank you for your imagination, your belief in Patient Voices and your determination to find new and wonderful ways to use stories to improve the quality of the learning and care you deliver.

To more than 1000 storytellers—patients, carers, relatives, staff, managers and commissioners—all those people who have shared stories with us: thank you for giving so graciously of yourselves; you are true heroes and heroines. We would be nothing without you.

To Paul Stanton: thank you for sharing our vision and finding funding for the very first Patient Voices stories and for continuing to recognise their value even after all these years!

To Monica Clarke and the late Ian Kramer—our very first two storytellers: we are deeply indebted to you for your intelligence, generosity and honesty in sharing your stories with us and for opening our eyes to the true meaning of consent.

To Cathy, Grete, Sissel, Kristin, Henrik, Darcy, Heather, Ragnhild, Veronique, Ann, Angeline, Heather, Steve, Karen, Michael, Burcu, Brooke, Tricia, Alex, Satu, Yuko, Akiko, Daniel, Amy, Emily, Rob, Stefani, Andrea and so many others in the international digital storytelling community: thank you for encouragement and enthusiasm, for making conferences so interesting and so much fun, for wonderful conversations, for sharing food, wine, hopes, dreams and, always, stories.

To Trish Greenhalgh, Iona Heath, Angela Coulter, Robin Youngson, Rita Charon, Brian Hurwitz and many others who have paved the way for patients, stories and the humanities to play their rightful part in making healthcare more humane and more compassionate: thank you.

To Ros Connelly: a very special thank you for rescuing us from a moment of despair, bringing your editing skills and your experience of our workshops to bear on the almost-final manuscript and guiding us to the finish for the first edition—and then doing it all again for the second edition!

To Fiona O'Neill: we are grateful for that much-needed nudge and for the reminder that: 'You owe it to the storytellers to get this book finished!'—and for so much else over the years.

To Dr Jo, a thousand thanks for being such a willing apprentice/accomplice, for always knowing what needs to be done and doing it, for your quiet and gentle wisdom, for so many gifts large and small, and for taking the lead in establishing the Patient Voices Advisory Board.

To aforesaid Advisory Board, thanks in anticipation of your wise counsel and support during the next phase of our journey.

To Joe Lambert, the father of digital storytelling, and to StoryCenter: thanks is inadequate to express our gratitude for your vision, inspiration and generosity. You have shared the gift of story in and with a world filled with the technology that makes it possible for anyone and everyone who is willing to take time, reflect and consider, to create a compelling personal story that can explore identities, create and strengthen relationships, break down boundaries and promote greater understanding within and between cultures—including the vastly different cultures of patients and professionals. Your work and your lives have inspired us and hundreds of thousands of others around the world.

And finally, to our grandchildren: Lola, Otis, Luna, Martha and Isaac, for giving us an excuse to fly kites, smell flowers, feed fish, swing on swings, inspect beetles, watch clouds, read stories—and for reminding us of the things that *really* matter.

Contents

List of Figures

List of Tables

Part I

A Tale of Two Decades

Pip Hardy and Tony Sumner

I keep six honest serving-men
(They taught me all I knew);
Their names are What and Why and When
And How and Where and Who. Rudyard Kipling. (Kipling 1902)

The impetus for this book was to document some of the Patient Voices projects that have taken place since the beginning of the programme, to share the experiences and learning from those projects and to explain the history and development of the programme.

In order to understand the projects described in Parts II–VI, there needs to be an understanding of, to use Kipling's "six good serving men and true", what the Patient Voices Programme is, why it was set up, when it came to be, how it works, where it operates and who created it.

Explaining the genesis, nature, purpose and benefits of the Patient Voices Programme has always been a complex task, despite the delivery of many presentations and keynotes (please see www.patientvoices.org.uk/present.htm), completion of research studies (Hardy 2007, 2016), articles and publications in journals (please see www.patientvoices.org.uk/articles.htm and www.patientvoices.org.uk/papers.htm), contributions to books on digital storytelling (Hardy and Sumner 2010, 2014, 2017; Hardy 2017; Jamissen et al. 2017; Dunford and Jenkins 2017) and the production of a documentary film (Patient Voices et al. 2017).

In this first part, Hardy and Sumner address these questions as they take us through the context and conception of Patient Voices, its establishment and consolidation, development and evolution, and methodology and approach.

Chapter 1 "The Journey Begins" explains the initial inspiration for the Patient Voices programme and the way in which technical, philosophical and educational factors and movements influenced early work.

Chapter 2 "Pilgrims' Progress" covers the period from 2004 to 2010, when the programme developed and refined its processes and approaches, coming to situate itself firmly with the Classical Digital Storytelling model created by StoryCenter.

From 2010 to 2017, covered in Chap. 3 "To the Far Horizon", the programme began to identify broad themes within its work and to look at more deeply and employ more directly the power of the process—rather than the product—to effect change in attitudes amongst healthcare staff.

Finally, Chap. 4 "The Patient Voices Approach" looks at the derivation of the approach, what happens within a Patient Voices workshop, and the processes that have been developed by the programme to provide appropriate consent and release of stories, protection of intellectual property and effective distribution of the stories.

References

Dunford, M., & Jenkins, T. (2017). *Digital storytelling: Form and content.* London: Palgrave Macmillan. doi:10.1057/978-1-137-59152-4.

Hardy, P. (2007). *An investigation into the application of the Patient Voices digital stories in healthcare education: Quality of learning, policy impact and practice-based value.* MSc dissertation, University of Ulster, Belfast.

Hardy, P. (2017). Physician, know thyself: Using digital storytelling to promote reflection in medical education. In Y. Nordkvelle, G. Jamissen, P. Hardy, & H. M. Pleasants (Eds.), *Digital storytelling in higher education: International perspectives.* London: Palgrave Macmillan.

Hardy, P., & Sumner, T. (2010). Humanizing healthcare: A conversation with Pip Hardy and Tony Sumner, Pilgrim Projects/Patient Voices. In J. Lambert (Ed.), *Digital storytelling: Capturing lives, creating community* (3rd ed., pp. 143–156). Berkeley, CA: Digital Diner Press.

Hardy, P., & Sumner, T. (2014). Our stories, ourselves: Exploring identities, sharing experiences and building relationships through Patient Voices. In H. Pleasants & D. Salter (Eds.), *Community-based multi-literacies and digital media projects: Questioning assumptions and exploring realities*. New York: Peter Lang.

Hardy, P., & Sumner, T. (2017). Digital storytelling with users and survivors of the UK mental health system. In M. Dunford & T. Jenkins (Eds.), *Story, form and content in digital storytelling: Telling tales*. London: Palgrave Macmillan.

Hardy, V. P. (2016). *Telling tales: The development and impact of digital stories and digital storytelling in healthcare*. Doctoral thesis, Manchester Metropolitan University, Manchester.

Jamissen, G., Hardy, P., Nordkvelle, Y., & Pleasants, H. (2017). *Digital storytelling in higher education*. London: Palgrave Macmillan. doi:10.1007/978-3-319-51058-3.

Kipling, R. (1902). *Just so stories*. London: Macmillan and Company.

Patient Voices, Stamm, R., & Alexandra, D. (2017). *Patient Voices: Three days in Cambridge*. Pilgrim Projects. www.patientvoices.org.uk/pvthedoc.htm

1

The Journey Begins

Pip Hardy and Tony Sumner

Introduction: The Lie of the Land

What we're experiencing is not simply the acceleration of the pace of change, but the acceleration of acceleration itself. In other words, change growing at an exponential rate. (Kurzweil and Van Dusen Wishard 2006)

The world today is a very different place from the world in which we began our Patient Voices journey, way back in the dawning years of the twenty-first century. The technology revolution has changed the way we live irrevocably: our grandchildren will not be able to imagine a world without mobile phones, instant access to the world wide web, and the ability to communicate with friends, family, and colleagues at anytime from anywhere in the world.

In the early years of the twenty-first century, compassion was something practised by Buddhist monks, and the voice of the patient was

P. Hardy (✉) • T. Sumner
Patient Voices Programme, Pilgrim Projects Limited,
Landbeach, Cambridgeshire, UK

© The Author(s) 2018
P. Hardy, T. Sumner (eds.), *Cultivating Compassion*,
https://doi.org/10.1007/978-3-319-64146-1_1

5

largely heard with scepticism at best and mistrust at worst. Education was, by and large, conducted in physical places in real time by experts in their subject. Stories were something you read to young children, and doctors were unquestioned in their knowledge and their position in health services everywhere, including in the UK National Health Service.

We would like to highlight some of the features of the landscape in which our journey began and that were particularly relevant to that journey, in particular, the political, educational, and technological aspects, which are inevitably also affected by social and economic factors.

The journey that the Patient Voices Programme has followed in the years since 2003 is, as so many journeys are, as much a journey *from* a place as a journey *to* a place. That place, in 2003, was set in a landscape that had been, just as the physical landscape is, shaped over time by a variety of forces of change. However, where the forces of wind, rain, and geophysics act on the landscape over millennia, the landscape from which our Patient Voices journey sets out was largely laid down in the seemingly antediluvian past of the years preceding and following the Second World War, then sculpted and shaped by technological, political, and social forces over the decade preceding 2003. Let us consider the impact of these various, interconnected forces, illustrated in Fig. 1.1.

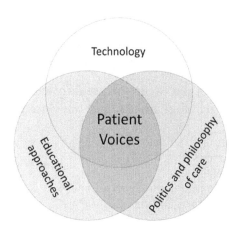

Fig. 1.1 Environmental forces shaping the landscape around Patient Voices

Educational Approaches

In the late twentieth century, open learning was still regarded by many academics as a threat to their expertise and centrality in the learning process. The majority of adult education still took place in classrooms and lecture theatres; research was done in libraries, and information was gathered from books and printed papers. The term 'Lifelong Learning' had yet to come into common usage; learning that was centred on the learner was still considered to be moderately radical, and approaches such as Malcolm Knowles' theory of 'andragogy' (Smith 2002) were far from the norm.

Gradually, appearing on the horizons of educationalists, instructional designers, and educational developers like us were the opportunities afforded by changes in technology to rethink the way educational opportunities were created and delivered, particularly in the field of distance and open learning. In the mid-1990s, computer-based learning meant either painfully slow interactions over modem or ISDN connections or laboriously created interactive materials delivered on CD-ROM. Even as late as 1999, organisations devoted to open learning, such as the Open University and the National Extension College in the UK, were still sending out boxes of weighty ring binders filled with printed materials, sometimes accompanied by video or audio cassettes, to their students.

Pilgrim Projects' work environment shifted with these forces. We went from producing print-based workbooks to creating interactive CD-ROMs containing the learning materials. Virtual Learning Environments (VLEs) appeared but when we developed 21 online accountancy courses in 2000, the limitations of the VLE technology at the time (such as Lotus LearningSpace) and the constraints of connection speeds (still mainly 56 kbit modems), meant that the creativity of our instructional designs was constrained to text and simple graphics.

By 2003, e-learning was no longer experimental but was becoming more common and millions were poured into the UK e-University, the NHS University, and other large e-learning programmes, including one that would be a key trigger for us, the UK Health Education Partnership.

The Politics and Philosophy of Care

Meanwhile, the first tremors of the seismic changes to come were rocking the world of health and social care provision. The rise of neoliberalism, the questioning and challenging of accepted European post-war norms about the primacy of social provision of health and social care, and the international drive towards greater safety and higher quality care, all resulted in the push for greater patient involvement, and the espousal, in UK policy, at least, of patient-centred care.

The deaths of an untoward number of babies at the Bristol Royal Infirmary triggered an inquiry that would irrevocably alter the landscape of healthcare and healthcare quality improvement. The Bristol Inquiry, chaired by Sir Ian Kennedy, highlighted the need for safer, higher quality care not only for babies with heart conditions but across the UK NHS.

In the UK and the US, there were several defining moments in this movement: the creation of the Picker Institute and the publication of *Crossing the Quality Chasm* (IoM 2001) and *The Bristol Royal Infirmary Inquiry Report* (Kennedy 2001) being among the most significant.

Policy drivers in healthcare in the UK became firmly centred on putting the 'patient' at the heart of care while improving quality and safety (DH 2001a, b).

Evidence-based medicine (EBM), the drive towards clinical excellence that is founded upon research (Sackett 1997), seemed to be the way forward, but an important balance was offered by Narrative Medicine and the recognition that people's stories offers important insights into their lives and their conditions (Hurwitz et al. 2004; Greenhalgh and Hurwitz 1999; Greenhalgh et al. 2004; Charon and Montello 2002).

The Expert Patient Programme acknowledged the crucial role that patients have to play in their own health and well-being. The 'patient experience', articulated by, among others, Angela Coulter and supported by research conducted by the Picker Institute, was recognised as forming an important aspect of healthcare delivery (Coulter and Dunn 2002).

The Database of Individual Patient Experience—now Healthtalkonline—the brainchild of Dr. Ann McPherson—was in its infancy. In certain circles, it was becoming desirable, if not always acceptable, to incorporate the patient voice in healthcare education and quality improvement initiatives.

The introduction into the UK health system of the concepts of the market and 'patient choice'; an increasingly elderly population with more complex and chronic health needs; changing approaches to the role of 'the patient' in healthcare education and service improvement programmes; the recognition of the need for inter-professional working and inter-professional education; and the ready availability of information to those able to search the internet—all pointed the way to a clear need for 'a patient voice'.

Technology

In the early 1990s, personal computing was not yet ubiquitous. Email was far from universal; mobile phones were rare and their sole purpose was making and receiving phone calls! The modern notion of social media had not been invented: there was no Facebook, Twitter, or YouTube. The internet existed, but data rates meant that access was limited to text-based email and searches. Most users still accessed services via dial-up modems and, while modem data rates steadily rose, within the limitations of the technology, from 1200 bits per second in the 1980s to 28 and 56 kbit/s by the mid-to-late 1990s, the fastest commonly available connections for most householders were delivered by 64 kbit ISDN lines. The technologies and software that would be used to access the services and caches of information connected together by the internet was still a race of many horses, with what were then frontrunners, such as Gopher, now long forgotten. Indeed, in 1994, what would become the winner—Tim Berner-Lee's World Wide Web—was still being described as:

> …*one of the contenders in the "be the Internet navigator-and-front-end sweepstakes"…* (Dern 1994)

The last years of the old millennium and the first years of the new saw momentous changes in personal communications and portable technologies. Widespread adoption of the internet, the dominance of the World Wide Web browsers, broadband connections, and smart(er) phones created a step change in how the population interacted with each other and with societal and governmental systems. With the arrival of graphic user interfaces, such as NeXTSTEP, GEM, Windows, and MacOS, and the advent of digital image, audio, and video-editing tools, more people could create their own multi-media pieces. With the introduction of powerful, low-power-consumption ARM (Advanced RISC Machines) processors, significant portable/hand-held computing became possible and, very quickly, ubiquitous. Connectivity has changed, too. In 2000, there were just under 150 million dial-up subscriptions in the 34 OECD countries (Wikipedia 2014) and fewer than 20 million broadband subscriptions. By 2004, broadband had grown and dial up had declined so that the number of subscriptions was roughly equal at 130 million each.

Meanwhile, unbeknownst to us, by 2003, StoryCenter (formerly the Center for Digital Storytelling (CDS)) in California had been helping people create personal stories about their lives, using new digital video-editing technologies, for nearly ten years. They came over to the UK to teach a group of people in Wales how to facilitate the creation of these multi-media nuggets of authentic community history to illustrate the richness of Welsh life and culture. The BBC Capture Wales digital storytelling project was in its infancy but would go on to spawn many talented and able converts to the process of digital storytelling.

You Wouldn't Want to Start from Here … or Would You?

So here we are, somewhere in the first few years of the new millennium. The patients are still in their (mostly) Nightingale wards; the doctors and nurses are still waiting for their pagers to beep; politicians are still creating policy documents that will, largely, be read on paper; technologists are creating cool new ideas and toys; educationists are gasping and grasping at new possibilities and challenges for open and distance learning and assessment; and the NHS is still somewhere between cradle and grave.

Against this backdrop of healthcare modernisation, we at Pilgrim Projects are conducting research into and developing e-learning materials about 'clinical governance', the ten-year journey towards clinical excellence that was to underpin and inform UK National Health Service modernisation initiatives during the first decade of the new millennium.

Pilgrim Projects is a bespoke education consultancy specialising in the development of open, distance, and e-learning resources with a focus on health and social care. One of our distinguishing characteristics has always been to create learning opportunities that were learner-centred, practical, real-world focused, reflective, and 'delightful'. Stories, vignettes, case studies, and other *realia* were always at the core of our learning and educational programmes.

Commissioned by the Royal College of Nursing to create a suite of e-learning modules on clinical governance that were *'engaging, innovative, creative, reflective, succinct and cognizant of the patient voice'*, we eagerly took up the challenge. It was a wonderful opportunity to immerse ourselves in the task of conducting research into best practice in healthcare—wherever that could be found—and searching for appropriate examples to illuminate important learning points and prompt reflection on practice.

Meanwhile, our own patient experiences, and those of our friends and family, were not necessarily characterised by high-quality clinical care, compassion, or humanity. We knew, from the evidence of experience, that things could be so much better—and that we were in a position to do something about it.

We knew that somehow this meant bringing in the voice of the patient, of the people who used healthcare services. The question was what would be the very best way we could do this?

Stories, Of Course!

Storytelling is the mode of description best suited to transformation in new situations of action. (Schön 1988)

The growing appetite for personal stories to illuminate the experience of service users of health and social care has, in recent years, resulted in a proliferation of methods designed to get to the heart of individual experience. Digital storytelling creates new possibilities for participatory and collaborative approaches to discovering and developing new knowledge, re-positioning participants as co-producers of knowledge, and, potentially, as co-researchers. It offers 'ordinary' people the opportunity to create a short video about an important life experience, weaving together a recorded voiceover with images, music, and other sounds, all chosen and edited by the storyteller.

The Patient Voices stories are valued for their brevity, succinctness, emotional power, flexibility, and versatility (Hardy 2007) and are now in wide use in virtual learning environments, lecture theatres, and conference venues throughout the English-speaking world and beyond. The Patient Voices website (www.patientvoices.org.uk) now receives nearly 2 million hits per year.

Stories themselves can also be used to heal, transform, deepen insights, promote understanding, and prompt reflection, and it is our belief in their potential to achieve these properties that puts stories at the heart of the Patient Voices Programme.

Clinical Governance

There is nothing so hard as having words in your heart that you can't utter.
(James Earl Jones 1931-)

Via the Clinical Governance Support Team (CGST) we were introduced to our first two storytellers, Ian Kramer and Monica Clarke. The CGST went on to sponsor the first series of some 20 or so stories to illuminate the values of clinical governance, that is, humanity, equity, justice, and respect (Stanton 2004a). These stories would be built into the United Kingdom Health Education Partnership (UKHEP Clinical Governance e-learning materials) and also incorporated in presentations to Primary Care Trust Board teams as a particularly effective way of prompting them to think about their raison d'etre and reflect on the extent to which the Trust was embodying those values of clinical governance. A year later, the stories made another appearance in *The Strategic Leadership of Clinical Governance* (Stanton 2004b).

We didn't even have to think about the choice of name: 'Patient Voices' laid claim and there was no contest. While acknowledging the patience of patients, it is even more important to listen carefully to *all* those voices waiting patiently to be heard. We wanted—and expected—to hear stories from patients, carers, nurses, doctors, physiotherapists, radiographers, and so on, in the hope that by listening to one another for just a few moments, better communication and greater understanding would be the result. Better care could not be far behind, we reasoned.

Learning from Storytellers: Ethics 101

We could not have been more fortunate in our first two storytellers: Ian Kramer and Monica Clark were great teachers and fantastic storytellers. They made our task easy and we learned so much from them. They gave us some insight into what it was really like to care for someone 24 hours a day, 7 days a week, and to have to take so many drugs each day that you feel too ill to do anything else. They showed us, by their passion and their commitment, that change can and does happen. They were unfailingly generous with their time, their insights, their wisdom, and, of course, their stories (Clarke 2004; Kramer 2004).

Both Ian and Monica had a strong sense of justice and had dedicated their lives to making healthcare better for everyone. They had also both been lawyers in their earlier lives and were easily able to articulate the sense of injustice that they had felt at having their stories 'taken' by researchers and others, 'dismembered' and incorporated in PhDs, books, papers, and publicity material, all the while ensuring their anonymity or, as Ian and Monica saw it, failing to acknowledge their contribution.

They told us that they didn't want to be anonymous or their stories to be 'edited' by editors or researchers taking the 'useful' bits and discarding the rest or anyone to profit from their stories. They helped us develop our first protocol and consent form, a two-sided agreement, incorporating assurances from us as well as consent from storytellers, with a large print version for those with visual impairment and to be read to people with other communication or literacy difficulties to ensure that they would understand what they were signing.

Our experiences with Ian and Monica laid the foundation for what have become three important principles of the Patient Voices Programme and informed the selection of the Creative Commons Licence under which all Patient Voices stories are released (once approved by the storyteller):

1. You must attribute the work in the manner specified by the author or licensor (but not in any way that suggests that they endorse you or your use of the work).
2. You may not use this work for commercial purposes.
3. You may not alter, transform, or build upon this work.

Creative Commons Licence Attribution-NonCommercial-No Derivs 3.0 http://creativecommons.org/licenses/by-nc-nd/3.0/

One Thing Leads to Another

Through Monica, we met Alison Ryan, another carer and then chief executive of the Princess Royal Trust for Carers, whose stories contrasted the incredible amount of caring work done by family carers with their invisibility and insignificance in the eyes of the system (Ryan 2004).

Monica introduced us to Emma Allen, whose stories illuminated the crucial role of communication, particularly where there may be communication difficulties, as when someone has had a stroke (Allen 2004).

Charles Bruce was our next storyteller; a doctor and a carer, his stories highlighted the paucity of support for those in caring roles and the almost absurd arrogance/negligence of some of his professional colleagues (Bruce 2005).

David Clark, another doctor, afflicted by heart failure in later life, told moving stories about the inequity of provision for those with different conditions while praising the NHS as a *wonderful institution* (Clark 2004).

We worked with each of these people individually or, in the case of Ian and Monica, in pairs. Brendan Routledge was our teacher, colleague, and companion during this time, generously sharing his knowledge and experience of digital storytelling in the context of education (which he referred to as *powerpoint for the soul* (Davitt 2004)) and working with us to refine the method for use in healthcare. We did, in fact, video these early storytellers—actually, Brendan wielded the video camera while Pip engaged in a conversation with them. The resulting video footage was intercut with still images, either provided by the storyteller or sourced from image libraries or, in most cases, a combination of both. When the editing of each video was complete, storytellers were invited to review the video and either (a) give the consent for it to be released or (b) request changes that would enable them to release the video.

We wanted the process to be one of co-production as far as possible, preferring to invite storytellers to tell us the most important thing in relation to a previously discussed prompt that touched on the values of clinical governance, rather than use a spine of questions. Typical early prompts included: 'Please tell us a story about communication'; 'Please tell us a story about respect/equity/justice…', and so on.

Because we intended to use these digital stories as educational resources to prompt reflection, many of these early stories have text on screen that restates the spoken word, reinforcing the key message of the story. Viewers indicated that this was helpful, allowing them time to absorb what the storyteller was saying and giving them both an audio and a visual opportunity to absorb key points in the story.

Process *and* Product

Looking back, we had much to learn about participatory media and digital storytelling. On the other hand, we already appeared to be shifting the balance of power from its customary residence in the mind of the interviewer/researcher/producer to the interviewee/storyteller/participant. We really wanted to hear what mattered to the people we were listening to, rather than getting answers to questions that mattered to us. We practised listening carefully, without interrupting, gently probing and encouraging only when something wasn't quite clear or it seemed that the storyteller had touched on something of particular importance. Pip drew on listening skills developed as part of training as a psychodynamic counsellor and was also greatly influenced by the work of Rachel Pinney—a Quaker and a doctor who had developed a practical attitude of heart and mind that she called *Creative Listening* (Pinney 1970).

Although we had set out to develop a reflective learning resource, from the earliest days we realised that the process of creating these stories might be as important as the product—the stories themselves. Starting with Monica and Ian, storytellers would invariably comment, after recording their stories, that they had found the process to be valuable, therapeutic, even cathartic. They commented on how rare it is to be really listened to. They appreciated being included in decisions about what images to use, which parts of the recording would go into the final story, and which would stay out; they liked having a say in what was happening and how it was happening. They liked working in a relaxed, informal atmosphere; we learned early on that food and hospitality played an important part in the process of creating digital stories!

Service Improvement and Clinical Microsystems

Meanwhile, working closely with Ross Scrivener of the Royal College of Nursing, we pressed on with the task of researching and writing the two UKHEP modules: *Clinical Governance Matters* and *Clinical Governance Works*. We continued to discover extraordinary pockets of excellence and utilised these examples to inspire our learners, leading them gently along the path of clinical governance until they were prepared to conduct their own quality improvement projects.

One of the examples of excellence was the Clinical Microsystems model propounded by Paul Batalden, Gene Nelson, and Margie Godfrey of Dartmouth Hitchcock Medical School (Nelson et al. 2002). Their work was attracting much attention in the American healthcare improvement world and, indeed, it seemed to us to be eminently sensible, practical, and doable. I wrote to Margie to request permission to quote from a paper that they had published. She emailed straight back mentioning that she was flying to London that night. We agreed to meet. I showed her a digital story or two. She was intrigued by what we were trying to do and invited us to submit our first series of stories to the annual Clinical Microsystems Conference Film Festival.

The conference setting was stunning: a beautiful New England lake at the height of the fall colours. The participants were equally impressive: a select group of the great and the good from the American healthcare improvement world, including Don Berwick and Maureen Bisognano from the Institute of Healthcare Improvement (IHI), complemented by participants from Europe, including Helen Bevan and Paul Bate from the UK, who were then looking at the characteristics of social movements, and Göran Henriks, who had been trialling the Clinical Microsystems model in Sweden with great success. Early morning swims in the lake, led enthusiastically by Helen, were balanced by thoughtful, reflective, stimulating, and inspiring small-group discussions with some of the most important people in the field of healthcare quality improvement. I was amazed, dazed, and delighted.

The last day of the conference arrived. The air of anticipation and festive atmosphere of the Film Festival was heightened by bags of popcorn and a stage lit as if for an Oscars ceremony Movies were shown, prizes awarded, speeches made. Patient Voices won the prize for 'Minimising Unnecessary Handoffs' and then there was a vote for the best movie.

The audience voted our little movies the best in the festival and Paul Batalden presented the 'People's Choice' award.

Before Moving On

And so, within a year of recording the first Patient Voices stories, we had won our first two awards. We were ready for anything, confident that we were on to something important, something that would make a difference. I had registered for an MSc in Lifelong Learning, studying via e-learning, eager to put theory into practice and vice versa. The first module, on policy and strategy, provided a wonderful opportunity to explore the benefits of the Expert Patient Programme as a Lifelong Learning opportunity, to discover what was happening in the world of patient involvement and patient empowerment and to conclude for myself that patients and clinicians needed to work far more closely together, respecting each other's areas of expertise (Hardy 2004). I was particularly influenced by a small book called *The Resourceful Patient* (Gray and Rutter 2002), which promoted the notion that the balance of power was shifting between patients and the clinicians who cared for them as information became more widely available. The work of Angela Coulter and others supported this view (Coulter et al. 1999) and argued that patients need high-quality information if they are to share decisions and be true partners in care (Coulter et al. 1998). She also reinforced what we were learning from experience, that patients (and carers) are often experts in their own conditions—and always in their own lives. Putting patients at the heart of care was the mantra of the UK Department of Health (DH 2001b) and that was exactly what we were trying to do.

Conclusion

The first stage of our journey had been a full and fruitful one. In addition to learning from desk research, we had also learned a great deal about listening; about what makes a good story; about working closely with people telling intimate personal stories; about trust, respect, and dignity; about the importance of hospitality and what co-production really means in practice; and about reflection. We learned a lot about technology (remember that broadband was nothing like as good as it is now!); about informed consent, copyright, ownership, and internet protocol; and about ethics and ethical behaviour. We were beginning to learn some difficult lessons in relation to negotiating the appropriate balance between supporting a storyteller to tell the story he or she needed to tell and, on the other hand, meeting the client's requirement for a story that would provide the 'right' kind of prompt for reflection. But perhaps most importantly, we were humbled by the stories of courage and resilience and good humour in the face of so much suffering.

We were ready for the next stage of our journey.

Key Points

- The process of creating a digital story is as important as the product—the resulting digital story.
- Walking in someone else's shoes for a few moments can bring about fundamental changes in understanding.
- As Dave Isay says: '*listening is an act of love*' (Isay 2007).

- Hospitality, in its fullest sense, is an important aspect of digital storytelling.
- Patients really do want to be regarded as people: respect, trust, justice, and dignity are crucial.
- Technology has a significant impact on creativity, learning, and reflection.

References

Allen, E. (2004). *Emma Allen's stories*. Pilgrim Projects Limited. Retrieved July 17, 2013, from http://www.patientvoices.org.uk/eallen.htm

Bruce, C. (2005). *Charles Bruce's stories*. Pilgrim Projects Limited. Retrieved March 2014, from http://www.patientvoices.org.uk/cbruce.htm

Charon, R., & Montello, M. (2002). *Stories matter: The role of narrative in medical ethics (reflective bioethics)*. New York: Routledge.

Clark, D. (2004). *Patient Voices: David Clark's stories*. Pilgrim Projects Limited. Retrieved March 2014, from http://www.patientvoices.org.uk/dclark.htm

Clarke, M. (2004). *Monica Clarke: Stories*. Pilgrim Projects Limited. Retrieved March 2014, from http://www.patientvoices.org.uk/mclarke.htm

Coulter, A., & Dunn, N. (2002). After Bristol: Putting patients at the centre: Patient centred care: Timely, but is it practical? *BMJ, 324*(7338), 648–651.

Coulter, A., Entwhistle, V., & Gilbert, D. (1998). *Informing patients: An assessment of the quality of patient information materials*. London: Kings Fund.

Coulter, A., Entwistle, V., & Gilbert, D. (1999). Sharing decisions with patients: Is the information good enough? *BMJ, 318*(7179), 318–322.

Davitt, J. (2004). Used in class. *The Guardian*.

Dern, D. P. (1994). *The internet guide for new users*. New York: McGraw Hill.

DH. (2001a). *The expert patient: A new approach to chronic disease management for the 21st century*. Great Britain: Department of Health.

DH. (2001b). *Shifting the balance of power within the NHS: Securing delivery*. Great Britain, London: Department of Health.

Gray, J. A. M., & Rutter, H. (2002). *The resourceful patient*. Oxford: eRosetta.

Greenhalgh, T., & Hurwitz, B. (1999). Narrative based medicine: Why study narrative? *BMJ, 318*(7175), 48–50.

Greenhalgh, T., Hurwitz, B., & Skultans, V. (2004). *Narrative research in health and illness* (Vol. Book). London: BMJ.

Hardy, P. (2004). *The expert patient programme: A critical review*. MSc in Lifelong Learning, University of Ulster, Belfast.

Hardy, P. (2007). *An investigation into the application of the Patient Voices digital stories in healthcare education: Quality of learning, policy impact and practice-based value*. MSc dissertation, University of Ulster, Belfast.

Hurwitz, B., Greenhalgh, T., & Skultans, V. (2004). *Narrative research in health and illness*. Malden, MA, Oxford: BMJ Books.

IoM. (2001). *Crossing the quality chasm: A new health system for the 21st century*. Washington, DC: National Academy Press.

Isay, D. (2007). *Listening is an act of love: A celebration of American life from the StoryCorps project*. London, New York: Penguin Press.

Jones, J. E. (1931–). *Source of quote unknown*.

Kennedy, I. (2001). *The report of the public inquiry into Children's heart surgery at the Bristol Royal Infirmary 1984–1995. Learning from Bristol* (pp. 325–332). London: Stationery Office.

Kramer, I. (2004). *Ian Kramer: Stories*. Pilgrim Projects Limited. Retrieved March 2014, from http://www.patientvoices.org.uk/ikramer.htm

Kurzweil, R., Van Dusen Wishard, W. (2006). Understanding our moment in history. *New Rennaisance Magazine, 11*(39).

Nelson, E. C., Batalden, P. B., Huber, T. P., Mohr, J. J., Godfrey, M. M., Headrick, L. A., & Wasson, J. H. (2002). Microsystems in health care: Part 1. Learning from high-performing front-line clinical units. *The Joint Commission Journal on Quality Improvement, 28*(9), 472–493.

Pinney, R. (1970). *Creative listening* (Rev. ed.). Loddington: Creative Listening.

Ryan, A. (2004). *Alison Ryan: Stories*. Pilgrim Projects Limited. Retrieved March 2014, from http://www.patientvoices.org.uk/aryan.htm

Sackett, D. L. (1997). Evidence-based medicine. In *Seminars in perinatology* (Vol. 1, pp. 3–5). Elsevier.

Schön, D. (1988). Coaching reflective teaching. In G. L. Erickson & P. P. Grimmett (Eds.), *Reflection in teacher education* (pp. 19–29). New York: Teachers College Press.

Smith, M. K. (2002). *Malcolm Knowles, informal adult education, self-direction and andragogy*. Retrieved from www.infed.org/thinkers/et-knowl.htm

Stanton, P. (2004a). *Clinical governance: An overview*. The Strategic Leadership of Clinical Governance in PCTs. NHS Modernisation Agency.

Stanton, P. (2004b). *The strategic leadership of clinical governance in PCTs*. NHS Modernisation Agency.

Wikipedia. (2014). Internet access. *Wikipedia*. Retrieved August 2014, from http://en.wikipedia.org/wiki/Internet_access#cite_note-OECD-countries-10

Dr Pip Hardy is a co-founder of the Patient Voices Programme and a director of Pilgrim Projects Ltd, an education consultancy specialising in open learning and healthcare quality improvement. She also serves as Curriculum and Learning Lead for NHS England's School for Change Agents. Pip has an MSc in Lifelong Learning and her PhD considers the potential of digital storytelling to transform healthcare.

Tony Sumner is a co-founder of the Patient Voices Programme and a director of Pilgrim Projects. With degrees in physics and astronomy and astrophysics, and many years' experience working in the software industry, he is particularly interested in how technology and storytelling can intersect to promote deep reflection.

2

Pilgrims' Progress

Pip Hardy

Quantity *and* Quality? (2004–2007)

The culture of the mind must be subservient to the culture of the heart. (Gandhi 1869–1948)

We had a programme, a purpose, a rationale (Hardy 2004) and a couple of awards. We felt we were doing valuable, important work—touching hearts and, hopefully, moving minds. We were optimistic that we could change the world. We carried on writing and editing, developing learning programmes, doing research, finding ways of sharing what we were learning, and encouraging others to make use of, and benefit from, these stories of experience as they were designing, developing and modernising healthcare.

P. Hardy (✉)
Patient Voices Programme, Pilgrim Projects Limited,
Landbeach, Cambridgeshire, UK

© The Author(s) 2018
P. Hardy, T. Sumner (eds.), *Cultivating Compassion*,
https://doi.org/10.1007/978-3-319-64146-1_2

23

Stories or Statistics?

Your stories are lovely—very moving—but they are, after all, only anecdotal.
And they certainly aren't statistically valid. A critical friend

Gradually it dawned on us that, despite our prizes, we were not going to rock the healthcare world with only 23 stories and no glossy marketing brochures. Furthermore, it seemed that people were not prepared to take us seriously unless we could support our aspirations with results from 'proper' research. According to the hierarchy of evidence, unless you can demonstrate results underpinned by statistics that have been gleaned from research that is both valid and reliable (that is, in other words, from a randomised control trial (RCT)), the evidence is considered to 'carry less weight' (Wikipedia 2013b). The strength of evidence provided by systematic reviews and RCTs is, of course, the foundation of evidence-based medicine (EBM). That is, best practice in clinical decision making is based upon an evaluation of risks and benefits resulting from treatment or the lack of it (Wikipedia 2013a; Sackett 1997).

In the list of types of evidence included in Wikipedia's entry, the evidence of experience does not even get a mention, and yet we were becoming aware that, even from the relatively small 'sample' of people that we had talked to, the evidence of experience was a crucial element of the body of evidence to be considered when making clinical commissioning or policy decisions.

Our stories were intended to provide a balance to the statistics. Each story represented 100% of that storyteller's experience, and it seemed to us, as Tony later wrote, *'Statistics tell us about the system's experience of the individual, while stories tell us about the individual's experience of the system'* (Sumner 2009a). Interestingly, around this time, Ben Page conducted a MORI (Market and Opinion Research International) poll revealing that *'patients care more about being treated with dignity and respect than they do about mortality rates'* (Page 2004); in other words, while clinical care was important, what really mattered to people was how they were treated as human beings.

Nevertheless, we clearly needed more stories if Patient Voices was going to have any impact.

A Snowball Effect: The First Workshops

Fortunately, digital storytelling can sometimes have a snowball effect. One of the other delegates at the 2004 Clinical Microsystems Conference (see Chap. 1) had also been impressed by the stories. Laura Hibbs invited us to run a short workshop for the North East Yorkshire and Northern Lincolnshire Strategic Health Authority (NEYNL). Forty people attended the half-day workshop; they were divided into smaller groups, each working together on a story. That workshop resulted in eight stories, told by the staff engaged in a range of quality improvement initiatives as a way of highlighting the human and collaborative aspects of their work. Their stories can be seen at http://www.patientvoices.org.uk/neynl.htm (Patient Voices 2006b).

One of the storytellers worked at the Heart Improvement Programme and commissioned us to run two more workshops with patients, nurses and the National Heart Improvement Programme (HIP) team, including the communications officer and the CEO (Patient Voices 2006a).

Before those two workshops, we had been working with people on a largely individual basis to create their stories through a combination of listening and questioning and trying to help people get to the very heart of their story. These workshops were our first forays into facilitating people to tell their stories in groups.

'Proper' Research

Your stories aren't collected using 'proper' research methods! A critical friend

Despite the growing number of stories, we were still met with varying degrees of scepticism. So, while creating more stories was necessary, it was obviously still not sufficient to convince some people of the value of our approach. Criticisms varied: you only seek out the bad stories (how, then to account for the 'good' stories?), stories from one place are not typical of stories in another place (our experience—and patient feedback and survey results—suggested remarkable similarities and shared concerns between people from different places) and the stories are still not statistically valid. We weren't 'proper' researchers, and the killer question we were asked not infrequently was: '*What difference do the stories really make in practice?*'

I hoped that doing an MSc might go some way towards making me a 'proper' researcher and that a research investigation into how the Patient Voices stories were being used would provide an answer to *that* question that kept popping up: what difference *do* the stories make?

The Center for Digital Storytelling (Now StoryCenter)

First, I needed to find out more about digital storytelling. I read everything I could find about digital stories and digital storytelling (which, in 2006, wasn't very much) and became even more convinced that we were doing work of vital importance. Early in my research, I came across the Center for Digital Storytelling (CDS)—now StoryCenter (www.storycenter.org)—an organisation responsible for inventing digital storytelling in what is now known as its 'classical' form. I became convinced that I needed to participate in a CDS workshop to learn to do what we were already doing, only better.

As it happened, they are based in northern California, where I visited my mother each year. The timing was perfect. I prepared a script and gathered some pictures, as instructed by *The Digital Storytelling Cookbook* (Lambert 2002). I hired a car in San Francisco and drove north to the little town of Ukiah, where the workshop was to be held—in a semi-derelict theatre, as it transpired.

The people I met and the things I learned there changed me—and the way we would work—forever. It was there that I discovered—and participated in—what is known in the digital storytelling world as 'The Story Circle' (Lambert 2002). We do not, after all, tell stories in isolation but rather as social beings, and so the comments, questions and feedback provided by others in the story circle are invaluable in the development and shaping of a story.

Putting It into Practice: NHS Heart Improvement Programme

Soon after my return from California, in April 2006, we facilitated the second Heart Improvement Programme workshop for a mix of clinicians, managers and patients. With some trepidation, I invited the storytellers to form a circle so that they could share their story ideas with one another and not only with me. Despite some initial reservations, and thanks to the example set by Adrian Pennington, the CEO, everyone participated. It worked well. People even said how much they had enjoyed the opportunity to share their stories, and what a good reminder it was that if we want things to be better, we have to work together. All those stories can be seen at http://www.patientvoices.org.uk/hip.htm (Patient Voices 2006a).

Consent and Control: Working in Partnership

Each new workshop, as well as creating more stories and a new bank of experiences, seemed to provide us with important lessons. We held two workshops, creating ten stories, with the Working in Partnership Programme (WiPP), another NHS Modernisation Agency initiative. WiPP stressed the benefits of self-care and acknowledged the crucial role that patients have to play in their own health and well-being. One of the workshops was attended by several Asian women who had taken part in the WiPP self-care programme, partly as a way of looking after themselves after living with domestic violence. They seemed keen to share their stories, although they had no pictures. So we recorded their voiceovers, talked with them about ways in which we might find suitable visual images for their stories and assured them that their stories would be completely anonymous.

This had not been an issue for us before, but clearly the identity of these women had to be protected, and we were certain that we could find ways around the problem. Our colleague, Brendan Routledge, did a masterful job of editing the stories using images of clouds and skies, plants and flowers, dark images contrasted with light images. Their names did not appear on the stories. However, when we showed the resulting stories to the storytellers, they decided that it was still too risky for the stories to be released. This was the first time this had happened, and of course, we respected their decision.

One of the participants in the second workshop also decided not to release her story *'for personal reasons'*, and so we realised that we would not always end up with as many stories as there were storytellers in a workshop, but it also confirmed the value and importance of placing storytellers in control of both the content and release of their stories before, during and after their completion. This experience would contribute to our thinking as we continued to develop and refine our three-stage consent and release process (Hardy 2015).

Unexpected Fruit

That workshop did, however, yield an unexpected story, which would figure in our research. It was made by the workshop organiser—neither clinician nor patient and, according to her, *not* someone with a story to tell.

My Friday afternoon invitation to '*tell us the story of why you do the work that you do*' must have piqued her interest, for, on the Monday morning, she showed me a short script accompanied by a picture of a gravestone. It was—and remains—one of the very few first drafts that didn't need any revising—it didn't even need shortening. We recorded it just as it was. She had four old photos—and the story was nearly complete. All that remained was to find a suitable piece of music. Our composer friend, Paul Connelly, came to the rescue. His song 'Don't go' fitted the piece perfectly and he was happy to give us permission to use it. (He has since composed music for very many Patient Voices stories, often in response to a particular request from a storyteller.)

For the love of Lee (McGlinchy 2006) became one of the stories that I showed at every opportunity and was a mainstay of the focus groups I ran as part of my master's programme research. That story, and the others from the project, can be seen at http://www.patientvoices.org.uk/wipp.htm (Patient Voices 2006c).

Walking the Talk: And Talking the Walk

This was a crucial and formative period in the development of the Patient Voices Programme. However, it also became obvious that if we wanted people to know what we were doing, we would have to go out and talk about it: a daunting prospect.

Liz Anderson, a lecturer (and now professor) in interprofessional learning at the University of Leicester Medical School and joint creator, along with Angela Lennox of the Leicester Model of Interprofessional Education (Anderson and Lennox 2009), had seen the potential of the Patient Voices stories for interprofessional education. On her suggestion, I submitted an abstract to the 2006 *All Together Better Health III* conference, which was accepted.

I found presenting terrifying, but at the conference dinner, I met Donna Wareham, a lecturer involved in interprofessional education at Staffordshire University, who thought I might be interested in '*an amazing website*' she had found that contained lots of short videos made by patients and carers. It turned out she had discovered, quite by chance, the Patient Voices website. She was using the stories to great effect in her interprofessional teaching to remind students about the humanity of every patient and encourage them to reflect on their own practice by watching and listening to the stories of other people's practice.

She loved the versatility of the stories. In fact, she used one particular story in several different lectures: about professionalism, health inequalities, patient safety, record keeping, corporate liability and clinical negligence, and she enthused about how fantastic it was to be able to use one short story to prompt discussion about all these important issues. The story she was using was *Jimmy's story* (Mauchland 2006). I was reassured that, perhaps, the stories were beginning to make a difference.

A few months later, I found myself at the 2006 *Nurse Education Tomorrow* conference, with a similar presentation, in the Service User Engagement theme but most notable for me for a fortuitous meeting. Carol Haigh, now Professor of Nursing at Manchester Metropolitan University, described herself as a 'quants chick' with little time for qualitative stuff. Nevertheless, she agreed to watch a digital story. I showed her *For the love of Lee* (McGlinchy 2006). She was silent.

That was the beginning of what has become a valued and valuable personal and professional relationship and Carol was the first person who articulated the potential for digital stories as qualitative data. Of course, that is exactly what they are. She was also to become the person who would supervise my PhD, as well as a loyal supporter of Patient Voices. As Carol is responsible for not one but two later chapters in this book, I will leave it to her to tell her side of the story.

Connecting to the Future: Seeing Things Differently

Towards the end of 2006, we were invited by the Royal College of Nursing and NHS Connecting for Health to tender to facilitate a large workshop/conference designed to help nurses envisage the future of nursing in the light of technological change. Our response was to *'provide a different kind of forum for critical reflection'* through the innovative use of reflection, stories and storytelling. Here is an extract from our proposal:

> *We are, after all, seeking to create the future story of healthcare, and this will, in turn, be shaped by the ongoing stories—both individual and collective—of those who deliver and receive healthcare. Indeed, it may be appropriate to consider nurses, in their future role, as keepers of the stories: both the personal stories of individual experience, as well as the careful documentation that will safeguard patients throughout their journey.*

We won the tender and then began the task of ensuring that we engaged participants in a process that we knew would have a greater impact than a one-off event. To that end, Paul Stanton and I worked together to develop a preparatory workbook to encourage delegates to bring their creativity, as well as their reflective skill, to bear on the task of creating the future (Hardy and Stanton 2007). This was the first of several workbooks on which Paul and I collaborated, designed to extend and enhance the learning from workshops and other events. Some of these workbooks can be seen at www.patientvoices.org.uk/workbooks.htm.

As our reputation grew, so the range of projects on which we worked expanded. Some of the workshops from this time are set out in Table 2.1.

As this phase of our work drew to a close, we were delighted when, in the spring of 2007, the Creating an Inter-professional Workforce Programme selected us as runners-up for the John Horder Award for Innovation.

Having been awarded a distinction for my master's dissertation (Hardy 2007), I was reassured that it was possible for valid research to be based on digital storytelling, although it was a few years before I was ready to undertake further study. Not long after that, StoryCenter invited me to

Table 2.1 Some projects and workshops (2004–2007)

Organisation	Brief description	URL
NHS Tayside	Stories about patient safety and risk from NHS Tayside	www.patientvoices.org.uk/nhstay.htm
Carers Resource	Stories told by carers about their experience of caring for loved ones suffering from a wide range of conditions intended to highlight both the importance and the needs of family carers	www.patientvoices.org.uk/hcr.htm
Royal College of Nursing	Stories created by nurses as part of their Professional Development Framework	www.patientvoices.org.uk/rcnpdf.htm
CINTRA Language Services Group	Stories created by professional interpreters and some of the people they work with to highlight some of the complex ethical and practical issues involved in interpreting, especially in healthcare situations	www.patientvoices.org.uk/interps.htm
Royal College of Nursing	Stories created as part of an e-learning programme intended to improve continence care in care homes; some of these stories have become Patient Voices staples, having been shown at conferences around the world	www.patientvoices.org.uk/rcnqip.htm
National Audit Office	Two important projects focused on gathering stories as qualitative data to accompany and enhance the range of data underpinning their Value for Money Healthcare reports: one about stroke care and one about neonatal services	www.patientvoices.org.uk/naoconn.htm www.patientvoices.org.uk/naoneo.htm

co-present at the *Chronic Disease Prevention and Management* conference in Calgary, Alberta. The convenor of our session, by way of introduction, said: *'I've heard about your stories, and so I have brought my own packet of tissues with me.'* I showed 'Getting to the bottom of things' (Bailey-Dering 2007), and yes, there were tears. Someone in the audience said: *'That story ought to be shown to every healthcare professional in the world.'*

Encouraged by these words, we moved to the next stage of our journey.

'There Is More That Unites Us Than Divides Us': From Saskatoon to Sheffield and Beyond (2008–2010)

Your stories are lovely but … people in Leeds are different from people in Sheffield. We need our own stories…

On the last day of the conference in Calgary, a woman sat down next to me with her cup of coffee. We got chatting, as you do, and she asked me what I did. I told her about Patient Voices.

'Hmm,' she mused, 'that might be just what we need to include in our evaluation of the Live Well™ project we've been doing with some First Nation peoples in Saskatchewan. I've been trying to find a way that would allow the participants to evaluate the project in their own words, their own stories.'

We exchanged cards. I fluctuated between thinking I would never hear from her again and being absolutely certain that the connection we had made would yield fruit. An email was waiting for me when I arrived home. Many emails and several transatlantic phone calls later, I found myself, in the spring of 2008, on a plane to Saskatoon.

In the University Hospital Board Room, ten First Nation people gathered at a joint StoryCenter/Patient Voices workshop to tell their stories of engagement with the Live Well™ with Chronic Conditions Programme (known in the UK as the Expert Patient Programme and in the US as the Stanford Chronic Disease Self-Management Programme). I had been well briefed about the storytellers and had acquainted myself with some of the particular issues facing First Nation peoples in Canada. I was aware that there might be issues of literacy—both technical and linguistic— quite apart from mental health issues and other problems resulting from generations of poverty.

I enlisted the help of Jenny Gordon, our colleague at the RCN, who had attended several Patient Voices workshops, first to make stories and later to help out, to co-facilitate the workshop with me. She had a way of putting people at ease and getting to the nub of the story, and she has warmth and enthusiasm in abundance. She was the ideal accomplice on this project and would go on to attend our first Facilitator Training Workshop later that year.

In Saskatoon, there were, as I had come to expect, some problems that could be anticipated—and some that could not (usually related to technology; in this case, it was to do with administrator passwords). With the gracious goodwill of our hosts and sponsors, Joy Adams and Suzanne Sheppard from the Saskatoon Health Authority, and the enthusiasm, commitment and humour of the storytellers, everyone had a good time and everyone finished a story—even those who had never used a computer before.

At the end of the workshop, as is our custom, we showed the stories. There were tears of joy and gratitude and tears of loss and regret. We celebrated with huckleberry pie and were honoured with speeches by the elders of the community and wonderful gifts—a traditional birch bark biting created by one of the storytellers and a wreath woven from some special scented grass, which still smells just as good today as it did then—but perhaps the best gift of all was when one of the storytellers said to me:

This has been the best three days of my life. I feel like I could do anything now.

The stories that were made in Saskatoon can be seen here: www. patientvoices.org.uk/sask.htm (Patient Voices and StoryCenter 2008).

One week after my return from Canada, we facilitated a workshop in Sheffield with a courageous group of service users and carers who were involved with the Faculty of Health and Wellbeing at Sheffield Hallam University.

The workshop was wonderful in many ways, and we were ably assisted by Julie Walters, who will write more about the Healing Journeys project in her chapter. One of the most important and memorable aspects of the workshop for me was in relation to assumptions. I had gone to Canada expecting there to be literacy issues of various kinds: computer, reading and writing, health ... and that there would be cultural differences. Naively, it hadn't occurred to me that I should expect to encounter the same issues in Sheffield as well.

During the first afternoon, after the story circle, the storytellers were busy—concentrating on drafting their stories and the scripts that they would record. We were watchful, offering help when asked and trying not to be intrusive. One of the storytellers beckoned Tony over. *'I have a question for you. I've been typing, like you showed me, but I can't seem to get the spaces between words.'* Tony showed her the space bar. We were suitably chastened and vowed not to make any further assumptions about storytellers anywhere.

At the end of the workshop, we always have a period for reflection and for storytellers to mention what they enjoyed (or didn't enjoy), what they feel they have accomplished and how they are feeling—a kind of debrief and check-out. We asked what had been the best thing about the workshop. *'Typing my own script!'* came the prompt reply from our storyteller.

The Sheffield workshop is the subject of Chap. 13 later in this book; the stories can be seen here: http://www.patientvoices.org.uk/shu.htm (Patient Voices 2008b).

There is more that unites us than divides us.

A Fortuitous Meeting—And the First Nurstory Workshop

Co-facilitating a workshop with Daniel Weinshenker from StoryCenter at the University of Colorado was another key moment for the Patient Voices Programme. Not only was it a fantastic opportunity to work with and learn from Daniel, who has a rare talent for creative writing and eliciting powerful stories, but that was where I met and worked with Cathy Jaynes on her 'Go around' story. Her story has travelled around the world and is one of the stories we always show when we want to impress people! Cathy and I have written papers (Hardy and Jaynes 2011) and presented together at a number of international conferences, and Cathy has gone on to lead an ambitious digital storytelling project aimed at improving safety in the air medical transport industry, which she describes in Chap. 7. That workshop was the first of what has become an impressive and long-running series of workshops for nurses to create reflective digital stories called *Nurstory* (http://www.nurstory.org/stories/).

Spreading Our Wings

By now, we had made several excellent relationships with people who had been infected by the digital storytelling bug. They came to make a story—usually as part of the preparation for organising a workshop in their organisation—and then they came back to make another story, and then another…. As their confidence grew, they started helping other people—they became our apprentices.

Facilitator Training

With the encouragement and support of Joe Lambert from StoryCenter, we held our first facilitator training workshop in June of 2008. This is a complex affair involving running a workshop within a workshop so that the trainee facilitators have some first-time storytellers on whom to practice. Joe came over from California to help out. We had four first-time storytellers, including three sisters from the Society of the Holy Child Jesus, and three enthusiastic trainees: Jenny Gordon from the Royal College of Nursing, Fiona O'Neill from Leeds University and Julie Walters from Sheffield Hallam University. We couldn't have hoped for a better mix of people and we all learned from one another. Here are a couple of comments from that workshop:

> I liked the clarity of the planning—allocating us tasks on each day that gave each of us an opportunity to have a go and also highlighted the myriad of hidden tasks that have to be done to ensure smooth running of a workshop.
> The process feels very sound and evidenced based. I learnt a lot more about the process and I trust it even more now.

We have continued to work, albeit infrequently, with all three of our newly trained facilitators, and two of them have contributed chapters to this book. That workshop remains the only time we have trained facilitators, other than the longer term 'apprenticeship' undertaken by our colleague, Jo Tait, who has become, over the course of ten years of diligent practice and dedication to digital storytelling, a trusted co-facilitator.

There remain some tensions for us between developing a pool of people who are able to help us facilitate workshops and training people who may, for a variety of reasons (including institutional pressures), become excellent competition!

Reflecting with Junior Doctors

Later that summer we were invited to develop a Student Selected Component (SSC) for final-year medical students at the University of Leicester called *Student Voices* (Patient Voices 2008c). This pilot programme was a new and welcome departure for us, and we were enthusiastic about the opportunity to investigate the use of digital storytelling as a reflective methodology. You can read about the project in Chaps. 10 and 11, but for us, working with intelligent, well-educated young people with an excellent grasp of the technology was both an interesting new challenge and a delight. Our hypothesis that creating a digital story would be a good way of learning how to reflect deeply on practice was confirmed both by the stories that were created and the comments made by the students. This project was an important trigger in our thinking, particularly for Tony, and he would go on to present about the project at the *Learning for a complex world* conference in 2009 (Sumner 2009b). The stories have been shown around the world now and are as useful for highlighting the need for compassion as for highlighting the power of reflection through digital storytelling.

Building Communities and Gaining Recognition

Year 2008 was when we began working with the *Communities of Health* project in East London (Patient Voices 2008a). Newham is one of the most diverse communities in the UK, with a high proportion of immigrants from around the world. The incidence of chronic conditions such as diabetes and heart disease is high. We were invited to work with some of these people to create stories about their conditions and how they manage them. The stories illuminate the wisdom of different cultures while giving a voice to people who are seldom heard, and guiding the design of services that can best meet the needs of a richly diverse society.

We were beginning to be more regular conference presenters, and in 2008, we led a symposium at the NETNEP (Nurse Education Today and Nurse Education in Practice) conference in Dublin. There we met Gemma Stacey, who embraced Patient Voices as a way of illuminating the *shock of reality* faced by newly qualified nurses. She managed to find funding for us to run one workshop, and then another …; she writes about the project in Chap. 12.

Celebrating the First Five Years: And Looking Ahead

Patient Voices was now well established and well respected, so we joyfully celebrated five years of success in late 2008 with a small retreat/master-class/conference focused on humanising healthcare and an invitation to think about the next five years. Many of the people who joined us for that event have contributed to this book, and all have continued to be sup-porters and friends of Patient Voices.

I have gone into some detail about the first five years to give you, the reader, a better understanding of the Patient Voices Programme, what we set out to do, how we did it and who we did it with. I don't propose to offer quite so much detail about the next five years, but a few highlights should be mentioned.

Since 2006, the NET conference (Networking for Education in Healthcare) had become an annual event where I presented something new each year and exchanged ideas with other people interested in health-care education from around the world. In 2009, I had the good fortune to meet Mandy Kenny from LaTrobe University in Central Victoria, Australia, who was to become another great supporter of our work.

Year 2009 saw an increasing number of workshops with a wide range of people in widely different places. We worked with people affected by stroke in the Isle of Wight (Patient Voices 2009b), with service-user edu-cators at the University of Liverpool, more workshops in Newham (Patient Voices 2008a) and an interprofessional workshop at the University of Nottingham (Patient Voices 2009c) with service users as well as health professionals. We were invited by Karen Taylor to work on a third project for the National Audit Office, this time to support her Value for Money report on end-of-life care (Patient Voices 2009a). 'Work in progress'

(Patient Voices 2009d) was a project designed to provide insights into the experiences of people with disabilities trying to get back to work. It taught us a great deal about working with people with a wide range of disabilities, from blindness to Asperger's. The Island of Bute in Scotland was the setting for a workshop to create stories about the uses of telehealth for people with chronic obstructive pulmonary disease (COPD) (Patient Voices 2010d), while a competition jointly run by the Royal College of Nursing and the National Patient Safety Agency led to a workshop for nurses to create stories about safety issues (Patient Voices 2010b).

Conference presentations were becoming a regular feature of our work, and it was an honour to be invited to give a keynote at the International Digital Storytelling Conference in Obidos, Portugal. There I met Grete Jamissen from Oslo and Akershus University College of Applied Sciences, among many other amazing people. She was, apparently, so taken with the presentation and the stories that she invited me to present at the next international digital storytelling conference to be held in Norway in two years' time.

In the meantime, we embarked on our own patient/carer journey. When our close friend, Steve Gee, was diagnosed with a terminal brain tumour in the summer of 2009, we decided to move our office to the converted barn at the bottom of his garden so we could help with his care. He deteriorated quickly, and we were pleased to be able to help with hospital visits and, increasingly, support at home. We gained huge insights into what it might be like to care for someone full-time and also into the psychological effects of pain and life-limiting illness. He died 15 months after diagnosis, but fortunately, he was able to come with us to two workshops, where he made two very important stories for his daughter, including 'For Issy'.

In 2010, I travelled to Australia, where I met Cathy Jaynes, to give a joint presentation at the NETNEP conference in Sydney and then to facilitate a workshop in Bendigo, Victoria, at Mandy Kenny's kind invitation. Mental health service users and staff gathered to create stories of recovery (Patient Voices 2010c), and we were especially delighted by one of the comments at the end of the workshop:

These three days have been better than years of group therapy—and I should know, because I've had plenty!

This idea of digital storytelling as therapy is of particular interest to me and is another area that could invite further investigation and research in the future.

In 2010, I registered to do a PhD at Cardiff University, investigating the potential of digital storytelling as a mindfulness practice. This focus was to change, along with my supervisor, but the work I did during those first 18 months laid a solid foundation for the rest of the PhD and gave me the opportunity to learn about phenomenology!

Also in 2010, we were shortlisted for two *British Medical Journal* awards: 'Health Communicator of the Year' and 'Excellence in Healthcare Education'. Friends and supporters joined us for the gala awards dinner, and we were delighted when they announced that we had won the 'Excellence in healthcare education' award (BMJ 2010). Sam Lister, the then Health Editor for *The Times*, nominated us for the Medical Journalists' Association 'Health Champion of the Year' award, and we were delighted to be shortlisted for that award also.

We returned to Australia in the autumn of 2010 to work with people who had worked as support workers during the bush fires in Central Victoria. This workshop was more an opportunity for storytellers to share and reflect on traumatic experiences than about creating a resource, although all commented on the enormous psychological benefits of having the chance to reflect on their experiences with others who had gone through a similar experience (Patient Voices 2010a).

We arrived back in Cambridge just a week before our friend Steve died. At his request, we gave the story he had made to his daughter. She cried, of course, and then said how wonderful it was to be able to hear his voice, a comment that echoed the words of Ian Kramer's mother, following his death. We were reminded of the timelessness and value of digital stories for families and future generations and of the similarities and parallels between all of our stories.

The Importance of Clinical Supervision

Just as our friend Steve's stories touched us and connected with us, so have and will all the stories we have heard. Luckily, several years earlier, my training as a counsellor had allowed us to see and understand the power and potential pitfalls of identification and transference that might affect us, the storytellers, and our relationship with the storytellers, and hence, ultimately, the safety and professionalism of the Patient Voices process. So, in 2007, we built into our practice a programme of regular clinical supervision based on the model used in counselling. We chose a very experienced and capable supervisor who had herself attended a Patient Voices workshop and so had a good understanding of our process. We have continued to have regular supervision ever since and have often marvelled at her ability to help us see what should have been obvious.

Conclusion

The years from 2004 to 2010 saw the consolidation of the Patient Voices programme. The collection of stories had grown substantially and research had revealed that they were being used in many and varied ways in education as well as service improvement programmes. We are eternally indebted to Joe Lambert, the father of digital storytelling, and to CDS for their vision, inspiration and generosity. They shared the gift of story in and with a world filled with the technology that makes it possible for anyone and everyone who is willing to take time, reflect and consider to create a compelling personal story that can explore identities, create and strengthen relationships, break down boundaries, and promote greater understanding within and between cultures, including the vastly different cultures of patients and professionals.

2010 was something of a turning point and Patient Voices entered a new phase of its development, as the next chapter reveals.

Key Points

- 'Story' is a word charged with meaning. The choice of the word 'story' has affected perceptions of their value. The distinction between story, anecdote, testimony and witness statement is a subtle one.
- There are many viewpoints to every experience, which means that there are many truths.

- Stories tell us how individuals experience the system, while statistics tell us how the system experiences the individual.
- A reflective story is a valid piece of auto-analysed data.
- Reflective digital storytelling is a powerful process and is often therapeutic.
- Facilitating the workshops in which the stories are created requires a skilful, professional and mindful approach to all aspects of the work, from technology, through ethical consent and release to the need for professional supervision.
- *Stories are always true; it's the facts that mislead.* (Winterson 2007)

References

Anderson, E. S., & Lennox, A. (2009). The Leicester model of interprofessional education: Developing, delivering and learning from student voices for 10 years. *Journal of Interprofessional Care, 23*(6), 557–573.

Bailey-Dering, J. (2007). *Getting to the bottom of things.* Pilgrim Projects Limited. Retrieved March 2014, from http://www.patientvoices.org.uk/flv/0110pv384.htm

BMJ. (2010). *Patient Voices: Excellence in healthcare education 2010 winners.* British Medical Association. Retrieved 2012, from http://groupawards.bmj.com/excellence-in-healthcare-education-2010-winners

Gandhi, M. (1869–1948). *Source of quote unknown.*

Hardy, P. (2004). *Patient Voices: The rationale.* Pilgrim Projects. Retrieved from http://www.patientvoices.org.uk/about.htm

Hardy, P. (2007). *An investigation into the application of the Patient Voices digital stories in healthcare education: Quality of learning, policy impact and practice-based value.* MSc dissertation, University of Ulster, Belfast.

Hardy, P. (2015). First do no harm: Developing an ethical process of consent and release for digital storytelling in healthcare. *Seminarnet: Media, Technology & Life-Long Learning, 11*(3).

Hardy, P., & Jaynes, C. (2011). Editorial: Finding the voices for quality and safety in healthcare: The never-ending story. *Journal of Clinical Nursing, 20*(7–8), 1069–1071. doi:10.1111/j.1365-2702.2010.03539.x.

Hardy, P., & Stanton, P. (2007). *E-health connections nursing workshop: Connecting to the future.* Pilgrim Projects.

Lambert, J. (2002). *Digital storytelling: Capturing lives, creating community* (1st ed.). Berkeley, CA: Digital Diner Press.

Mauchland, B. (2006). *Jimmy's story*. Pilgrim Projects Limited. Retrieved March 2014, from http://www.patientvoices.org.uk/flv/0047pv384.htm

McGlinchy, Y. (2006). *For the love of Lee*. Pilgrim Projects Limited. Retrieved March 2014, from http://www.patientvoices.org.uk/flv/0054pv384.htm

Page, B. (2004). What they really really want. *Health Service Journal, 114*(5900), 16–19.

Patient Voices. (2006a). *Stories from the NHS Heart Improvement Programme.* Pilgrim Projects Ltd. Retrieved May 2017, from http://www.patientvoices.org.uk/hip.htm

Patient Voices. (2006b). *Stories from the North and East Yorkshire and Northern Lincolnshire Strategic Health Authority (NEYNL)*. Pilgrim Projects Ltd. Retrieved May 2017, from http://www.patientvoices.org.uk/neynl.htm

Patient Voices. (2006c). *Stories from the Working in Partnership Programme (WiPP)*. Pilgrim Projects Ltd. Retrieved May 2017, from http://www.patientvoices.org.uk/wipp.htm

Patient Voices. (2008a). *Communities of Health: Stories from NHS Newham.* Pilgrim Projects Ltd. Retrieved May 2017, from http://www.patientvoices.org.uk/newham.htm

Patient Voices. (2008b). *Healing journeys*. Pilgrim Projects Ltd. Retrieved May 2017, from http://www.patientvoices.org.uk/shu.htm

Patient Voices. (2008c). *Stories from junior doctors in training*. Pilgrim Projects Ltd. Retrieved May 2017, from http://www.patientvoices.org.uk/lssc.htm

Patient Voices. (2009a). *End of life care*. Pilgrim Projects Ltd. Retrieved May 2017, from http://www.patientvoices.org.uk/naoeol.htm

Patient Voices. (2009b). *Stories from the Isle of Wight Stroke Club*. Pilgrim Projects Ltd. Retrieved May 2017, from http://www.patientvoices.org.uk/iowsc.htm

Patient Voices. (2009c). *Stories of inter-professional working from the University of Nottingham*. Pilgrim Projects Ltd. Retrieved May 2017, from http://www.patientvoices.org.uk/unip.htm

Patient Voices. (2009d). *Work in progress*. Pilgrim Projects Ltd. Retrieved May 2017, from http://www.patientvoices.org.uk/exdra.htm

Patient Voices. (2010a). *After the fires*. Pilgrim Projects Ltd. Retrieved May 2017, from http://www.patientvoices.org.uk/bchs.htm

Patient Voices. (2010b). *Stories from the National Patient Safety Agency*. Pilgrim Projects Ltd. Retrieved May 2017, from http://www.patientvoices.org.uk/npsa.htm

Patient Voices. (2010c). *Stories of recovery from La Trobe University.* Pilgrim Projects Ltd. Retrieved May 2017, from http://www.patientvoices.org.uk/latrobe.htm

Patient Voices. (2010d). *Telehealth stories.* Pilgrim Projects Ltd. Retrieved May 2017, from http://www.patientvoices.org.uk/telehealth.htm

Patient Voices and StoryCenter. (2008). *Stories from the Saskatoon health region live well™ with chronic conditions program for aboriginal people.* Pilgrim Projects Ltd. Retrieved May 2017, from http://www.patientvoices.org.uk/sask.htm

Sackett, D. L. (1997). Evidence-based medicine. In *Seminars in perinatology* (Vol. 1, pp. 3–5). Elsevier.

Sumner, T. (2009a). *Inspiring innovation through Patient Voices: Presentation at innovation expo.* London: Edexcel London.

Sumner, T. (2009b). *The power of e-flection: Using digital storytelling to facilitate reflective assessment of junior doctors' experiences in training.* Paper presented at the learning for a complex world, University of Surrey, 31 March 2009.

Wikipedia. (2013a). Evidence based medicine. *Wikipedia.* Retrieved from http://en.wikipedia.org/wiki/Evidence-based_medicine

Wikipedia. (2013b). Hierarchy of evidence. *Wikipedia.* Retrieved from http://en.wikipedia.org/wiki/Hierarchy_of_evidence

Winterson, J. (2007). *The stone gods.* London: Hamish Hamilton.

Pip Hardy is a co-founder of the Patient Voices Programme and a director of Pilgrim Projects Ltd, an education consultancy specialising in open learning and healthcare quality improvement. She also serves as Curriculum and Learning Lead for NHS England's School for Change Agents. Pip has an MSc in lifelong learning and her PhD considers the potential of digital storytelling to transform healthcare.

3

To the Far Horizon

Pip Hardy and Tony Sumner

Introduction

Life is eternal; and love is immortal; and death is only a horizon; and a horizon is nothing save the limit of our sight. William Penn (Wikipedia 2016)

By 2011, the Patient Voices Programme had grown from a twinkle in our collective eye—an added dimension to the educational materials we designed—to being our main source of work and revenue. We were facilitating around ten workshops each year around the UK and elsewhere and hundreds of stories had been recorded. We had welcomed a number of international visitors, including storytellers from China, Norway, Denmark, Sweden, the USA and Canada. Several hundred stories have been released to the Patient Voices website, which was receiving the best part of one million hits per year and the stories were being viewed throughout the English-speaking world. Clearly, interest in Patient Voices

P. Hardy (✉) • T. Sumner
Patient Voices Programme, Pilgrim Projects Limited,
Landbeach, Cambridgeshire, UK

© The Author(s) 2018
P. Hardy, T. Sumner (eds.), *Cultivating Compassion*,
https://doi.org/10.1007/978-3-319-64146-1_3

was growing. We have travelled around the world, for conferences as well as workshops. We have worked with people from all walks of life, tried to find ways of enabling those who are disabled to tell their stories, learned about rare and unusual illnesses. We have published papers and written proposals and carried out research into the ongoing effectiveness of Patient Voices. Pip had registered to do a PhD, looking at the potential of digital storytelling to transform healthcare—a personal journey that was to finish in late 2016 to the welcome comment *no corrections* from her examiners (Hardy 2016).

Expanding Our Horizons: 2011–2014

By 2011, our roles were becoming more clearly demarcated: Tony in charge of all things technical, including the website and post-production work on stories; Pip generally the one who travels to meetings and conferences, makes presentations, does research and tries to 'market' Patient Voices. We were rarely developing learning materials, although an exception was the creation of an e-learning package about Motor Neurone Disease (MND) for clinicians, augmented by digital stories about MND.

Making Contacts Around the Globe

We were becoming part of a growing global network of people leading the way in digital stories.

Early in 2011 we travelled to Norway to present a keynote at Create—Share—Listen, the 4th International Conference on Digital Storytelling in Lillehammer, meeting up with familiar faces from Portugal and creating new friends and contacts.

In 2012 our travels took us back to Norway to facilitate a reflective digital storytelling workshop for staff at Oslo University College and Oslo Technical Museum using iPads rather than our normal laptops.

We returned to Australia in 2012 to facilitate two workshops. Again using iPads, these workshops were part of the 'Building Healthy Rural Communities' project, which aimed to contribute to a future-oriented, community-relevant, efficient and effective model of providing rural health and human service. Key to this was working with communities to create stories that would assist in establishing health and service priorities and engender actions that would address these needs.

We welcomed a group of clinicians from Hong Kong, including the CEO of a large hospital cluster, who were following up best practice from the 2010 BMJ awards. We invited colleagues (some of whom have contributed chapters to this book) to spend the day with us to give our visitors a fuller flavour of Patient Voices. Later, we received an invitation to present the keynote at their Annual Quality Conference in Hong Kong, and three of their colleagues came to a workshop here in the UK so that they could experience the digital storytelling process through making their own stories.

The visit to Hong Kong was a valuable learning experience, reminding Pip once again that humanity is universal. When she showed 'Getting to the bottom of things' and invited reflections on the story, she was intrigued by one response: *That's not really a story about rheumatoid arthritis—it's a love story.* Interestingly, when she showed that same story to a group of doctors back in London a few weeks later, one of the audience proclaimed it to be *a crime story.* You might like to watch it and decide for yourself!

Now we were becoming well known and well regarded in the international digital storytelling community as the leading practitioners in digital storytelling in healthcare. Pip gave keynotes at the next two international digital storytelling conferences, in Ankara in 2013 and Athens in 2014. It was something of a challenge to come up with, something new that would delight a familiar audience and so it came as a huge relief when one regular attendee at these conferences commented that 'you always give us something new to think about.' And of course, every conference gives us an opportunity to think about something new or to think about things differently.

Workshops Abounding

Meanwhile storytelling workshops were continuing to explore new avenues.

We had become more convinced than ever of the importance of hospitality in digital storytelling workshops—that is, the provision of comfortable, congenial, welcoming surroundings away from the usual place of work; nourishing and plentiful food; and a warm welcome—and we have convinced most of our workshop partners of the key role hospitality plays in putting people at their ease and enabling them to tell the stories they need to tell.

Table 3.1 shows the 2011–2014 workshops not mentioned elsewhere in this chapter.

During this period, we learned a great deal about the creativity of people with dementia, their capacities to engage with the storytelling process and our own need to be able to provide 'agile, nimble, adaptive facilitation' (Sumner and Hardy 2013).

We also learned, from our work at Mid Staffordshire hospital that, even though the failings at Mid Staffs were the subject of a major inquiry (Francis 2010, 2013), many people do not wish to complain—they simply want someone to listen to—and acknowledge—their experiences (Patient Voices 2012c).

Working with young people affected by liver disease was a new departure for us, necessitating checks by the Criminal Records Bureau and risk assessments. Support workers were also available during the workshop, something we have, by and large, avoided on the basis that having more people around can be distracting and, where these people are sponsoring the workshop, they often want to have input into the stories. This can sometimes—although certainly not always—have a detrimental effect on the stories, potentially turning them into promotional videos rather than the stories that need to be told by the storytellers. However, the workshops went well and we were amazed by the courage, maturity and resilience of these young people.

Getting It Down on Paper

Joe Lambert invited us to write a chapter for the third edition of his book, *Capturing Lives Creating Community* (Hardy and Sumner 2010; Lambert 2013), and our list of published papers and book chapters grew,

Table 3.1 Some projects and workshops (2011–2014)

Organisation	Brief description	URL
NHS Lothian	Stories exploring the way telehealth can enable service users to change their life stories and, as in the first telehealth-themed workshop in 2010, to give staff a chance to share their experience of how technology can change care-giving	www.patientvoices.org.uk/sth-htm
Sheffield City Council	Stories told by carers from Sheffield with experiences of many conditions. But one in particular, 'The day the singing stopped' (Wood 2011), was prescient for work to come	www.patientvoices.org.uk/sheffcc2.htm
University of Abertay	Stories from people with early-stage dementia—the first Patient Voices workshop explicitly intended to address the issues facing people with dementia	www.patientvoices.org.uk/dc.htm
Health Foundation	Stories intended to investigate ways of improving the complaints service, as part of the Speaking Up project at Mid Staffordshire Hospital.	www.patientvoices.org.uk/speakingup.htm
University of Nottingham	Stories from allied health professionals in Nottingham, deepened our engagement with interprofessional working and education	www.patientvoices.org.uk/unahp.htm
Department of Health	Stories from patients who have been involved in research, 'getting involved in research,' took our earlier work on patient and public engagement onto an arc that would lead us more deeply into the use of digital storytelling in a range of aspects of research	www.patientvoices.org.uk/ppires.htm
Children's Liver Disease Foundation	Stories from young people affected by severe liver disease to raise awareness of the conditions	www.patientvoices.org.uk/ttt.htm
South Tees NHS Foundation Trust	A pair of workshops looked at the effects on, and experiences of, members of a team—in this case an oncology ward—who had faced intense professional and personal challenges	www.patientvoices.org.uk/ht.htm

as did the list of papers we would like to write … but from 2010 to 2017, so did our output.

In 2013, colleagues and friends suggested that, to celebrate the tenth anniversary of the programme, we should work together to produce a book detailing the genesis and development of the Patient Voices Programme and describing some of the projects that had filled that decade. Drafts became a book, which in turn needed a launch, and a launch became a conference and—with the support of NHS England, Deloitte and Kingsham Press, we ran our first Patient Voices conference at the Kings Fund in London in December 2014. It was a fine celebration with keynote talks by Neil Churchill from NHS England's Patient Experience team, Helen Bevan from NHS England's Horizons team, Iona Heath, former chair of the Royal College of General Practitioners and, of course, Joe Lambert from StoryCenter. A number of storytellers were able to attend and participate in a panel, thanks to a generous contribution from Deloitte UK, and many friends from the international digital storytelling community joined us to share the joyous occasion.

In addition to completing the first edition of this book (Hardy and Sumner 2014), we have now contributed chapters to books about new media literacies (Pleasants and Salter 2014), and the theory and practice of digital storytelling (Dunford and Jenkins 2017), and edited and contributed to a volume on digital storytelling in higher education (Jamissen et al. 2017).

Mental Health in Manchester

During this period, we also worked on what has become, to date, the only long-term Patient Voices project with Manchester Mental Health and Social Care NHS Trust, now a part of Greater Manchester Mental Health NHS Trust. It began with one workshop, late in 2011, to highlight issues of dignity and respect with a view to improving care in the Trust. There have now been 12 workshops and growing interest in the impact the stories are having at every level of the Trust—as you will learn in Chap. 8. This work has resulted in short listings for several awards, including the *Health Service Journal's* Innovation in Mental Health award.

In 2012, Patient Voices were part of a winning team in the NHS Institute for Innovation and Improvement's *Patient Feedback Challenge*.

For the Patient Voices team, the project involved facilitating a series of workshops for patients and staff in The Princess Alexandra Hospital, Harlow; NHS Manchester Mental Health and Social Care Trust; and Bart's Health, London, looking at particular issues from both sides in three different organisations. Those stories can be seen here:

http://www.patientvoices.org.uk/learningtogether.htm
http://www.patientvoices.org.uk/workingtogether.htm
http://www.patientvoices.org.uk/comingtogether.htm

2014–Present: All the Stories Are One

We began this period with one of the most personally affecting and challenging workshops we have ever facilitated.

Risk and Ethics: Tanzania

Malaria exacts a heavy toll from millions of families across the world. Handeni is one of the poorest districts in Tanzania. There is little infrastructure and mechanisation is minimal. The majority of the population live a very hand-to-mouth existence, living in mud huts and subsisting by growing maize, beans and, perhaps, a few vegetables. Malaria is very common. Babies and young children are particularly susceptible to the worst effects of malaria. When it rains, the mud huts collapse…And the mosquitos emerge.

So reads the introduction to the Saving Brains digital stories (Patient Voices 2014b).

This project, in conjunction with the World Health Organization and funded by Grand Challenges Canada, allowed one group of families in rural Tanzania whose children had been brain damaged as a result of contracting malaria when they were very young to express how it has affected their lives. The digital stories were intended to form part of the communication strategy to disseminate the results of research that had been carried out over the previous 10 years.

The project aimed to share those stories, which it did very successfully, but the stories that emerged also served to communicate priorities for potential future research into the economic experiences of those people and prompted us to think even more deeply about the ethical issues in relation to particularly vulnerable people and children. One of the challenges of this project was to weigh the benefits and risks of revealing the identity of the storytellers through their pictures and spoken words, in a culture where the potential for stigma is great. Although the parents/storytellers were very happy for their pictures to be included in the digital stories they created, the ethics committee remained concerned. Having seen the stories and discussed at length the issues with the clinicians involved, the ethics committee ultimately decreed that the likely benefits of increased understanding and global awareness of the impact of malaria were greater than the possible risks arising from storytellers being identified and the decision to show the children's faces was upheld.

Reflection and e-Flection

One of the recommendations in Pip's MSc dissertation was that digital storytelling be used with medical and healthcare students to promote reflection. The work we began in 2008 with final-year medical students at the University of Leicester (Patient Voices 2008) (described in Chaps. 10 and 11) has grown into a highly effective and adaptable reflective module for medical students, 'Physician know thyself,' which ran in 2014 and 2016 at King's College London Medical School (Patient Voices 2014a). It has proved immensely rewarding to us as facilitators and reminded us again of the need for agile and adaptive facilitation.

Education and storytelling have been entwined within our work from the very beginning of the Patient Voices Programme in 2003, and so, in 2013, when Pip was asked to become the Curriculum and Learning Lead for the School for Change Agents (formerly the School for Health and Care Radicals), it was inevitable that she would weave the power of digital stories through the learning materials to prompt reflection and motivate action, but also to help participants understand the power of storytelling as a force for transformational change (Hardy 2015).

Becoming Servant Facilitators

Our work in mental health continued in Manchester and was joined by work in Telford on the Positively Different project and in South London for the Power of Story project. One story in particular from South London, The book of Stephan, reminded us again of the complexity of caring for people with dementia. This was a theme that came out strongly in workshops for Lancashire County Council, Dementia Insights and NHS South Staffordshire and Shropshire Foundation Trust, Living with Dementia, where people with dementia and their carers/partners created stories about their shared experiences.

While we centre our working process firmly on the classical digital storytelling model developed by StoryCenter, some projects and some groups of storytellers have always needed us to shape our process to them, rather than forcing them to fit to 'our' process. Our work during this period with people with learning disabilities, funded by NHS England (Patient Voices 2015), was no exception to that rule. Shifts to workshop patterns, excellent and knowledgeable organisation by the people 'on the ground,' enhanced facilitation levels—and the determination, good humour and creativity of the storytellers—made the creation of affecting stories possible. The stories were intended to illuminate what good care can look like for people with learning disabilities and, in the words of one of workshop organisers, 'If we can get care right for people with learning disabilities, we can get care right for everyone.'

The DNA of Care: Staff and Patient Care

Staff stories have played a part in the work of the Patient Voices Programme since the earliest stages. After our initial work with patients, in 2006 we ran several workshops involving staff. Presciently, given the aims of the DNA of Care project, story number 25 in our catalogue was made by the nurse in charge of a Coronary Care Unit and entitled 'Caring for staff as well as patients' (Kent 2007). When, after we had worked with NHS England on the Learning Disability stories, we were asked to run a major project using digital storytelling to help NHS staff share their experiences, we were reminded again that staff and patient experiences within health and social care are entwined like a double helix of experience, with the stories being the links between them. And so, the DNA of Care project began. By the time it finished, we would have run five workshops and helped 33 members of staff tell 34 stories (Patient Voices 2016b). The stories that emerged were testament to the care, commitment, integrity and resilience of the people who made them. You can read about the project and several other projects that have been sparked by it, in Chap. 22.

Further Stories from Both Sides

Informed by their experiences as storytellers on the *DNA of Care* project, several members of staff formed new projects. The first two of these looked again, as we had with the *Patient Feedback Challenge* Both Sides Now! workshops in 2012 (Patient Voices 2012a, b, d), at how stories about the same experience told from different perspectives can inform and illuminate each other. The *Terrific Teens* project used Patient Voices Reflective digital stories to explore the experiences of teenagers with long-term conditions and the experiences of their parents. The project was conceived by a DNA of Care storyteller, a paediatric allergy consultant from Imperial College NHS Trust. Held in October 2016, the first stage explored the experiences of teenagers with life-threatening allergies and their parents. Further workshops addressing other long-term conditions are planned. For each condition, the model is to run two Patient Voices workshops in parallel—one for parents and one for teenagers—and then bring the groups together after the 3-day workshop, to share, experience and reflect upon each other's stories.

Another DNA of Care storyteller, this time a consultant anaesthetist from University College London NHS Hospital Trust, saw the potential for a pair of workshops, one for staff and one for patients, to illuminate what it is like to work in, and be cared for by, a specialist complex pain team. This team works with patients who have persistent or chronic pain and aims to improve people's quality of life and manage pain, whether in hospital or transiting back to living at home (Patient Voices 2017).

Cultivating Compassion in End of Life Care

During this period we brought our experiences of developing learning programmes, interprofessional working, personal and professional experience of end of life care and digital storytelling together for the Cultivating Compassion in End of Life Care project (Patient Voices 2016a). Working for Health Education North East and in collaboration with the Centre for the Advancement of Interprofessional Education, reflective digital stories about end of life care were created in a series of workshops attended by family carers and professionals as varied as lawyers and palliative care physiotherapists, healthcare assistants and consultants, paramedics and community nurses. From the stories, learning themes were developed and a series of learning materials constructed around them to develop an interprofessional learning resource intended to cultivate compassion in end of life care. This project is the subject of Chap. 21.

Digital Storytelling: Future Research

Since the publication of the first edition of this book, which contained a chapter specifically focused on the use of digital storytelling in research (please see Chap. 17), there has been growing recognition of the uses of digital stories and of digital storytelling in research, both in terms of Patient Voices' work and in the wider academic digital storytelling community (Jamissen et al. 2017). 2017 began with two more projects in the broad research stream, one to help nurse researchers and academics at the University of Hertfordshire to reflect on, create and share their own stories of research processes and motivation and another with the Nursing and Midwifery School of King's College, London, to look at ways in which digital storytelling can enhance the dissemination of the results of academic research into the effectiveness of Schwartz Rounds.

The Story of the Process

Over the years, one of the quotes that we have used most often to explain the importance of sharing stories has been 'One of the hardest things in life is having words in your heart that you cannot utter' (James Earl Jones 1931–). Ironically then, for us, one of the greatest challenges for all digital storytelling projects is in explaining to prospective participants the nature of the process. We have created briefing materials, run pre-workshop sessions and yet, still, it is difficult to separate the fact that the delivery medium for a digital story is a video file from the idea that a storyteller will be videoed or interviewed. For the DNA of Care project, we created a brief introduction to the process, which was used in webinars and from the website to inform prospective DNA of Care storytellers about the nature of the Patient Voices process. For the Patient Voices team, it became apparent during our reflection on the project that the video created had been of great value, and so we commissioned the creation of a professional 30-minute documentary about the process. The making of the documentary incorporated a workshop at which several storytellers returned to make second stories and some came to make their first stories. This film is believed to be the first documentary film to be made about the digital storytelling process.

The documentary was premiered in July 2017 at Un/Told—An Un/ Conference about digital storytelling at the University of East London.

Looking Ahead: To the Far Horizon

The quotation that opens this chapter seems particularly appropriate as we look ahead to the next phase of Patient Voices. While we hope that death is not imminent, either for us or for the Programme, we have become more aware in recent years of the need for both sustainability and managed growth. To that end, the Patient Voices website, which was showing its age, received a complete overhaul in 2016, with a more modern look and what will become a more efficient database, improving ease of searching—to date, this is still a work in progress.

Towards the end of 2016, perhaps our busiest year ever, we were encouraged by colleagues and friends to think about the future. Accordingly, the Patient Voices Advisory Board has been established. A wonderful group of people from the worlds of healthcare, academia and digital storytelling met for the first time in London to engage in some appreciate inquiry about the future of Patient Voices. We feel honoured to have such a wise group of people who are prepared to roll their sleeves up and become involved in the work of Patient Voices, providing skills and knowledge in research, marketing, blogging, bid-writing, social media and other talents yet to be revealed. We look forward to sharing the next stage of our journey with them and are confident that, with their wise and gentle guidance, the work of Patient Voices will continue 'to the far horizon.'

Conclusion

Every workshop teaches us something new and we strive to be reflective practitioners, as well as practitioners of reflection. We have made it our practice to take time at the end of each day and after the end of every workshop to reflect on what we have done and what we have learned. We write down our reflections, as well as those of the workshop participants. Over and over again, we are humbled by the courage of the people who share their stories with us and by the extraordinary challenges people overcome. We laugh and we cry with storytellers. We share painful experiences with them—and sometimes joyful ones. We get to know them in ways that few other people ever do. Many groups we work with think they have the monopoly on suffering. Many people we work with have suffered greatly, whether they are affected by mental illness or malaria, by the pain of rheumatoid arthritis or the disabling effects of a stroke, whether they are a carer or a newly qualified nurse. And so we have reached the conclusion that suffering is universal—and our ability to share stories about it is one of the things that makes us human and offers what we might call redemption.

Over and over again we are reminded of our shared humanity and the overwhelming need for respect and compassion. Although we have now heard so many stories of tragedy, hardship and suffering that we are rarely shocked, we are still, sometimes, surprised by the depth of compassion that we see in the workshops and in the stories, such as the story told by a security guard on night shift (Vaitkunas 2013).

There are two quotations that appear in almost every presentation we have given. They remind us not only of why we tell stories but of who and what we are as human beings. The first is about our need to face, and overcome, our dragons or challenges, to demonstrate our courage, our strength, our cleverness—our humanity:

> *No matter what form the dragon may take, it is of this mysterious passage past him, or into his jaws, that stories of any depth will always be concerned to tell.…* (O'Connor 1969)

Please see Chap. 4 for more about dragons.

The second is about the transformation that can occur when we do tell our stories:

> *People reach greater maturity as they find the freedom to be themselves and to claim, accept and love their own personal story, with all its brokenness and its beauty.* (Vanier 2004)

And now, please enjoy the stories told by the people we have worked with, each chapter a tribute to the vision and persistence of the person who wrote it. We hope that, by the time you have finished reading this book, you will agree with us that 'Each affects the other and the other affects the next and the world is full of stories and the stories are all one' (Albom 2003).

Key Points

- *There is more that unites us than divides us*—people around the world value the same things: health, family, safety, belonging and so on.
- Reflection plays a key part in the work of digital storytelling facilitation as well as in digital storytelling.
- Compassion is everywhere—and in unexpected places.
- Sharing and hearing stories about the same thing from multiple perspectives can provide valuable insights as well as healing.
- Collaboration and the wisdom of others is necessary to secure the future of Patient Voices.

References

Albom, M. (2003). *The five people you meet in heaven* (1st ed.). New York: Hyperion.

Dunford, M., & Jenkins, T. (2017). *Digital storytelling: Form and content.* London: Palgrave Macmillan. doi:10.1057/978-1-137-59152-4.

Francis, R. (2010). *Independent inquiry into care provided by Mid Staffordshire NHS Foundation Trust January 2005—March 2009* (Vol. 1). London: The Stationery Office.

Francis, R. (2013). *The Mid Staffordshire NHS Foundation Trust Public Enquiry.* Press Statement.

Hardy, P. (2015). The power of storytelling as a force for transformational change. *NHS Horizons.* Retrieved 2017, from http://theedge.Nhsiq.Nhs.uk/the-power-of-storytelling-as-a-force-for-transformational-change/

Hardy, V. P. (2016). *Telling tales: The development and impact of digital stories and digital storytelling in healthcare.* Doctoral thesis, Manchester Metropolitan University, Manchester.

Hardy, P., & Sumner, T. (2010). Humanizing healthcare: A conversation with Pip Hardy and Tony Sumner, Pilgrim Projects/Patient Voices. In J. Lambert (Ed.), *Digital storytelling: Capturing lives, creating community* (3rd ed., pp. 143–156). Berkeley, CA: Digital Diner Press.

Hardy, P., & Sumner, T. (2014). *Cultivating compassion: How digital storytelling is transforming healthcare.* Chichester: Kingsham Press.

Jamissen, G., Hardy, P., Nordkvelle, Y., & Pleasants, H. (2017). *Digital storytelling in higher education.* London: Palgrave Macmillan. doi:10.1007/978-3-319-51058-3.

Jones, J. E. (1931–). *Source of quote unknown.*

Kent, D. (2007). *Caring for staff as well as patients.* Pilgrim Projects. Retrieved June 2017, from http://www.patientvoices.org.uk/flv/0025pv384.htm

Lambert, J. (2013). *Digital storytelling: Capturing lives, creating community* (4th ed.). New York; London: Routledge.

O'Connor, F. (1969). *Mystery and manners; Occasional prose.* New York: Farrar.

Patient Voices. (2008). *Stories from junior doctors in training.* Pilgrim Projects Ltd. Retrieved May 2017, from http://www.patientvoices.org.uk/lssc.htm

Patient Voices. (2012a). *Coming together.* Pilgrim Projects Ltd. Retrieved 2017, from http://www.patientvoices.org.uk/comingtogether.htm

Patient Voices. (2012b). *Learning together.* Retrieved 2017, from http://www.patientvoices.org.uk/learningtogether.htm

Patient Voices. (2012c). *Speaking up*. Pilgrim Projects Ltd. Retrieved 2017, from http://www.patientvoices.org.uk/speakingup.htm

Patient Voices. (2012d). *Working together*. Pilgrim Projects Ltd. Retrieved 2017, from http://www.patientvoices.org.uk/workingtogether.htm

Patient Voices. (2014a). *Physician, know thyself*. Pilgrim Projects Ltd. Retrieved May 2017, from http://www.patientvoices.org.uk/lssc.htm

Patient Voices. (2014b). *Saving brains*. Pilgrim Projects Ltd. Retrieved 2017, from http://www.patientvoices.org.uk/savingbrains.htm

Patient Voices. (2015). *Champions*. Pilgrim Projects Ltd. Retrieved 2017, from http://www.patientvoices.org.uk/champions.htm

Patient Voices. (2016a). *Cultivating compassion in end of life care*. Pilgrim Projects Ltd. Retrieved May 2017, from http://www.patientvoices.org.uk/ipeineolc.htm

Patient Voices. (2016b). *DNA of care*. Pilgrim Projects. Retrieved May 2017, from http://www.patientvoices.org.uk/dnaoc.htm

Patient Voices. (2017). *Complex pain, complex teams*. Pilgrim Projects. Retrieved May 2017, from http://www.patientvoices.org.uk/complexpainteam.htm

Pleasants, H. M., & Salter, D. E. (2014). *Community-based multiliteracies and digital media projects: Questioning assumptions and exploring realities*. New York: Peter Lang.

Sumner, T., & Hardy, P. (2013). *Dangling conversations: Digital storytelling—Age, vocation and value*. Paper presented at the Silver Stories, University of Brighton.

Vaitkunas, D. (2013). *Night shift*. Pilgrim Projects Limited. Retrieved June 2014, from http://www.patientvoices.org.uk/flv/0685pv384.htm

Vanier, J. (2004). *Drawn into the mystery of Jesus through the Gospel of John*. New York: Paulist Press.

Wikipedia. (2016). *Rossiter W. Raymond*. Retrieved from https://en.wikipedia.org/wiki/Rossiter_W._Raymond#.27Death_is_Only_an_Horizon.27

Wood, S. (2011). *The day the singing stopped*. Pilgrim Projects Ltd. Retrieved June 2017, from http://www.patientvoices.org.uk/flv/0545pv384.htm

Dr Pip Hardy is a co-founder of the Patient Voices Programme and a director of Pilgrim Projects Ltd, an education consultancy specialising in open learning and healthcare quality improvement. She also serves as Curriculum and Learning Lead for NHS England's School for Change Agents. Pip has an MSc in Lifelong Learning and her PhD considers the potential of digital storytelling to transform healthcare.

Tony Sumner is a co-founder of the Patient Voices Programme and a director of Pilgrim Projects. With degrees in physics and astronomy and astrophysics, and many years' experience working in the software industry, he is particularly interested in how technology and storytelling can intersect to promote deep reflection.

4

The Patient Voices Approach

Pip Hardy and Tony Sumner

Introduction: Digital Storytelling: What It Is—And What It Is Not

The term 'digital storytelling' was first used to describe the workshop process designed by Joe Lambert, Dana Atchley and Nina Mullen in California in the 1990s to teach ordinary people how to use new media tools and technologies to create short videos about their lives. The history and methodology of what was to become StoryCenter (formerly the Center for Digital Storytelling) is described in detail in *Digital storytelling: capturing lives, creating community* (Lambert 2002), and so I will not go into that here.

The workshop model derived from the Freirian process of building critical consciousness and promoting social justice (Freire 1973); both the workshop and the stories that are created therein are wonderful examples of what Ivan Illich referred to as 'convivial tools' (Illich 1973;

P. Hardy (✉) • T. Sumner
Patient Voices Programme, Pilgrim Projects Limited,
Landbeach, Cambridgeshire, UK

© The Author(s) 2018
P. Hardy, T. Sumner (eds.), *Cultivating Compassion*,
https://doi.org/10.1007/978-3-319-64146-1_4

Meadows 2003). Workshops both offer a potentially meaningful process to participants and yield a set of outcomes (the produced digital stories) that can be analysed and shared in many useful ways (Gubrium et al. 2014).

Digital storytelling has now become a generic—almost ubiquitous—term used to describe the use of new media technologies for new or innovative narrative forms, ranging from well-funded journalistic projects such as the *New York Times' Snowfall* (Branch et al. 2012) to the provision of a .pdf or an audio file containing a 'story'—usually the transcript of an interview. Projects and outcomes vary in their relative emphasis on the 'digital' or the 'story' element. Digital storytelling projects in schools can provide creative ways for young people to learn about new technologies and to improve their writing skills. Other digital storytelling projects, such as Amy Hill's *Silence Speaks* (www.silencespeaks.org), focus on enabling storytellers to find meaning through voicing difficult stories about painful, often traumatic, experiences. However, as Pleasants and Salter remind us, 'as media-making tools become increasingly ubiquitous, it is CDS's ethos and approach to storytelling as life-affirming and transformative as much as it is their technological savvy and expertise that continues to draw newcomers to their approach'(Pleasants and Salter 2014).

When we refer to a digital story, we do not mean a talking head video, a *vox pop*, a podcast, a recorded interview or a Facebook post. We will use the term 'digital storytelling' to refer to the workshop-based process defined and described by StoryCenter (www.storycenter.org) in which ordinary people use multimedia tools to create their own short autobiographical videos, which can be disseminated via the internet (as in the Patient Voices Programme) or shown on television (as in the BBC's *Capture Wales*). Still images, usually drawn from the storyteller's personal collection, are combined with a recorded voiceover, scripted and read by the storyteller, sometimes with added music, resulting in a rich tapestry that is at once '*effective, affective and reflective*' (Sumner 2009a).

The StoryCenter workshop process grew out of community theatre and community development work and consists of an intriguing blend of personal reflection, creative writing, drama and speaking, art and narrative therapy, multimedia production and facilitated small-group work. Intensive work is done on the script: refining and distilling the story to

250–300 words requires deep reflection on the meaning of the story and careful choice of just the right words. Attention needs to be paid to the selection of appropriate images to tell parts of the story; consideration must be given to pacing and use of voice and, at last, viewing the finished piece. Every stage of the workshop prompts reflection and often evokes new learning for storytellers and viewers alike. In addition, storytellers are offered a wide range of skills to investigate, learn, enjoy and demonstrate. Learners of all kinds, all ages, all backgrounds, all levels of skills are able to engage with the process and find a comfortable way of expressing themselves.

It is this model that has informed the Patient Voices approach to digital storytelling, together with a deep desire to address what philosopher Miranda Fricker has termed 'epistemic injustice' (Fricker 2009). Epistemic injustice takes two forms:

- testimonial injustice, 'when prejudice causes a hearer to give a deflated level of credibility to a speaker's word…' and
- hermeneutic injustice, which '…occurs at a prior stage, when a gap in collective resources puts someone at an unfair disadvantage when it comes to making sense of their social experiences.' (Fricker 2009)

People who come to our workshops are almost always familiar with the first of these forms of injustice and many are well acquainted with the second.

It's About the Story…

The Patient Voices approach to digital storytelling places a firm emphasis on the story, and the reflection that supports good storytelling. The 'digital' part of the process is simply a tool—much like a pen—to help the storyteller express the story in the most appropriate way to the intended audience. This approach is founded on years of experience that support the belief that stories are a laboratory in which students and others can construct meaning from their experience (Paulson and Paulson 1994; Sumner 2009b).

We also draw heavily on the idea of 'story' as distinct from narrative, or anecdote, or case study or history or data. In recent years, the burgeoning popularity of 'patient stories' has led to a situation in which almost anything that comes out of a patient's mouth is deemed to be a story. For us, a story is something more than that.

A story needs conflict, crisis and resolution. It needs characters and plot. It needs time, pace and place. Louise Aaronson helpfully distinguishes story from anecdote, focusing on the meaning inherent in the story, as opposed to a simple exposition of events:

> In contrast to anecdote, story—at least in the literary sense—offers so much more: narrative arc, movement, unification of action, irrevocable change. Meaning. (Aronson 2013)

Every Story Needs a Dragon

When Joe Lambert left a copy of the late Jo Carson's *Spider Speculations* (Carson 2008) on the table after one of his visits, we didn't foresee how that book would affect our understanding of stories and their potential for healing in individuals, communities and societies. That book has had a profound influence on the way we think about and articulate the shape of stories and the need for a dragon, for it was within its pages that we first encountered these words of Flannery O'Connor, the twentieth-century American novelist:

> No matter what form the dragon may take, it is of this mysterious passage past him, or into his jaws, that stories of any depth will always be concerned to tell…. (O'Connor 1969)

The dragon is an essential component of any story that is worth hearing (or telling). The dragon, as we understand it, is the challenge that is faced by the hero or heroine of the story—the illness, the accident, the despair, the grief, the loss—that must be overcome in order for the hero or heroine to demonstrate his or her courage, strength, wit, wisdom, kindness, resourcefulness or whatever quality it is that contributes to that person's humanity (Hardy 2016).

Storytellers at the Centre of the Process

Underlying the Patient Voices' reflective digital storytelling process is what we refer to as 'the ultimate open-ended question': 'Tell us a story about something that really matters to you.' This places the storyteller firmly at the centre of the process and ensures a spirit of co-operation and collaboration that may not be familiar to many who come to share their stories with us. They may be more accustomed to the probing questions of researchers who have their own agendas to follow, whereas it is our intention to ensure that control of the story remains, as far as possible, with the storyteller.

It would be disingenuous to suggest that there are not several power dynamics inherent in a storytelling workshop. Many storytellers regard us—the facilitators—as 'the experts'. We take great care to remind them that while we may know about the theory and practice of making digital stories, they are the experts in their own lives, in their own stories. We are simply present as facilitators to enable the telling of their story in a particular format. Perhaps, rather than a power imbalance, what is actually present are several expertise gradients. This is why we emphasise the facilitative aspect of our role in the workshop rather than the didactic. Working closely together with storytellers to co-produce their stories ensures that our expertise as digital storytelling facilitators is used to best effect to bring out their expertise in their own lives and result in the most effective—the best possible—story, in much the same way that clinicians working closely with patients can ensure the most effective, co-produced care.

Empowering storytellers by placing them in control of the edit results in an even more radical departure from more conventional forms of data gathering. While we, as facilitators, may offer suggestions and help with shortening, refining and distilling the script and in the selection and arrangement of images, ultimately it is the storyteller who decides what will be included and what will be left out. The integrity of the story is thus preserved and storytellers need have no fear that their words will be taken out of context, misquoted or misconstrued. They retain ownership of the story throughout and can rest assured that their story will not be 'dis-membered' once they leave the workshop (Hawkins and Lindsay 2006).

Consent as Process

Over the years, we have developed a robust, three-stage consent and release process that affords storytellers time to consider their participation in the Patient Voices Programme, and the possibility of deciding not to make their stories public at any stage of the process.

The first 'formal' stage is when we invite storytellers to read and sign our Protocol and Consent form soon after they arrive at the workshop. This is only after we have contacted storytellers by email and/or phone to introduce ourselves and explain the workshop process. The form is simply an expression of intention to participate in the workshop, together with an understanding of the Patient Voices Programme, the aims and the focus of the particular workshop in which they are participating and any possible risks. It also sets out what the storyteller can expect from us in terms of support.

Once a storyteller has completed a draft story, on the last day of the workshop, we invite him or her to complete an Interim Release form. At this stage, storytellers may decide to keep their story private or release it only to others in their workshop group, or they may express the intention to make it fully public after they have had time to reflect further on their story outside the workshop and following any necessary post-production work. All storytellers leave the workshop with a DVD of their draft story so that they can reflect on it at leisure and show it to friends and relatives.

When post-production work has been completed (this may include substitution of different images provided by storytellers, e.g., a photo of a sister or brother or parent or grandparent that they couldn't find before the workshop, or different music composed or licensed specifically for the story, or other small changes that have been requested and agreed), storytellers are invited to sign a Final Release form. Once finalised and approved by the storyteller, stories are released under a licence stipulating that they cannot be changed or sold and that they must be correctly attributed (Creative Commons 2013).

Our ethical consent and release process has, by and large, been developed by us at the Patient Voices Programme, with help from our earliest storytellers, as described in Chap. 1. In recent years, we have been delighted to contribute to Amy Hill's work to develop a *Bill of Rights for Storytellers*, and we are proud to use the ethical framework for facilitators that she has created (Gubrium et al. 2012) as a way of further strengthening our process. The development and implementation of the Patient Voices consent and release process has also been considered more fully in a paper entitled 'First do no harm: developing an ethical process of consent and release for digital storytelling in healthcare' (Hardy 2015).

Copyright and Distribution

One of our primary goals—reinforced by the wishes of storytellers from the start of the programme—was to make as many stories publicly viewable as possible, with the informed consent of storytellers. Our aim in doing this was to maximise the social capital that would result from the viewing of the stories in which storytellers had made emotional and intellectual investments.

This immediately brought into play much experience from Tony's previous work in software development and Pip's in publishing. We were aware that we had to help storytellers create stories that respected the intellectual property of others.

There are several resource and intellectual flows within the Patient Voices process (Fig. 4.1). For each of these, we had to develop guidelines that would ensure that images, music, video and sounds used in the story did not violate the copyright of others. Hence, we encourage the use of storyteller-created artefacts where possible. Where that is not possible, we purchase images or video clips from stock image libraries, license or have music composed for use in stories.

Responses to issues around intellectual property and copyright from storytellers have been enlightening. In general, they see the issue as one of respect for the work of others, just as they wish others to respect their stories.

Establishing respect for the story amongst viewers was a key factor in the choice of a 'no derivatives' licence when we release stories, in order to prevent stories being dismembered or embedded within another creation. This has required careful consideration of aspects of both sourcing material for use in stories and distribution of the stories.

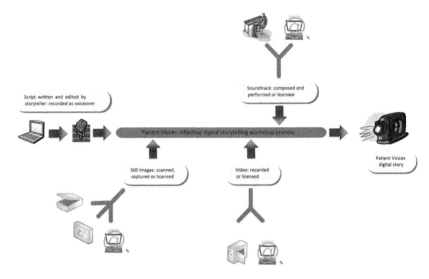

Fig. 4.1 Resource and intellectual flows in the Patient Voices reflective digital storytelling process

It is tempting for storytellers to use images they have found through an internet search, and this initially requires clarification that, even if not stated, images found in this way will almost always be someone's copyright. The next hurdle comes when a storyteller searches for images released under a creative commons licence. The issue that affects the story then is most commonly that the image will have been released by its creator under a 'sharealike' licence. These images are unsuitable for use in a Patient Voices digital story, as using them would mean granting 'sharealike' rights to everything else used in the story—that is, other images (whether the storyteller's or licenced), music, sounds and so on.

We are often asked why the Patient Voices stories are not available on sites such as YouTube, for example. The issue here that needs careful consideration is that, in uploading a video to a sharing site, the uploader usually consents to giving the site owners some sort of licence to display the video. Whether they can or not depends on the licence conditions under which the elements of the digital story were sourced and the terms of the licence that must be granted to the site.

These are often in conflict. The YouTube terms of use, for example, state under 'Rights you Licence' in Clause 8.1 that:

"8.1 When you upload or post Content to YouTube, you grant:

- to YouTube, a worldwide, non-exclusive, royalty-free, transferable licence (with right to sub-licence) to use, reproduce, distribute, prepare derivative works of, display, and perform that Content in connection with the provision of the Service and otherwise in connection with the provision of the Service and YouTube's business, including without limitation for promoting and redistributing part or all of the Service (and derivative works thereof) in any media formats and through any media channels;
- to each user of the Service, a worldwide, non-exclusive, royalty-free licence to access your Content through the Service, and to use, reproduce, distribute, prepare derivative works of, display and perform such Content to the extent permitted by the functionality of the Service and under these Terms." (YouTube 2017)

There is obviously a clash here between the terms and conditions and protecting the intellectual property of all those who have contributed to the story—the storyteller, musicians, photographers etc. The key issues are the preparation of derivative works and the ability to sub-licence the uploaded materials.

This has been a major factor in choosing, so far, to host the Patient Voices stories ourselves—we do not wish to risk the possibility of an image being taken from a story, the music extracted or snippets of audio used out of context. There are patient- and staff-related materials on video-sharing sites such as YouTube, and we are yet to understand whether they have been uploaded in full knowledge of the licence implications.

Creating Safe Space

Establishing and sustaining a space that is both safe and creative is key to ensuring that storytellers have a good experience and are able to tell the stories they need to tell.

A number of factors contribute to this sense of safety, including a strong ethical framework (Hardy and Sumner 2008; Gubrium et al. 2012) and a robust consent process, such as that alluded to above (Hardy 2015).

We try to meet storytellers several weeks before a workshop, usually in an introductory briefing session, often accompanied by tea and a sandwich. This meeting gives everyone a chance to get to know one another in a more 'normal' situation, before coming together to share very personal stories. If meeting in person is not possible, we talk to people by phone or Skype so that they can ask questions, seek reassurance and resolve anxieties.

Hospitality

Hospitality forms one of the cornerstones of the Patient Voices approach. In our experience of modelling the values to which we aspire in the health service, we have found that people particularly value the broad notion of hospitality. By hospitality, we have in mind the ancient Greek word *xenia*, that is, a basic generosity and courtesy to those far from home. It relies on mutual respect and understanding of the reciprocal roles of guest and host, mutual giving and receiving and, interestingly, on the ritual of a parting gift. This expression of hospitality recognises the interconnectedness of all of humanity, acknowledging that there is no guest without a host and no host without a guest; in this sense, it is perhaps more like the African concept of *Ubuntu*, as Archbishop Desmond Tutu describes it:

> *Africans have this thing called UBUNTU. It's about the essence of being human, it is part of the gift that Africa will give the world. It embraces hospitality, caring about others, being able to go the extra mile for the sake of others. We believe that a person is a person through another person, that my humanity is caught up, bound up, inextricably, with yours.* (Battle 1997)

Indeed, Don Berwick, formerly of the Institute of Healthcare Improvement, had this to say about hospitality in relation to healthcare:

> *We are guests in our patients' lives; and we are their hosts when they come to us. Why should they, or we, expect anything less than the graciousness expected by guests and from hosts at their very best? Service is quality.* (Berwick 1999)

We place great value on the physical surroundings. Workshop sponsors are asked to ensure that the venue is pleasant, comfortable, calm, peaceful and safe, and that there is always someone ready with a warm welcome and a cup of tea to greet storytellers—even those who arrive early! We know that digital storytelling is hard work, and so we ensure plentiful and nourishing food and drink, and there is always a parting gift of a DVD of each storyteller's story.

Attending to people's physical needs as well as their emotional needs can often be challenging, especially when working with patients affected by long-term conditions or staff affected by traumatic events. Significant adaptations to the workshop format may be necessary to accommodate people with low energy levels, poor mobility, cognitive impairment, limited communication functioning and reduced literacy levels (Hardy and Sumner 2014; Stenhouse et al. 2013). Some of these situations are described in later chapters in this book; see, for example, Chap. 6, Fiona O'Neill's chapter about working with people with rheumatoid arthritis in the Arthur and Co. project, and Chap. 19, Rosie Stenhouse and Jo Tait's chapter about working with people with dementia in the Dangling Conversations project.

We keep things simple. We use ordinary, everyday language, avoiding the often pompous language beloved of many researchers and academics. We avoid jargon. We ensure that technology teaching is kept to a minimum—just what's necessary to produce the story. We make sure that the technology works so that it is facilitative in much the same way as our role is facilitative.

Principles underpinning the Patient Voices work include a deep respect for all individuals and the stories they want to tell, whatever their age, race, gender, educational background, social or health status or sexual orientation (O'Neill and Hardy 2008). We remind ourselves, during almost every workshop when one of us is struggling with a storyteller or finding someone difficult to work with, of Joe Lambert's immortal words of wisdom: *'You just have to love them to bits.'*

Digital Storytelling: A Reflective Process

In the Patient Voices approach, based upon the StoryCenter workshop model, the creation of a digital story normally takes three consecutive days, but the particular format can be adapted to suit the needs and characteristics of the storytellers. The process is highly reflective, intellectually stimulating, emotionally demanding and technologically challenging.

Careful planning and mindful facilitation are crucial to success. Workshop numbers are small—between 6 and 10 participants—to ensure sufficient individual support. Each participant is provided with a named PC laptop pre-loaded with the appropriate image and video editing software—in our case, usually Adobe Photoshop Elements and Adobe Premier Pro. However, we sometimes switch to other software packages where, for example, they integrate better into assistive technologies to make it easier for people with disabilities to create their own stories.

Stages in the workshop process are described below, while a typical three-day workshop programme is illustrated in Table 4.1.

What Happens in a Patient Voices Digital Storytelling Workshop?

Getting to Know One Another: Introductions

The first step in creating a safe space in which personal stories can be shared is by getting participants to share, understand, learn and trust themselves and one another. This is also the first stage of reflection, as people get to know one another through the process of thinking deeply about why they want to create this particular story at this particular time.

What Makes a Good Story?

The Seven Elements and the Seven Steps of digital storytelling (Lambert 2002, 2006, 2009, 2013) provide the basis for a discussion about what makes a good story and inform the deconstruction of some digital stories. We do this in an informal and inclusive way, showing and talking about selected digital stories and encouraging everyone to express a view.

Sharing Stories: Story Circle

The story circle provides a safe space, place and opportunity (like the Greek *temenos* or 'sacred place') for participants to share their stories,

Table 4.1 Patient Voices workshop: three-day programme

Day 1	
10.00–10.30	Welcome and introductions
10.30–11.30	What makes a good story? Deconstructing stories
11.30–11.45	BREAK & REFRESHMENTS
11.45–13.15	Story circle: share and develop story ideas
13.15–14.15	LUNCH
14.15–15.15	Script development
15.15–15.30	BREAK & REFRESHMENTS
15.30–17.15	Working with images: Photoshop tutorial
17.15–17.30	Check-in and review of the day
Day 2	
09.00–09.15	Check-in and review goals and schedule
09.15–11.00	Scripting, storyboarding, image editing, record voiceovers
11.00–11.15	BREAK & REFRESHMENTS
11.15–12.15	Digital video editing tutorial part 1: the basics (Premiere Pro)
12.15–13.15	Continue recording voiceovers, scanning and editing images, preparing storyboards
13.15–14.15	LUNCH
14.15–17.15	Production time: voiceover recording, image editing, beginning the rough edit
17.15–17.30	Storytellers' check-in and review of the day
Day 3	
09.00–09.15	Check in and review goals and schedule
09.15–12.00	Digital video editing tutorial part 2: special effects in Premiere pro
12.00–12.30	Production time: complete rough edit
12.30–13.15	LUNCH
13.15–15.15	Production time: special effects, music, titles, final edit
15.15–16.00	Preparation for screening of stories (BREAK for storytellers)
16.00–16.45	Premiere of stories (accompanied by celebratory food and drink!)
16.45–17.15	Review and reflection, evaluation and consent forms
17.15	Farewell and close

Note: On the afternoon of day 2 and on day 3, when people are working at their own pace, breaks are taken as and when needed!

often for the first time, and to gain feedback from their peers. We place great emphasis on listening, sometimes commenting that perhaps these workshops should be called 'Story listening' rather than 'Story telling' workshops. This is the most sensitive and emotional part of the process and we place guidelines around it to ensure confidentiality, respect and mindful attention to one another. These guidelines, which we agree with the storytellers, also promote deep listening, constructive questioning, appreciative comments and creative silence.

Refining Stories: Developing a Script

The focus of the storytellers' process now shifts from the outward focus on the group, to an inward focus on personal reflection—akin to what Wordsworth described as *'emotion recollected in tranquillity'* (Wordsworth et al. 1969)—as storytellers work individually and with us to develop, distil and refine their scripts down to 250–300 words. This task requires the ability to listen carefully and question appropriately, as well as the skills needed to edit sensitively. It can be difficult for people who have learned to write formally (in the third person passive voice) to write as they would speak, and it often requires gentle probing and questioning to help them to speak as they are thinking and feeling—and then encouragement to write it down that way!

Editing Images: Photoshop Tutorial

This session provides a change of pace and introduces a bit of technical wizardry. Storytellers are encouraged to think visually, as well as verbally, through learning some of the basics of an image-editing software programme and focusing on the imagery of emotion. When time is limited, we often just demonstrate some of the possibilities afforded by Photoshop so that people can ask for help if they want to create a particular effect. Since the first edition of this book was published in 2014, we have had the good fortune to work closely with Darcy Alexandra, a visual anthropologist, digital storyteller and documentary film-maker (www.darcyalexandra.com/). We have learned much from her about the value of a visual strategy that will contribute to the integrity of the story, as well as the possibilities afforded by consideration of the relationship between words and pictures as a kind of conversation or even a dance, not duplicating one another or going off at a tangent but responding and extending understanding.

Recording the Voiceover

Many storytellers conquer the all-too-common fear of hearing their own voice as they practise reading their scripts, first to each other and then to us and, finally, record the voiceover for their stories. This is often a time for new insights and confidences to be shared—storytellers are alone with a facilitator and the intimacy of the recording room can prompt explanations and new explorations as we concentrate on how the words will sound.

Planning the Edit: Storyboarding

Preparing a plan for the digital story helps storytellers to decide which parts of the story will be told in words, and which in pictures, and helps to avoid the dangers of getting lost in their story when it's time to edit the video. Once again, we encourage storytellers to think visually, imagining the mental image that accompanies the words. We include storyboards in each storyteller's pack and remind them that completing a storyboard is like having a map before setting out on a journey or a recipe before beginning to cook—without it, you may get somewhere, but it will probably take longer, and there may be a number of wrong turns along the way.

Bringing It All Together: Premiere Pro Tutorial

Words and pictures come together as storytellers learn how to use video editing software to bring the ingredients of their story together in a wonderful synthesis of words and pictures and take charge of directing their own movie. Excitement and exhilaration vie with frustration and the pressure of time as storytellers deepen their understanding of their story by hearing their voice repeatedly and concentrating on how images can tell the parts of the story that words cannot. This is a time of particular challenge for some people—especially elders—and particular delight for those who enjoy technology or relish learning new things. Adding music—if the storyteller wishes—is the final step.

Celebration: Premier of Stories

After the intensity of individual concentration and contemplation, the group re-forms. This celebration of the creation of all the stories is often a very moving experience, when storytellers watch what they, and others, have produced in such a short time and have the opportunity to see and reflect on their stories outside of their own heads. This session underlines, through the sharing of experiences as digital stories, the similarities of experience and the connections between storytellers in the group. Depending on the group, we may invite storytellers to reflect and comment on each other's stories as they are shown. This is particularly relevant for educators who are considering using digital storytelling with their students and for students who can learn valuable lessons about giving and receiving feedback as well as the power of reflection.

Reflection and Debrief

An important part of every Patient Voices workshop, and key to our own development as reflective practitioners, is the opportunity to share what went well and what didn't, what people have learned about themselves and others. Storytellers often reach important new insights and come to accept themselves and their stories in new ways, 'in all their brokenness and beauty' (Vanier 2004). We also learn what went well and what we could do better!

The Reflective, Adaptive Process of Facilitation

Facilitating a digital storytelling workshop is a bit like managing a three-ring circus. Lots of different things are going on, often at the same time, with people of different capabilities and at different stages in the process. Safe, competent digital storytelling facilitators need to have a complex set of skills and qualities, including (but not necessarily limited to):

- writing and editing
- group facilitation

- individual facilitation
- time management
- listening skills
- image editing
- video editing
- technology skills
- problem solving
- tact and diplomacy
- self-awareness
- emotional resilience
- patience

Above all, facilitators need to be flexible, adaptable, agile, responsive and reflective. We have found that the ability to reflect on our practice, the discipline of writing down our own reflections after each workshop and taking the time to review storytellers' comments and feedback have all helped us to adapt to each new group and to make changes, where necessary, during a workshop.

We are also fortunate in having a very wise and experienced clinical supervisor, who helps us to reflect after each workshop on issues or content that may have been difficult for us. We regard this practice as an essential aspect of professional facilitation, ensuring the safety of story-tellers, as well as safeguarding our own mental and emotional wellbeing. This is particularly important when working with storytellers who are affected by mental health issues (Hardy and Sumner 2017).

Our commitment to ongoing research, professional development, supervision and reflective practice has also helped us to address the issues of testimonial and hermeneutic injustices mentioned earlier in this chapter. In our attempt to redress testimonial injustice, we are committed to hearing all the voices in the world of healthcare that have been waiting patiently to be heard, not just those of patients or carers but also, and increasingly, those of the people who deliver care, from surgeons to speech and language therapists, from porters to paediatricians. To that end, it is our practice to:

- seek out and recognise the stories of all storytellers in the group.
- recognise that all stories have their own relevance.

- acknowledge that the epistemic authority of each storyteller is inherent in their story and its telling.

It has been helpful for us to think of this approach as 'reflexive facilitation'. Drawing on the ideas of Valerie Yow, we have drawn up this list of things to consider in relation to storytellers and workshops:

1. What am I feeling about this storyteller?
2. What similarities and differences affect this interpersonal situation?
3. How does my own ideology affect this workshop?
4. What group(s) outside the workshop am I identifying with?
5. Why am I facilitating this workshop in the first place?
6. In selecting storytelling prompts and offering editorial suggestions (textual/visual/audio), what alternatives could I have employed and why did I reject them?
7. What are the effects on me as I facilitate this story?
8. How do my reactions to the story affect my facilitation? (Yow 1997; Sumner and Hardy 2014)

In order to address hermeneutic injustice, we have to address the disadvantages. For us, this relies on an 'adaptive facilitation' process, including (but not limited to):

- appropriate technology
- adaptations to workshop scheduling
- adequate levels of facilitation support
- access
- awareness of and sensitivity to cultural differences
- interpreting and translation services

We have worked diligently over the years to ensure that the Patient Voices digital storytelling process is resilient and transferable across different contexts, different countries and different cultures, but it relies on the willingness and ability of facilitators to respond, adapt and work long hours and go the extra mile.

Conclusion

The development of the Patient Voices Programme has come to be characterised by the quality of both its product—the digital stories—and the process of creating those stories. This process, now referred to as 'classical' digital storytelling, is a powerful process, a process that requires thoughtful planning, careful facilitation, expert knowledge, a wide range of skills and mindful attention to all stages of the process. It relies on respect for everyone involved in the creation of the stories underpinned by a strong ethical framework. It is this careful attention to detail that can contribute to healing and transformation, as well as education and improvement.

Key Points

- The Patient Voices approach is firmly based on the StoryCenter model of 'classical' digital storytelling.
- Stories differ from narratives and anecdotes in significant ways.
- Working in healthcare requires adaptive, agile and reflexive facilitation to meet specific needs of patients and staff.
- An ethical process of consent and release is necessary to safeguard storytellers and all who contribute to a digital story.
- Hospitality, and the recognition of our interconnectedness as human beings, is a fundamental characteristic of the Patient Voices approach.
- Supervision is essential to ensure the emotional safety and wellbeing of digital storytelling facilitators working in the healthcare context.

References

Aronson, L. (2013). *A history of the present illness: Stories* (1st U.S. ed.). New York: Bloomsbury.

Battle, M. (1997). *Reconciliation: The Ubuntu theology of Desmond Tutu.* Cleveland, OH: Pilgrim Press.

Berwick, D. (1999). *The Permanente Journal, 3*(1), 9.

Branch, J., Miller, E., & Spangler, C. (2012). *Snowfall: The Avalanche at Tunnel Creek.* New York: The New York Times.

Carson, J. (2008). *Spider speculations: A physics and biophysics of storytelling* (1st ed.). New York: Theatre Communications Group.

Creative Commons. (2013). *Attribution-NonCommercial-NoDerivs 2.5 Generic.* Retrieved from http://creativecommons.org/licenses/by-nc-nd/2.5/

Freire, P. (1973). *Education for critical consciousness* (Vol. 1). New York: Continuum.

Fricker, M. (2009). *Epistemic injustice: Power and the ethics of knowing.* Oxford: Oxford University Press.

Gubrium, A., Hill, A. L., & Harding, L. (2012). Digital storytelling guidelines for ethical practice, including digital storyteller's bill of rights. *StoryCenter.* Retrieved November 2015, from https://www.storycenter.org/s/Ethics.pdf

Gubrium, A. C., Hill, A. L., & Flicker, S. (2014). A situated practice of ethics for participatory visual and digital methods in public health research and practice: A focus on digital storytelling. *American Journal of Public Health,* e1–e9. doi:10.2105/AJPH.2013.301310.

Hardy, P. (2015). First do no harm: Developing an ethical process of consent and release for digital storytelling in healthcare. *Seminarnet: Media, Technology & Life-Long Learning, 11*(3). http://seminar.net/volume-11-issue-3-2015/256-first-do-no-harm-developing-an-ethical-process-of-consent-andrelease-for-digital-storytelling-in-healthcare

Hardy, P., & Sumner, T. (2008). Digital storytelling in health and social care: Touching hearts and bridging the emotional, physical and digital divide. *Lapidus Journal, 3*(3), 24–31.

Hardy, P., & Sumner, T. (2014). Our stories, ourselves: Exploring identities, sharing experiences and building relationships through Patient Voices. In H. Pleasants & D. Salter (Eds.), *Community-based multi-literacies and digital media projects: Questioning assumptions and exploring realities.* New York: Peter Lang.

Hardy, P., & Sumner, T. (2017). Digital storytelling with users and survivors of the UK mental health system. In M. Dunford & T. Jenkins (Eds.), *Story, form and content in digital storytelling: Telling tales.* London: Palgrave Macmillan.

Hardy, V. P. (2016). *Telling tales: The development and impact of digital stories and digital storytelling in healthcare.* PhD by publication, Manchester Metropolitan University.

Hawkins, J., & Lindsay, E. (2006). We listen but do we hear? The importance of patient stories. *Wound Care, 11*(9), S6–14.

Illich, I. (1973). *Tools for conviviality.* New York: Harper and Row.

Lambert, J. (2002). *Digital storytelling: Capturing lives, creating community* (1st ed.). Berkeley, CA: Digital Diner Press.

Lambert, J. (2006). *Digital storytelling: Capturing lives creating community* (2nd ed.). Berkeley, CA: Digital Diner Press.

Lambert, J. (2009). *Digital storytelling: Capturing lives creating community* (3rd ed.). Berkeley, CA: Digital Diner Press.

Lambert, J. (2013). *Digital storytelling: Capturing lives, creating community* (4th ed.). New York; London: Routledge.

Meadows, D. (2003). Digital storytelling: Research-based practice in new media. *Visual Communication, 2*(2), 189–193.

O'Connor, F. (1969). *Mystery and manners; occasional prose.* New York: Farrar.

O'Neill, F., & Hardy, P. (2008). *Designing patient-shaped healthcare: Hearing patient voices.* White Rose Health Innovation Partnership Technology Bulletin. Retrieved May 2017, from http://www.patientvoices.org.uk/pdf/articles/wrhip14.pdf

Paulson, F. L., & Paulson, P. R. (1994). Paper presented at the Annual Meeting of the American Educational Research Association in New Orleans, LA.

Pleasants, H. M., & Salter, D. E. (2014). *Community-based multiliteracies and digital media projects: Questioning assumptions and exploring realities.* New York: Peter Lang.

Stenhouse, R., Tait, J., Hardy, P., & Sumner, T. (2013). Dangling conversations: Reflections on the process of creating digital stories during a workshop with people with early stage dementia. *Journal of Psychiatric and Mental Health Nursing, 20*(2), 134–141. doi:10.1111/j.1365-2850.2012.01900.x.

Sumner, T. (2009a). *Inspiring innovation through Patient Voices: Presentation at innovation expo.* London: Edexcel London.

Sumner, T. (2009b). *The power of e-flection: Using digital storytelling to facilitate reflective assessment of junior doctors' experiences in training.* Paper presented at the Learning for a complex world, University of Surrey, 31 March 2009.

Sumner, T., & Hardy, P. (2014). *Raising voices: A reflective and reflexive look at the interdependencies of crisis, injustice, voice, storytelling, justice and facilitation!* Paper presented at the Digital storytelling in times of Crisis, Athens, Greece, 8th May 2014.

Vanier, J. (2004). *Drawn into the mystery of Jesus through the Gospel of John.* New York: Paulist Press.

Wordsworth, W., Coleridge, S. T., & Owen, W. J. B. (1969). *Lyrical ballads, 1798* (2nd ed.). London: Oxford University Press.

YouTube. (2017). *Terms of service.* Retrieved June 2017, from https://www.youtube.com/t/terms

Yow, V. (1997). Do I like them too much?: Effects of the oral history interview on the interviewer and vice-versa. *Oral History Review, 24*(1), 55–79.

Pip Hardy is a co-founder of the Patient Voices Programme and a director of Pilgrim Projects Ltd, an education consultancy specialising in open learning and healthcare quality improvement. She also serves as Curriculum and Learning Lead for NHS England's School for Change Agents. Pip has an MSc in lifelong learning, and her PhD considers the potential of digital storytelling to transform healthcare.

Tony Sumner is a co-founder of the Patient Voices Programme and a director of Pilgrim Projects. With degrees in physics and astronomy and astrophysics, and many years' experience working in the software industry, he is particularly interested in how technology and storytelling can intersect to promote deep reflection.

Part II

Involvement, Impact and Improvement

Pip Hardy and Tony Sumner

Storytelling is the mode of description best suited to transformation in new situations of action. (Schön 1988)

The history of system improvement has, in general, been one of quantitative and statistical approaches. Where qualitative approaches to gathering patient and staff experience have been used, the analysis rapidly regresses to a pseudo quantitative one, driven by the goal of creating and using a numerical metric, which may or may not relate effectively to an individual's experience.

The chapters in this part reflect, at a particularly challenging time for healthcare around the world and the UK National Health Service (NHS) in particular, on how the Patient Voices Programme can provide timely reminders of the core values of empathy and compassion, relating the uniqueness of individual experiences to the humanity of all, and to underpin quality and safety improvement programmes. Drivers for change in the NHS in the last decade have included the Francis Report into the events in mid-Staffordshire (Francis 2010) and the 6Cs programme adopted by the NHS to drive compassion in nursing practice (Cummings 2012).

One of the motivations for developing the Patient Voices Programme was our belief in the power of stories to carry meaning and effect changes in behaviour. The use of stories to underpin safety and quality improvement programmes is not new—an early adopter was the National Aeronautics and Space Administration through its Aviation Safety Reporting System incorporating a succinct monthly newsletter containing stories from pilots called 'Callback' (Hardy 1990), but the emerging digital and Internet technologies made the creation and distribution of the stories vastly more powerful.

As we watched the projects described in this book unfold, we came to believe that the power of stories to do this is because 'Statistics tell us the system's experience of the individual, whereas stories tell us the individual's experience of the system…' (Sumner 2009a) and to understand that 'The ability to tell, hear and share stories of experience and aspiration is a pre-requisite for the development of a learning organisation of reflective individuals' (Sumner 2009b).

The stories themselves do not provide solutions but provoke positive and reflective debate that can lead to practical improvements, more holistic care, awareness of shortcomings and the fundamental involvement of health service users in all aspects of healthcare through really listening to each other's experience and attending to the insights that emerge.

In Chap. 5 'Towards Compassionate Governance: The Impact of Patient Voices on NHS Leadership', Paul Stanton reflects on his experience of using Patient Voices stories to help address the need for compassionate governance by NHS Boards. He stresses the importance of listening to and reflecting on patients' stories both for governance of safety and quality and to promote inclusive and co-productive caring, citing the empathic sensitivity, compassion and co-productive nature of the Patient Voices method, where the locus of control remains with the storyteller, as a parallel model for NHS working.

In Chap. 6 'Arthur and Co: Digital Stories About Living with Arthritis', written collaboratively with the storytellers, Fiona O'Neill examines new ways of involving patients and carers in health professional education using patients' stories. From her own therapeutic experience of creating a digital story to working in Leeds with volunteers who work with people with arthritis, she outlines the process of creating stories in a gentle, affirmative and truly reflective environment. The theme of journeying was carried into the transformative potential of the experience, and then further, as the stories were taken to health professionals and families to help them 'walk in another's shoes'.

Cathy Jaynes, in Chap. 7 'Safety Stories: Creating a Culture of Safety with Digital Stories', relates her search for a 'culture of safety' and 'what safety looked like' in air medical transport to her transformative discovery of the impact of digital storytelling told in 'our' language. She describes the genesis of the Safety Story project and the efforts required for fundraising, backing and attending the workshops. She also considers the feedback from educators using the stories as an educational resource, the theoretical foundation for the stories' effectiveness, and the impact on individuals and organisations when safety and humanity are prized.

Chapter 8 'Working with Dignity and Respect: Improving Mental Health Services with Digital Storytelling', written by Patrick Cahoon, Carol Haigh and Tony Sumner, explores how the Patient Voices reflective digital stories were created and used by a mental health and social care trust over several years to enhance training and awareness of dignity, privacy and respect amongst service users and service providers. Workshops for service users, carers and health professionals have resulted in stories being shown, with consent, in places as diverse as a Manchester shopping centre and NHS Board rooms, and used in recruitment for positions up to Chief Executive. The stories are driving change and innovation in care and awareness in the health service and community groups and amongst the wider public—and saving money!

In Chap. 9 'Breathe Easy: Digital Stories About COPD', Matthew Hodson discusses a Patent Voices project undertaken with a group of patients with Chronic Obstructive Pulmonary Disease to help understand the personal impact of this debilitating condition and capture patients' experience of engagement with the Acute COPD Early Response Service (ACERS) service. The workshop, described in detail, was shared by clinicians and patients with a high degree of openness and transparency. He describes how the stories demonstrate the workings of the 6/7 Cs of the core values of nursing care (Cummings 2012) and are a powerful tool for listening to patients' experiences in order to promote change.

References

Cummings, J. (2012). *Compassion in practice. Nursing, midwifery and care staff, our vision and strategy*. London: Department of Health. Retrieved from www.dh.gov.uk/health/2012/12/nursing-vision/

Francis, R. (2010). *Independent inquiry into care provided by Mid Staffordshire NHS Foundation Trust January 2005 – March 2009* (Vol. 1). London: The Stationery Office.

Hardy, R. (1990). *Callback: NASA's aviation safety reporting system*. Washington, D.C.: Smithsonian Institution Press.

Schön, D. (1988). Coaching reflective teaching. In G. L. Erickson & P. P. Grimmett (Eds.), *Reflection in teacher education* (pp. 19–29). New York: Teachers College Press.

Sumner, T. (2009a). *Inspiring innovation through Patient Voices: Presentation at Innovation Expo*. London: Edexcel London.

Sumner, T. (2009b). *The power of e-flection: Using digital storytelling to facilitate reflective assessment of junior doctors' experiences in training*. Paper presented at the Learning for a Complex World, University of Surrey.

5

Towards Compassionate Governance: The Impact of Patient Voices on NHS Leadership

Paul Stanton

Introduction

The NHS stands at a crossroads. Under coincident pressures of an accelerative increase in demand and of protracted public sector austerity, it will only survive if the development of new models, patterns and forms of care can make it fit for twenty-first-century purpose.

In preparing for a workshop on the need for health and social care transformation, I recently watched again a couple of the very first Patient Voices stories that I had commissioned from Pilgrim Projects almost a decade ago. The stories are told by my late colleague and friend, Ian Kramer. I first used them embedded into a series of dry PowerPoint slides, with the Board of an NHS Trust in the Midlands that I had been sent to visit.

The Board was struggling, in the face of the insistent pressure of central targets, financial stringency and an extensive hospital rebuilding programme, to grasp the central contribution of 'Clinical Governance'

P. Stanton (✉)
Southminster Consultancy Associates Ltd,
Scarborough, North Yorkshire, UK

© The Author(s) 2018
P. Hardy, T. Sumner (eds.), *Cultivating Compassion*,
https://doi.org/10.1007/978-3-319-64146-1_5

(see below) in securing the safety, dignity and quality of care. The Board in question did not welcome yet another Department of Health (DH) outsider's instructions on how it should conduct its own business. Ian's brief story, *Introduction* (Kramer 2004b), changed the nature of our discourse. Its transparent sincerity and immediacy, its clarity, dignity and quiet authority reminded them (as it reminded me on that day and still reminds me now) of the need to still the ever-present clamour of the urgent and to focus and reflect upon the essence of the caring task and the need constantly to learn. Indeed, it is worth taking a moment to consider whether you think that the NHS could be better at learning from other healthcare systems, as Ian suggests.

Later that day, non-executives and executive Board members talked reflectively about the range of ways in which patient contributions might have a practical impact on the safety and quality of care. Their debate was illuminated and enlivened by Ian's story about how patient input could help to quality assure clinical audit procedures. The story is called *Another pair of eyes* (Kramer 2004a).

Although there has been an increased understanding of the need to involve patients more directly in the design of healthcare services since Ian created his digital stories in 2004, I am not certain about the extent to which patient perspectives have been incorporated into clinical audit processes and I sometimes reflect upon whether Ian's experiences could be repeated today.

Clinical Governance

The term 'clinical governance' has mostly now been superseded. The emphasis within policy and guidance is now upon the 'governance of safety and quality'. Though neither safety nor quality are simple notions, this evolution is admirable. 'Clinical governance' needed elaborate explanation to Boards and clinical staff. It did not facilitate inclusive discussions with patients or carers about the safety or quality of their own care and was incomprehensible to social workers and social care staff. Explicit emphasis on 'safety and quality' places both at the heart of an NHS Board's governance agenda and provides the basis for inclusive discourse with patients and communities and with all of those who commission and provide local care. This is an essential prerequisite for a long overdue move from preoccupation with discrete 'episodes of care' to whole-system attention to safety and quality throughout the 'journey of care'.

Impact of Patient Voices Stories

Before I describe the range of ways in which, over more than a decade, Patient Voices have contributed to my work with NHS Boards and senior clinicians, I want to reflect upon the nature and origin of the distinctive impact that Ian's stories and a host of others in the ever-expanding library of Patient Voices have upon me and upon other audiences.

First, I believe that the creation of each individual Patient Voices story is a 'parallel process' to that which generates the safest and best forms of NHS care—that is, when a patient and an expert clinician work together in a partnership characterised by reciprocal respect. In the same way, each Patient Voices story is a co-production between an individual storyteller and Pip and Tony at Pilgrim Projects. A storyteller brings her/his memories and experiences of care in all of their unique spiritual, psychological, emotional and physical complexity. Pip and Tony contribute refined technical expertise and an experience-based understanding of the 'digital narrative art'. Crucially, the relationship with individual storytellers and with groups is characterised by an empathic sensitivity and compassion that is expressed through the active way in which Pip and Tony listen (in Simone Weil's phrase) 'with their whole being' to what is said (and sometimes left unsaid) and through the tenderness with which they treat each and every individual in the groups with whom they work.

The power of this quiet process is explicitly described in Pep Livingstone's *Tell me your story* (Livingstone 2009). Pep consciously reflects on the process that led to the creation of her first *Once upon a time* story (Livingstone 2008). Just as Pep describes, Pip and Tony facilitate (but do not direct) a process in which the locus of control—in the creation of the narrative, choice of images and selection of music—remains with the storyteller, albeit they reflect with Pip and Tony (and often with other members of the group) on the pros and cons of alternative courses of action.

The maintenance of 'locus of control' is a key reason that so many storytellers find the process of telling their story to be a comforting or even a healing one. Something of this sense of healing is conveyed subtly in even the most anguished of the stories that are told. It is also one of the reasons that many of them are imbued with a powerful poetic quality. In his 1802 *Preface to The Lyrical Ballads*, William Wordsworth (Wordsworth and Coleridge 1968) defined a poem as 'the spontaneous overflow of powerful feelings' but noted that poems take their 'origin from emotion recollected in tranquillity'. The same is true of Patient Voices stories—many derive from powerful episodes of loss, trauma or joy but, like poems, they are conscious artefacts where words, images and sounds are crafted together, so that, in Alexander Pope's phrase, the 'sound becomes an echo to the sense', through a tranquil process of reflection and distillation. Please take a few moments, if you can, to listen to Mia's story *I love you more* (Bajin 2009). This story seems to me to possess many poetic qualities, beautifully conveying a powerful and bitter/sweet message about the enduring power of love. I wonder what feelings it evokes in you?

Like poems, a story has no single or definitive 'meaning'. Meaning is created afresh each time a story is viewed—through the interaction between the objective digital artefact and the subjective viewer/listener with whom the story resonates—both consciously and subconsciously. The poet Gerard Manley Hopkins (1844–1889) (Hopkins 1967) grappled with this phenomenon in relation to 'rainbows':

> *It was a hard thing to undo this knot.*
> *The rainbow shines but only in the thought*
> *Of him that looks. Yet not in that alone,*
> *For who makes rainbows by invention?*
> *And many standing round a waterfall*
> *See one bow each, yet not the same to all,*
> *But each a hand's breadth further than the next.*
> *The sun on falling waters writes the text*
> *Which yet is in the eye or in the thought.*
> *It was a hard thing to undo this knot.*

This unique response (*each a hand's breadth further than the next*) to the 'same' digital narrative (which *writes the text*) is one reason why these stories provide such a powerful stimulus to reflection and discussion in groups—whether these groups are the diverse members of an NHS Board, a group of senior clinical specialists or NHS team colleagues. Each person is exposed to the same stimulus, but each one actively perceives it from her/his own perspective. In sharing their perspectives and exploring both the commonalities and difference in individual response and the insights that are triggered, people learn more about each other, more about themselves and more about the (often submerged or unconscious) emotional dynamic of the group. The story becomes a common starting point from which tacit assumptions about the nature of the caring task can be safely explored.

If you watch Fiona O'Neill's story about her father, *Only connect: a life in stories* (O'Neill 2007), it may not cause you to cry, but for me it touches on still unresolved grief at the loss of my own father more than 40 years ago. Many of us may take some comfort from the sense of quiet dignity that Fiona conveys, and I hope that all of us can applaud the sensitivity and the tenderness displayed by the hospice staff and perhaps ponder why such sensitivity and tenderness is so often absent when an old person dies (as too many of us and of those we love will) in a hospital (rather than a hospice) bed.

Using Digital Stories with NHS Boards

One of the reasons I have used Patient Voices extensively in my work with NHS Boards is that, in the face of so many coincident pressures, the NHS has not always put patient safety and quality at the top of its performance and regulatory agenda. Urgent political and target-led demands and a plethora of data can often obscure the most important task of governance: to promote and assure the safety and the quality of individual patient care. In his report on the failings at Mid Staffordshire Hospital, Robert Francis observed, among many other thoughtful reflections, that:

> *an unhealthy and dangerous culture pervaded not only this Trust ... echoes of the cultural issues found in Stafford can be found throughout the NHS system.* (Francis 2013, 1361)

Aspects of a negative culture have emerged at all levels…These include: a lack of consideration of risks to patients, defensiveness, looking inwards not outwards, secrecy, … acceptance of poor standards … [and] failure to put the patient first in everything done. (Francis 2013, 1357)

As the (then) NHS CEO accepted, "the performance management system at the time was not focused on, or sensitive to, issues of quality." (Francis 2013, 70)

Reflecting upon the avoidable deaths of so many patients at Mid Staffs Hospital, Robert Francis concluded that there had been 'a dangerous abrogation of directors' fundamental duty to protect the safety of those who come to the Trust for care and treatment' (Francis 2013, 68).

When he reflected upon the first phase of the Inquiry, Francis drew attention to the distinctive impact that listening to the personal testimonies of the relatives of patients who had died avoidably had upon him, his Inquiry colleagues and observers: 'The experience of listening to so many accounts of bad care, denials of dignity and unnecessary suffering made an impact of an entirely different order to that made by reading written accounts' (Francis 2010a, b). Overwhelmingly it is written accounts, complemented by verbal reports from executive directors, that are presented to Boards. While it is not easy for a patient (or relative) to appear before an NHS Board and give a personal account of their experience, a Patient Voices story can convey a similar immediacy and spark reflective focus on the essence of the Board's collective governance task.

When, for example, in 2008 the Corporate Manslaughter and Homicide Act became law, I wanted to ensure that every Board member understood not just the onerous legal responsibility that was placed upon their collective shoulders but kept at the forefront of their mind that such a charge could only arise where an individual patient, not a mortality statistic, had died in their care. I used Betty's story about the death of her brother, Jimmy, (Mauchland 2006) to illustrate this point. Please take a moment to listen to her reflections, called *Jimmy's story*, and consider what you regard as the key issues in relation to the safety and quality of care that this bleak and chilling account raises.

Among other things, my discussions with Boards and their members have identified the following implications for a Board's governance scrutiny of the safety and quality of their own provision:

- Staff culture
- Evidence of adherence to policy in the way that staff initially deal with a clinical emergency
- Action that should be taken to follow-up on the absence of proper case records
- The sharing of learning from a serious untoward incident
- The need to listen and to act upon information from family and other carers
- Issues of safe transfer of full information and the need to govern the transition of care between different organisations

Eloquently and movingly, Jimmy's story shows how:

> *risks express themselves most forcefully at points of transition—that is, at the interfaces between organisational sub-systems (e.g. between the ward environment and theatre), at the boundary between different organisations (e.g. between primary and secondary care providers) and at the frontier between different sectors (e.g. between health and social care or housing) in an escalating hierarchy of dislocation and potential harm.* (Stanton 2004)

The Role of Carers

People who care at home for friends or for family members are the bedrock of care, yet, too often the NHS seems reflexively to undervalue the insights of a patient's own carer. This is beautifully underlined by Alison Ryan's story, *Who cares?* (Ryan 2004), about her husband's experience in the lead-up to his liver transplant. Apart from emphasising the crucial role of carers—and the need for them to remain as full and active partners in the 'care team' at all points of a patient journey—this story reveals the ambivalence and sometimes aggressive/defensive response that carer contributions can evoke in all but the most expert and sensitive professionals. By their training and their daily experience, many professionals have grown used to the exercise of (unquestioned) authority and control. Not all of them welcome the culture shift that is necessary to accept that the best care is a co-production. As Sir Ian Kennedy commented, more than a decade ago, in the light of his 2001 Inquiry into the avoidable deaths of babies at Bristol Royal Infirmary:

> ...*we should help professionals through the barriers that prevent them seeing their patients as interactive partners. A mature culture will settle on sharing power and responsibility, on a subtle negotiation ... between professional and patient as to what each wants and what each can deliver. This is the culture we should work towards—helping each other as we go.* (Kennedy 2001)

Not everyone in the professions has yet reached that point of 'maturity'. When I worked for the DH, a General Practitioner, who both then and now occupied a highly influential position in the professional hierarchy, objected to my use of Patient Voices on the grounds that he/she '*had no time for professional whingers*'. Apart from the deep insecurity that this conveyed, it also told me with certainty that this GP had never looked at the story we were discussing (nor, I suspect, any others). The story in question was Ian's *Measured innovation: working together* (Kramer 2004c) which is a celebration of the expertise of professional staff and of their willingness to respond with sensitivity and imagination to what this particular GP might have dismissed as 'a failure to comply with prescribed treatment'.

I use Ian's story frequently in my work with senior clinicians and with GPs to exemplify what I mean when I talk about the (somewhat clumsy) term 'the co-production of care' and when I try to ensure that 'informed concordance with treatment' receives as much attention as does accurate prescribing. I am delighted to say that I have never heard Ian's story described as 'whinging'. You might care to consider the question: what lessons, if any, does this story hold for you?

Using Stories to Highlight the Need for Dignity and Respect

Alongside their contribution to reflection on the overarching themes of compassionate governance and expert clinical practice, sometimes a particular story can provide the perfect introduction to a specific thematic conference or workshop. When I organised a consultation day for the

Department of Health on Non-Heartbeating Organ Donation, I was able to use the moving story told by Grace and Joe Desa about the loss of their son, Daryl—*Giving someone a second chance* (Desa and Desa 2004). This provided a powerful and hopeful introduction to this vital, painful and seldom-discussed topic and ensured that the highly technical discussions that followed, about the importance of rapid organ retrieval, also reminded clinical staff of the need for the deepest sensitivity in their approach to relatives who are themselves in the grip of psychological and spiritual trauma.

It is significant that many Patient Voices stories, such as Ian's *Introduction* (Kramer 2004b) and Betty's story about her brother's death *Jimmy's story* (Mauchland 2006), end with an open question. No Patient Voices story can provide answers to the complex challenges of expert clinical care or of the governance of the patient journey. What they can do is help individual professionals and clinical teams to formulate evermore thoughtful and focused questions about how, for example, they can ensure that every patient is treated with respect and dignity and that individual patients' and their own carers' expertise is acknowledged, so that they are truly full and active partners in their own care. Equally, Patient Voices can help Boards to reflect on how their 'duty of care' is discharged; the appropriateness of risk identification policies that the executive has put in place, and the robustness of the assurances that they, as Board members, receive about the day-to-day safety and quality of care. Had these questions been posed forcefully and persistently by Board members (executive and non-executive alike) at Mid Staffs, it is impossible to believe that 'deficiencies [that] were systemic, deep-rooted and fundamental [and] had existed for a long time' could have gone unchallenged—nor that year after year patients could have been 'routinely neglected by a Trust that was preoccupied with cost cutting, targets and processes and lost sight of its fundamental responsibility to provide safe care' (Francis 2010b).

At the end of his exhaustive Inquiry into some profound NHS system failures, Francis concluded that it was vital to learn from the individual experiences of patients and 'to allow their voices to be heard by those with responsibility for delivering care at these and other hospitals' (Francis 2010b).

There can be no single way in which the seldom-heard voices of the most frail and vulnerable patients and of marginalised groups can be heard and acted upon. All organisations and all professionals need, imaginatively, to consider how they can ensure that their own practice is illuminated and challenged by the lived experience of those to whom they have a duty of care.

Similarly, those of us who work with the care system as educators and facilitators of learning need to imbue our own practice with these insights. I hope you will give some thought as to how you might use Patient Voices stories in your own work.

Capturing the Lived Experience of Dementia Patients and Their Carers

A few years ago, I had the privilege of conducting an appreciative inquiry into the impact of dementia on patients and carers in Essex (Stanton 2013), spending time in their own homes and learning to admire their courage, their strength and their resilience in the face of the corrosive and debilitating impact of dementia. I strove to capture the reality of their lived experiences in the report and recommendations that I wrote for Healthwatch Essex and have since shared with local NHS and social care commissioners. When I re-read my own report, I knew that much of the immediacy of the impact that the inquiry had made on me—and more importantly the impact that dementia had on patients and the lives of those who cared for them—had been lost in the written presentation. In preparing to write this chapter, I came across again Barbara's elegiac story about the impact of Alzheimer's disease in *The real Malcolm* (Pointon 2009) and was captivated afresh. When I meet with commissioners, I often show this Patient Voices story to them to illuminate and add impact to recommendations in my report. Barbara speaks to these recommendations with more force and eloquence than I can ever muster.

Conclusion

These are turbulent and dangerous times for the NHS. In a twenty-first-century context characterised by exponential change, the accelerative needs of an ageing population, the constraints imposed by economic downturn and the looming shadow of 'Brexit', it appears to be caught up in a storm that is only partially of its own making. Thankfully, after decades of denial, a new central leadership regime in the NHS has explicitly recognised the urgent need for system-wide transformation. Boards and NHS professionals need imagination and persistence to embark upon the challenging journey of change that lies before them. They can draw courage and inspiration from the patients and carers they serve, whose stories are often imbued with hope and deep wisdom.

There it is; the light across the water. Your story. Mine. His. It has to be seen to be believed. And it has to be heard. In the endless babble of narrative, in spite of the daily noise, the story waits to be heard … every light was a story. And the flashes themselves were the stories going out over the waves, as markers and guides and comfort and warning. (Winterson 2004)

As this chapter ends, please pause to consider this question: if you were to tell your own story as a provider or recipient of care, where would this story take you and how might it help others to reflect on the caring task?

Key Points

- Patient Voices digital stories do not provide solutions to the complex dilemma of providing compassionate and safe care. They do, however, act as a powerful stimulus to reflective and patient-focused consideration and debate about elements of the dilemmas of care and how practice can be improved.
- Because of their 'poetic' qualities, Patient Voices digital stories evoke powerful feelings and stimulate personal reflection on the core values of the caring task and of its essential humanity.
- A carefully chosen thematic story can illuminate debate on a specific aspect of care, as well as touching upon overarching commonalities.
- The litany of Patient Voices contains examples of inspiring care, as well as cautionary tales. In turbulent times they provide what Jeanette Winterson described as 'markers and guides, comfort and warning' (Winterson 2004) to all of those engaged in caring.

- Listening to the voice of patients and carers can prompt each of us to reflect and begin to formulate our own 'story of care'—whether as a recipient or as a provider.

References

Bajin, M. (2009). *I love you more*. Pilgrim Projects. Retrieved May 2017, from http://www.patientvoices.org.uk/flv/0400pv384.htm

Desa, G., & Desa, J. (2004). *Giving someone a second chance*. Pilgrim Projects Limited. Retrieved March 2014, from http://www.patientvoices.org.uk/flv/0008pv384.htm

Francis, R. (2010a). *Final report of the independent inquiry into care provided by Mid Staffordshire NHS Foundation Trust*. Retrieved January 15, 2011.

Francis, R. (2010b). *Independent inquiry into care provided by Mid Staffordshire NHS Foundation Trust January 2005–March 2009* (Vol. 1). London: The Stationery Office.

Francis, R. (2013). *The final report of the Mid Staffordshire NHS Foundation Trust Public Inquiry*.

Hopkins, G. M. (1967). *The poems of Gerard Manley Hopkins*. Oxford: Oxford University Press.

Kennedy, I. (2001). *Learning from Bristol: The report of the public inquiry into children's heart surgery at the Bristol Royal Infirmary 1984–1995*. London: The Stationery Office.

Kramer, I. (2004a). *Another pair of eyes*. .Pilgrim Projects Limited. Retrieved July 17, 2013, from http://www.patientvoices.org.uk/flv/0017pv384.htm

Kramer, I. (2004b). *Introduction*. Pilgrim Projects Limited. Retrieved March 2014, from http://www.patientvoices.org.uk/flv/0015pv384.htm

Kramer, I. (2004c). *Measured innovation: Working together*. Pilgrim Projects Limited. Retrieved March 2014, from http://www.patientvoices.org.uk/flv/0016pv384.htm

Livingstone, P. (2008). *Once upon a time*. Pilgrim Projects. Retrieved May 2017, from http://www.patientvoices.org.uk/flv/0208pv384.htm

Livingstone, P. (2009). *Tell me your story*. Pilgrim Projects. Retrieved May 2017, from http://www.patientvoices.org.uk/flv/0402pv384.htm

Mauchland, B. (2006). *Jimmy's story*. Pilgrim Projects Limited. Retrieved March 2014, from http://www.patientvoices.org.uk/flv/0047pv384.htm

O'Neill, F. (2007). *Only connect: A life in stories*. Pilgrim Projects. Retrieved May 2017, from http://www.patientvoices.org.uk/flv/0132pv384.htm

Pointon, B. (2009). *The real Malcolm*. Pilgrim Projects Limited. Retrieved March 2014, from http://www.patientvoices.org.uk/flv/0394pv384.htm

Ryan, A. (2004). *Who cares?* Pilgrim Projects Limited. Retrieved March 2014, from http://www.patientvoices.org.uk/flv/0003pv384.htm

Stanton, P. (2004). *The strategic leadership of clinical governance in PCTs*. NHS Modernisation Agency.

Stanton, P. (2013). *Understanding the experience and choices of those dealing with the impact of dementia*. Healthwatch Essex Patient Involvement Projects (PiPs). Healthwatch Essex.

Winterson, J. (2004). *Lighthousekeeping*. London: Harper perennial, (2005 printing).

Wordsworth, W., & Coleridge, S. T. (1968). *Lyrical ballads 1805*. London; Glasgow: Collins Publishers.

Paul Stanton was formerly director of NHS Board Development and a Senior Adviser on Strategy in the Department of Health. He currently works with NHS provider Boards and Clinical Commissioning Groups and leads a project on Health and Social Care Sustainability and Transformation implementation. He has been a Visiting Professor at Newcastle Business School and Northumbria and De Montfort Universities.

6

Arthur and Co: Digital Stories About Living with Arthritis

Fiona O'Neill, Gill Bowskill, Carole Carter, Brian Clark, Karen Hoffman, and Jools Symons

Introduction and Background

This project has opened my eyes to the suffering others go through, mainly in silence, on their own, invisible to outsiders. I cannot recommend strongly enough that people should take time out and listen to the stories of people with problems, who could be your neighbours and you would never know. (Brian Clark, storyteller)

Note: This chapter is the result of a collaboration. It was written only after getting together once again with the storytellers to discuss their experiences and views about what should be included here.

My professional career as a nurse began in the 1970s. Early experiences were shaped by a nursing culture characterised by getting things done. I remember clearly the day I was taught how to do a bed bath. I felt that the young man recovering from a fairly minor surgery would much rather

F. O'Neill (✉) • G. Bowskill • C. Carter • B. Clark • K. Hoffman • J. Symons
Otley, UK

© The Author(s) 2018
P. Hardy, T. Sumner (eds.), *Cultivating Compassion*,
https://doi.org/10.1007/978-3-319-64146-1_6

103

have taken himself down to the bathroom for a wash. Instead he got the full works and I was left feeling puzzled. This notion that care should be negotiated between the giver and the receiver appeared in those days to mark me out as different. There seemed to be little time to listen and the role of the patient was largely passive, to receive gratefully the wisdom, expertise and, as in the case of the bed bath, the often unasked-for interventions of professionals.

In 2001, the recommendations of the Bristol Inquiry that patients must be treated by health professionals as partners and 'equals with different expertise' really resonated (Kennedy 2001). A key recommendation from the response to the Inquiry was for a much greater focus on patient-centred practice in the education and continuing professional development of health professionals (DH 2002). Now working as a researcher and teacher at Leeds University, I started on a continuing journey to embed patient knowledge and expertise at the heart of professional learning. Through this chapter, I came across Patient Voices and was encouraged to attend a workshop and make a story. I attended the workshop with colleagues, including Jools Symons, a carer who was leading the development of a very vibrant and innovative patient and carer community across our local universities.

Our own understanding of the importance of patients and carers having opportunities to tell their own stories in a supportive learning environment had become embedded at the heart of the development model. Working with patients and carers, we developed 'patient learning journeys' as a framework for preparing people to get involved. We found that being able to reflect on and develop new insights and learning about their own journey as patients and carers enabled people to move on from the often painful and traumatic experiences that had motivated them to get involved. Coming to terms with these experiences and finding ways of turning their insights into positive and powerful learning for students had become one of the organising principles of our work. We had learnt that providing opportunities for patients and carers to tell their stories and to reframe their experiences was a valuable and often missed aspect of preparing for involvement. We went to the Patient Voices workshop confident that we could further develop our understanding of stories in our own work.

Following the careful instructions on how to prepare for the workshop, I had assembled some photographs. Looking through the old photo drawer, I was drawn to photos of my dad and put them in my bag, not really knowing why. My dad was a great storyteller and his stories were one of the many things I missed about him since his death. Sitting in the story circle, there was no place to hide and my story was about how much I missed him and how sadness had become part of my life. The experience of making my story was transformative. I rediscovered my dad through making the story, and the simple acknowledgement of this, facilitated by the gentle encouragement of my fellow storytellers, was the start of a process of healing. I left the workshop changed forever, proudly clutching my finished story that I still love to watch and share with my children, who have new insights into a granddad they never knew: *Only connect: a life in stories* (O'Neill 2007).

Designing Patient-Shaped Healthcare

Determined to stay involved with Patient Voices, an opportunity came through a Leeds University-led initiative to promote interactions between academia, industry and the NHS through open innovation. We secured funding to work with Patient Voices to explore ideas about the value of incorporating patient experiences and knowledge into the process of innovation and design in healthcare. An emphasis on 'co-production' and 'co-design' focuses on the value of unleashing and working with the skills, knowledge and capacities of individuals and communities to find better solutions to the complex challenges of twenty-first century healthcare. Working with Patient Voices enabled us to explore the value of storytelling as a vehicle for improving understanding of the needs and experiences of patients and to build this knowledge into the process of innovation in healthcare.

Arthritis affects one-fifth of the UK population. Often misrepresented as a disease of older people, arthritis can have a devastating impact across all ages. According to Arthritis Research UK (www.arthritisresearchuk. org), of those diagnosed with arthritis, 72 per cent meet the definition of 'disabled' outlined in the Disability Discrimination Act 1995 (Disability

Rights Commission 2002). We identified a small group of local people who were all working as volunteers with Arthritis Care. Arthritis Care is the UK's largest charity working with and for all people who have arthritis. As we valued the very productive relationship with volunteers from the local branch who had played an instrumental role in the development of Patient Learning Journeys at Leeds University, it was a natural progression to invite this group to be our partners in this project.

Five volunteers came forward to participate, and we worked together with Patient Voices to design a flexible process that attended to the specific requirements of the group. The principles underpinning the Patient Voices work include a deep respect for individuals and the stories they want to tell, and this helped to define our collaborative process. Working with the energy levels of the group and making sure we gave attention to creating a convivial and nourishing environment were important parts of the overall approach.

We spaced the workshops over a number of weeks. The workshops were held at Leeds University and we ensured we had attended to things like access, parking and also the timings of the workshop to shorten the days in keeping with the participants' energy levels. The first workshop introduced the group to Patient Voices and digital storytelling and included a writing exercise that played an important role in shaping the stories and getting the group started. Using the prompt 'my favourite appliance', the storytellers wrote short stories that helped us to focus on the role that often the most simple technology can have in daily life with arthritis. The stories included one about a walking stick, a dishwasher and an i-Pod and how important these items are to daily life. The next time we met, the group had already formed close bonds and the interval between the two workshops had been used to refine and develop ideas for stories. The next workshop day started with a story circle where we helped to further refine the stories in preparation for drafting and editing their scripts. Having four facilitators—Pip, Tony, Jools Symons and myself—meant there was lots of time to help individuals with their scripts and with the technical aspects of making the actual digital stories. The third day included a celebratory premiere of everyone's stories. We also arranged a public launch of the stories and invited friends and families as well as invitees from across the patient and public involvement community at Leeds University and other interested parties, including colleagues from Arthritis Care.

The Stories

The five stories created are all different and powerfully illustrate how a long-term illness like arthritis is experienced in a unique way by each individual. The title that the group adopted as fitting for the project came from the story told by Karen Hoffman: *My dear friend Arthur* (Hoffman 2008). 'Arthur' is the name Karen gives to her arthritis—an unwelcome and unknown arrival in her life that stopped her from doing the things she loves. Karen tells the story of her gradual acceptance and understanding of Arthur through their journey together. This metaphor of journeying and acceptance and progression from dark times to finding ways of accepting and moving on was a theme in all the stories. The dramatic question, the tension that good stories set up and that holds us until the end, is described as one of the seven elements that need to be attended to in the design of good digital stories (Lambert 2006). In their own way, each of the stories reflected the deep need to tell stories about this struggle and reconciliation. Pip Hardy quotes Flannery O'Connor to remind us of this challenge and how we come out the other end of our encounter with dragons:

> No matter what form the dragon may take, it is of this mysterious passage past him, or into his jaws, that stories of any depth will always be concerned to tell…. (O'Connor 1969)

This determination and resilience of the storytellers is evident in a number of ways. In her story *I'm Back* (Bowskill 2008), Gill tells of how she and her family adapted, finding easy ways of doing things until the day she gets fed up of thinking about what she can't do and gets her 'sparkle' back by finding things she *can* do. Gill has become involved in campaigning, and through her work with Arthritis Care, she is able to help and support others. In his story *Max and me* (Clark 2008), Brian provides a powerful insight into the unseen pain that accompanies arthritis and the relief provided by the companionship of his dog Max and his trusty walking stick Lyca. The role that simple technology plays is also illustrated in Carole's story *Magic light switches* (Carter 2008). The sensor-driven switches allowed Carole to stop sitting in the dark when psoriatic arthritis prevented her from switching on her lights. The need for more sensible product and service design featured in other stories; Gill Bowskill observed that she cannot operate disabled lifts due to the poor design of the operating button! Patient involvement in the early stages of design is essential if we are to achieve step changes in accessibility and make our world a better place for all.

The stories allowed us to develop clearer insights into what it is really like to live with a long-term illness, including the pain and fatigue that are often present. The common themes that emerged from the stories can be summarised as follows:

- the importance of being believed and listened to by health professionals on the (often) prolonged journey to a diagnosis
- the creativity and resourcefulness of individuals in finding ways of adapting their lives to their changed circumstances while remaining true to themselves
- the value of getting involved in volunteering and a strong motivation to help and support others
- the invisibility of pain to others and different coping strategies that are used

My young daughter watched the stories and captured her new insights perfectly when she proclaimed, 'just because you can't see pain doesn't mean that people aren't in pain'. Brian Clark reflected on his own story at the public launch saying:

> Arthritis and its associated pain is like the three letter 'I's:
> Isolated—when you are first diagnosed, you feel you are the only one who feels like you do.
> Invisible—because you cannot see arthritis or feel someone else's pain.
> Individual—as everyone has different types of the disease and different thresholds of pain.

The stories had made these experiences accessible to others. We can walk alongside the storytellers and access their wisdom and knowledge to help change our perceptions and increase understanding. While our focus for the project was on the role of technology and innovation, the stories helped us to understand that technology can be both an enabler and, if thoughtlessly designed, a barrier, to individuals living with arthritis. What is important is to hear about what it is really like from those that know. Listening to these unique experiences reminds us of our common humanity and shared purpose to co-design services and develop new technologies in ways that involve and engage the expertise and experiences of patients so we can achieve truly patient-shaped healthcare.

What Happened Next: Reflections Five Years On

As part of the preparation for the first edition of this book, four of our storytellers met with Jools and me to reflect on and share what we had individually and collectively learnt from our experiences as part of 'Arthur and Co'. We were all happy to meet up again and there was a very noticeable energy and readiness to talk about an experience that all of us had been touched by and remember with clarity and a real sense of value, undiminished by the years. A number of themes emerged from our discussion and these are summarised below.

The Process

We discussed the process of making the digital stories. Everyone appreciated the group aspect of the process and found the pace and gentle encouragement of facilitators and fellow storytellers very valuing and affirming. It was described as a truly reflective process because careful facilitation and the time taken allowed people to get to the core of their story. This was contrasted with less facilitative and reflective approaches to capturing patient perspectives through video interviews. The technical skills developed through making the stories were also appreciated by some members of the group in particular.

Transformative Experiences

We discussed what impact making the stories had on us as individuals. Although this hadn't always been recognised at the start, being part of the group had had a positive impact on all the storytellers and this was described in various ways. Karen described this as part of a healing process, helping her to accept 'Arthur', her arthritis. She no longer refers to Arthur anymore, feeling that there is no need for the separation of something that she now accepts. Carol talked about how empowering she found the process, allowing her to 'grab' control that she felt had been lost. Reflecting on making her own story about caring for her boyfriend (Symons 2007), Jools described that, although she didn't know she needed to, making her story allowed her to put a painful and still raw experience 'to bed'. This sense of being weighed down and then released by a group process resonated across the group.

Another aspect of the transformative potential of storytelling is the opportunity to reflect on the 'dark times' that inevitably accompany a diagnosis of a long-term illness and to be able to turn this into something much more positive. It was felt that telling stories can be an integral part of coming to terms with a life-changing illness and help the individual to 'turn the corner'.

Walking in Another's Shoes: A Resource for Learning

The group had used the stories in various ways. This included showing the stories to student doctors, nurses and radiography students. The stories were incorporated into a structured session, looking at issues such as understanding what it is like to live with chronic pain. These sessions evaluated well. Students commented on how the stories helped them to understand what it is really like to live with arthritis. It was also felt that the stories help to dispel common misconceptions, including that arthritis does not affect younger people. The stories allow the viewers to develop a sense of empathy and understanding of the real experiences of storytellers, their journey through the health system and how best to support people who have arthritis and similar long-term health conditions. The message of hope, that receiving a difficult diagnosis isn't the end but rather the beginning of a journey of coming to terms with it, and to live well, despite the difficulties, is all part of encouraging health professionals not to make assumptions but rather to listen and find opportunities to learn. Gill felt the stories helped to get the message across that health professionals need to 'engage their brain before they speak' and to recognise the individuality and experiences of the patients they serve.

The stories had also been shared with others. Carol spoke of how she had encouraged her own healthcare team to watch the stories and how they had appreciated the opportunity. Sharing the stories with family members has also been important. Karen shared her story with her parents. Her father was clearly moved and reflected that until now he hadn't realised quite how tough it had been for Karen. A note of caution was sounded in being sensitive about the impact of the stories on close family and colleagues who may have previously been unaware of the thoughts and experiences so clearly articulated in the stories.

Helping Others

All of the storytellers had used the stories in their various volunteering activities, supporting their clear motivation to help others come to terms with and find positive ways of living with arthritis. Karen, who has gone on to achieve a counselling qualification, voiced her view that the stories can help people to really understand disability and provide hope about 'life at the other side'.

A Timeless Resource

Eight years on, the storytellers all agreed that the stories are timeless and as real and relevant today as they were when first made. Furthermore, the positive energy and enthusiasm for the process, including the transformative aspects of participation, underlines the truly powerful and transformative quality of our involvement in Patient Voices.

Conclusion

In his report for the National Advisory Group on Patient Safety, Donald Berwick included the need to *'engage, empower, and hear patients and carers throughout the system and at all times'* as one of four main principles that would build an even better 'learning NHS' (Berwick 2013).

It is hard to gather substantial evidence about the impact 'Arthur and Co' has had in terms of our objective of promoting patient involvement in the design and development of new technology. What we can say without doubt is that we all benefited from our experience and real learning took place. This learning is not restricted to the storytellers and includes and extends to those who have watched the stories and had the opportunity to walk in another's shoes for a while. There must be many different approaches if we are to meet the challenge so clearly articulated by Donald Berwick. Patient Voices provides an effective way of unleashing the wisdom and knowledge of patients and carers and making this accessible as part of a learning NHS. The fact that this happens through a process that can enable very significant personal change and development and build communities of support and friendship like our 'Arthur and Co' group is truly remarkable and needs to be celebrated.

To come out of any learning intervention changed and transformed is the ambition of all good teachers. So much of what we call learning gets left at the classroom door; this is emphatically not the case with Patient Voices. We have all grown and changed through Arthur and Co and hope that others have too. The last word rests with Gill who observes:

> *If you could bottle it [Patient Voices] everyone should take a spoonful at some time in their lives.*

Postscript for the Second Edition

My daughter Laura, who had attended the launch of 'Arthur and Co', is now a student nurse. One evening she phoned me and said: 'Guess what Mum, they showed one of "your" stories today in our lecture theatre'. And so, in a fitting postscript to this chapter, Laura told me about how watching *Eric's first fifty years* (Moorhouse 2008) had stimulated a lengthy and insightful discussion about the impact of chronic illness and the value of patient-led initiatives (in this case, the Expert Patient Programme and Challenging Arthritis) in giving back hope and control.

I asked Laura what resonated most about watching the story. She thought it enabled the students to really feel the despair that Eric experienced as his well-made plans fell apart. She also reflected on the importance of nurses understanding and really supporting patients to find out and connect with patient groups. The students had also agreed how valuable it is for patients to be able to help each other and share their experiences and knowledge.

I put the phone down and smiled, grateful to be reminded once again about the value of Patient Voices, and ready to tell this new story….

Each affects the other and the other affects the next, and the world is full of stories, but the stories are all one. (Albom 2003)

Key Points

- The Patient Voices stories are timeless; they can be used for many years afterwards.
- The process of storytelling, including the group dynamics, expert facilitation and attention to the needs of storytellers, allows people to get to the core of their story.
- The opportunity to reflect as part of the process helps storytellers to move on in their own journey and this transformative aspect of the process is very valuable and has healing properties.
- The stories are real and contain the heartfelt and authentic experiences of storytellers. The emotional heart of the stories is what resonates with people who watch the stories and get to walk alongside the storytellers. This plays a role in helping people to have empathy with the needs of those living with pain and the effects of long-term health conditions.
- The approach allowed storytellers to articulate the value of getting involved in voluntary work and move on past the often difficult journey from initial diagnosis, thus demonstrating our human capacity for change and growth.

Note About the Collaborators Gill Bowskill, Brian Clark, Carole Carter and Karen Hoffman all took part in the Arthur and Co digital storytelling workshop. They are all affected by rheumatoid arthritis and were all volunteering for Arthritis Care at the time of the workshop. They have all subsequently gone on to become more deeply involved as patient educators, and Karen has qualified as a counsellor.

Jools Symons is Patient and Public Involvement Manager at Leeds Institute of Medical Education. She has been instrumental in the involvement of patients and carers in medical education and, along with Fiona, she set up the Patient Learning Journeys in Leeds and Bradford. She is currently leading the Lived Experience Network (LEN).

References

Albom, M. (2003). *The five people you meet in heaven* (1st ed.). New York: Hyperion.

Berwick, D. (2013). *A promise to learn—A commitment to act: Improving the safety of patients in England*. London: Department of Health.

Bowskill, G. (2008). *I'm back!* Pilgrim Projects. Retrieved May 2017, from http://www.patientvoices.org.uk/flv/0225pv384.htm

Carter, C. (2008). *Magic light switches*. Pilgrim Projects. Retrieved May 2017, from http://www.patientvoices.org.uk/flv/0222pv384.htm

Clark, B. (2008). *Max and me*. Pilgrim Projects. Retrieved May 2017, from http://www.patientvoices.org.uk/flv/0221pv384.htm

DH. (2002). *Learning from Bristol: The Department of Health's response to the report of the public inquiry into children's heart surgery at the Bristol Royal Infirmary 1984–1995*. London: Stationery Office.

Disability Rights Commission. (2002). *Disability Discrimination Act 1995: Code of practice for providers of post-16 education and related services*. London: Stationery Office.

Hoffman, K. (2008). *My dear friend Arthur*. Pilgrim Projects. Retrieved May 2017, from http://www.patientvoices.org.uk/flv/0226pv384.htm

Kennedy, I. (2001). *The report of the public inquiry into children's heart surgery at the Bristol Royal Infirmary 1984–1995. Learning from Bristol* (pp. 325–332). London: Stationery Office.

Lambert, J. (2006). *Digital storytelling: Capturing lives creating community* (2nd ed.). Berkeley, CA: Digital Diner Press.

Moorhouse, E. (2008). *Eric's first fifty years*. Pilgrim Projects. Retrieved May 2017, from http://www.patientvoices.org.uk/flv/0224pv384.htm

O'Connor, F. (1969). *Mystery and manners; Occasional prose*. New York: Farrar.

O'Neill, F. (2007). *Only connect: A life in stories*. Pilgrim Projects. Retrieved May 2017, from http://www.patientvoices.org.uk/flv/0132pv384.htm

Symons, J. (2007). *CPR*. Pilgrim Projects. Retrieved May 2017, from http://www.patientvoices.org.uk/flv/0131pv384.htm

Dr Fiona O'Neill is a nurse and has worked in a number of education and practice development roles across the NHS. She remains passionate about the value of bringing the patient voice into health professional education and creating opportunities for people to tell and listen to stories as an integral part of a learning NHS.

7

Safety Stories: Creating a Culture of Safety with Digital Stories

Cathy Jaynes

Introduction and Background to the Project

We can't create a culture of safety—we don't know what it looks like.
(Anonymous HEMS pilot, 2007)

The early years of this millennium saw an increasing number of air medical crashes in the United States and a doubling in fatalities of 'souls on board'. We had been in this position before, in the 1970s. At that time, the air medical transport industry was young and besieged by an

---

Although the subject of this chapter is not a Patient Voices project, the author has worked closely with Patient Voices and has collaborated with Pip Hardy on several papers and conference presentations. Her work is important in the development of digital storytelling in healthcare and warrants inclusion in this volume.

C. Jaynes (✉)
Monarch Medical Technologies,
Charlotte, NC, USA

© The Author(s) 2018
P. Hardy, T. Sumner (eds.), *Cultivating Compassion*,
https://doi.org/10.1007/978-3-319-64146-1_7

alarming rate of crashes. United States federal regulators and the industry both responded with rules and processes that drove a surge of vigilance in the air medical community. The incidences of crashes dropped significantly for many years.

But here we were again. Despite a marked increase in safety technologies and strategies, the crash rate had increased and we were mourning the loss of too many colleagues and friends.

I'd begun my own career as a flight nurse in the late 1980s. My orientation was filled with cautionary tales of fatigue and the mission mentality that drove flight crews to accept flights despite less than favourable weather conditions—the chief culprits blamed for the early industry's struggle with safety.

In the fall of 2005, Dr John Wish asked if I would help with a research project designed to gather ideas about how to improve the air medical industry's safety record. John was something of a rare bird in our industry. A retired economics professor, he had never been officially affiliated with any air medical programme, but he worked passionately and tirelessly for better utilisation and safety.

His granddaughter had been injured on a rural stretch of a beach in the American Northwest. Response issues had seriously delayed her arrival at a trauma centre, and John had talked his way into the operating room so he could be there when she arrived. He was still there as she died.

The research project distributed a survey to every transport company belonging to the Association of Air Medical Services (AAMS)—the organisation that forms the backbone of the transport community. The response was enormous: 832 pilots returned the survey, about 31 per cent of Helicopter Emergency Medical Services (HEMS) pilots in the industry at the time (Dery et al. 2007). The pilots responded to multiple-choice questions rating the effectiveness of training, operations, and various types of equipment used to improve safety. But three open-ended questions allowed for a narrative response to what was, basically, the same question asked in subtly different ways:

What do we need to do to create a culture of safety in our industry?

In 2007 I had the opportunity to analyse those narrative responses. Many important themes emerged and I was struck by the articulate comments made by many pilots, but one statement stuck with me:

We can't create a culture of safety—we don't know what it looks like.

Creating a Culture of Safety

Culture is defined as 'the attitudes, feelings, values, and behaviours that characterize and inform society as a whole or any social group within it' (Collins English Dictionary 2012). That anonymous pilot had triggered a set of key questions for our industry, our 'social group':

What does safety look like?
What are the attitudes, values and behaviours that are believed to form the foundation of safe operations?
What made us unsafe?

The emphasis for so many years had been on putting good rules and guidelines in place, getting the right safety equipment and providing training for our medical crews as well as our pilots. But we still weren't seeing the results we wanted—we were far away from zero accidents, zero fatalities, or zero injuries.

Interestingly, the healthcare industry as a whole was wrestling with the same issues. In the United States, one of the most dangerous things that could happen to someone in the healthcare system was to become a patient in a hospital. Medication errors, wrong-site surgeries, and other issues were outcomes of the system's inability to treat patients safely.

Leaders like Lucian Leape and James Reason (Buerhaus and Leape 2004; Peltomaa 2012) were promoting theories of safety in an effort to give us tools and insight into solutions. Ironically, many healthcare safety 'best practices', such as crew resource management concepts, checklists, and the development of safety regulations, were developed from the culture and processes of the aviation industry, yet we were at the exact point where those two industries blended together—air medical transport—and we were still not keeping our crews and patients safe.

Learning the Art and Science of Digital Storytelling

In 2007, I was invited to participate in a digital storytelling workshop to be held at the University of Colorado's College of Nursing and jointly facilitated by The Center for Digital Storytelling and Patient Voices. The workshop, initiated by Dr Sue Hagedorn and Dr Vicki Erickson, was designed to explore the potential of digital storytelling as a method of reflective practice—to start a project called 'Nurstory'. Several of us on faculty were invited to be guinea pigs for the project and to tell a story about a compelling experience in our nursing careers, something that sustained us as a nurse.

Before the workshop, Sue and I had spent many a late afternoon at the College talking about our nursing careers—what was meaningful to us. I had been a flight nurse for almost 17 years and I loved the work. I loved being in that sacred, caring space with people in what was often a horrific time for them. I also missed the close-knit working relationship of a flight crew. I'd left my clinical practice after completing a PhD in 2004 to take a faculty position at the University of Colorado. My doctoral work had focused on quantitative methods of evaluating the healthcare system with an eye towards quality improvement and equity. I wanted to improve the system I had worked in for so many years. I had instinctively known all along that it wasn't just about the numbers or the statistics, but now I was about to learn a way to capture and distil narrative evidence, the stories of healthcare, and air medical transport. This would be transformative for me.

I came to the workshop not knowing what story I wanted to tell. I had so many rich experiences of the special connections between patient and nurse, and I thought that would be the focus. But, as I sat in the story circle, I realised that a near miss during one of my final shifts as a flight nurse was a story ready to be told, a story about 'what safety looked like'.

Go around (Jaynes 2007) was the result. It describes safety as a combination of training and trust, teamwork, and communication but warns that it is always played out against the inseparable background of our personal lives.

I worked closely with two of the facilitators leading the workshop. Daniel Weinshenker, from StoryCenter, did a great job at coaching my initial writing and helping me edit the video with effects that brought the right emotion into the story I *wanted* to tell. Pip Hardy from Patient Voices was the other. She came right alongside me in the process, asking me why this story meant so much to me. She pushed me to struggle to make it the deeper story I *needed* to tell. We've laughed about it since—when people ask me how the story became so personal, I just say, 'Pip made me!'

Plotting the Course

Some months after the storytelling workshop, I was invited to attend the Humanising Healthcare symposium at Bowen Island in British Columbia. Pip was also there, facilitating the work, and we began to discover our mutual interest in the stories of patients and practitioners. We talked for hours about everything from andragogy to how stories from miners in Alberta were changing the culture of safety in that industry. Surprisingly, as we talked, I learned that Pip's father, Rex Hardy, had implemented a publication for pilots to share safety information in a way that was fairly radical in the late 1970s. In his book *Callback*, Rex Hardy wrote about the Aviation Safety Reporting System (ASRS) and the monthly newsletter, *Callback*, that he developed and edited, and described the approach he used to improve safety:

> *As a working pilot, I had been exposed for many years to a formidable barrage of well-intentioned literature dealing with safety (as Mark Twain remarked about the weather, everybody talks about it, but nobody does anything about it), but much of it consisted of well-intentioned but dull exhortations, scholarly dissertations, pedantic lectures, or detailed accident reports … if we expected the troops in the field—the pilots and controllers—to pay any heed, something*

brief and catchy was required … pilots talk to pilots, controllers to controllers, we speak your language. (Hardy 1990)

This seemed incredible to me, that Pip and I were meeting back at that intersection of aviation and healthcare in our own histories. We decided then and there that we would have to continue as friends and colleagues, looking for opportunities to work together to help the stories be heard.

Part of our discussion was talking through the idea of using digital storytelling to teach safety. It was at this symposium where I resolved to gather 100 Safety Stories—brief and catchy and in 'our' language, to help us recognise what safety does—and does not—look like. Pip and her colleague Tony Sumner have been—and continue to be—a huge encouragement to me in my own work, and Pip came to San Jose in 2009 to help facilitate our first Safety Story workshop. The workshop was fragmented, with people disappearing from time to time to attend the Air Medical Transport Conference (AMTC). Despite this, the stories that emerged were all powerful, some unexpected, a few shocking. A bond formed between those storytellers, and they have gone on to become ambassadors for our Safety Story project—and the process by which the stories are created.

Rod Crane, the CEO of MedFlight of Ohio, was the first to support our fundraising efforts for digital storytelling workshops. He understood the importance of this project to the industry and worked tirelessly to promote it. The MedEvac Foundation International and the Air Medical Operators Association have made generous financial contributions to the project and have provided promotional support. Krista Haugen, co-founder of the Survivors Network, has helped us find storytellers and also helps us hold the vision of what this project can offer to the industry. Workshops are small—just six to eight people—but we still struggle to fund and fill them as busy transport folks juggle tight budgets and time to attend.

I know that there are crew members who have travelled to workshops with full financial and emotional support from their programme and others who have come on their own dime, but there are also storytellers who have been silenced when their programmes or vendors have forbidden them to come.

What's Happened to the Stories?

The reaction to the Safety Stories as tools for safety education in the air medical transport industry has been stunning. The outcomes are, so far, narrative only—and the field is ripe for effectiveness research. Safety educators across the industry are using the stories to teach safety from the inside out. A colleague in the Federal Aviation Administration's Helicopter Safety team has called the stories 'the new face of safety education'.

The MedEvac Foundation International continues to fund a workshop annually and has embedded the stories in their website (www.medevacfoundation.org/safety-stories), so they continue to be publicly accessible. Many of the stories also live on the Nurstory website (www.nurstory.org).

Narrative and Culture

I never intended a theoretical approach to our Safety Stories project. It was based on my own experience—and on my intuition that sharing stories about safety would help us change thinking and practice. However, the literature addresses many educational constructs that are met through digital storytelling. There is a good theoretical foundation for these stories' effectiveness as educational tools. Jerome Bruner focuses on the process of meaning making and proposed that narratives or stories create space for that to happen. Getting to meaning is the heart of the storytelling workshop. It is also at the heart of what makes the digital story such a powerful educational tool (Mattingly et al. 2008; Bruner 1986, 1996).

Narrative and culture are inextricably linked in Bruner's thinking and form the foundation from which cognitive processes are developed. Behaviours are formed by both left and right brain processes, so that meshing of emotion and cognition is an important part of learning. As we have seen in the telling of the *Safety Stories*, and in their use in trying to describe 'what safety looks like', we are taken back to Bruner's observation that:

It is only in the narrative mode, that one can construct an identity and find a place in one's culture. (Bruner 1996)

My experience has been that at the front lines of healthcare—whether you are the patient or the practitioner—there is often a wounding struggle. Research, prescriptions, surgeries, therapies, and hard work are all key elements that construct the science of healthcare. But healthcare is constructed of art as well—communication, meaning, emotion, and presence—life and death.

Narrative and Healing

What has been something of a surprise and a blessing in the midst of this work is to see the kind of healing it is bringing to those in the air medical community whose voices are waiting to be heard. About half of the attendees in our workshop have been referred to us by the Survivors Network—air medical crew members who have survived a crash or other serious incidents. A quote from a recent participant's email mirrors what many have said after the Safety Story workshop:

> *I can't tell you how much it means to me to have support and understanding! That was an area of huge deficit after my incident that left me searching, even within myself for understanding of it all. I am so thankful that you and the others were brave enough to come forward, speak out, and tell your stories to lead the way for everyone else! Although I didn't know it at the time, the workshop was exactly what I needed and was extremely healing for me. I am forever grateful to everyone who provided me the opportunity to participate. And as a bonus, what a blessing it was to have had such amazing people in my group. I am positive the relationships formed made all the difference in the world.*
> (Personal communication, July 18, 2013)

Conclusion

A routine built into the work of air medical transport is the shift report or briefing. These change-of-shift sessions are meant to be the time for review of an operational checklist in order to assure adequacy of supplies and to pass on information about weather, maintenance, or pending patient care issues. But often the sessions become a time to debrief, to talk things through, to compare notes, and learn from each other. It's where we traditionally share our stories. But many stories have never been shared beyond the debrief or remain tucked away inside our psyches.

John's story—that of a grandfather's painful loss of his grandchild—moved him to a work far beyond his career. That work sparked a shift in the thinking of how we might view safety. His story, like all of our stories, matters. His willingness to share the story that changed his actions eventually led to my rethinking how to reformulate my approach to improving safety.

The Safety Story project is just beginning to help our community tell its stories so that they can be shared beyond our briefings or our silence and help us choose our future. In his story, *Breathless* (Duncan 2010), David repeats the mantra that helped him survive his crash: 'Find your reference point and don't let go'.

These Safety Stories are our reference points. We need to find them and not let go.

Key Points

- We set out to gather air medical Safety Stories, but the stories have expanded to fill a void around the topic of safety in any setting.
- The people who told the stories found connection and healing.
- The process of creating the stories has been as important as the digital stories themselves.
- The ability to share these, and other stories like them, is critical if organisations are to learn from mistakes and develop a just culture in which every voice can be heard.
- Stories are essential in creating a culture where safety and humanity are prized and the values of intellectual, emotional, and spiritual intelligence inform 'the way we do things here' (Hardy and Jaynes 2011).

References

Bruner, J. (1986). *Actual minds, possible worlds*. Cambridge, MA; London: Harvard University Press.
Bruner, J. (1996). *The culture of education*. Cambridge, MA: Harvard University Press.

Buerhaus, P., & Leape, L. (2004). Patient safety in US hospitals. *Journal of Nursing Scholarship, 36*(4), 366–370.

Collins English Dictionary. (2012). *Collins English dictionary—Complete & unabridged* (10th ed.). William Collins Sons & Co Ltd. Retrieved May 2017, from http://www.dictionary.com/browse/culture

Dery, M., Hustwit, J., Boschert, G., & Wish, J. (2007). Results and recommendations from the helicopter EMS pilot safety survey 2005. *Air Medical Journal, 26*(1), 38–44.

Duncan, D. (2010). *Breathless*. The Center for Medical Transport Research. Retrieved May 2017, from http://medevacfoundation.org/safety-stories/#

Hardy, R. (1990). *Callback: NASA's aviation safety reporting system*. Washington, DC: Smithsonian.

Hardy, P., & Jaynes, C. (2011). Editorial: Finding the voices for quality and safety in healthcare: The never-ending story. *Journal of Clinical Nursing, 20*(7–8), 1069–1071. doi:10.1111/j.1365-2702.2010.03539.x.

Jaynes, C. (2007). *Go around*. Retrieved May 2017, from http://medevacfoundation.org/safety-stories/#

Mattingly, C., Lutkehaus, N. C., & Throop, C. J. (2008). Bruner's search for meaning: A conversation between psychology and anthropology. *Ethos, 36*(1), 1–28.

Peltomaa, K. (2012). James reason: Patient safety, human error, and Swiss cheese. *Quality Management in Healthcare, 21*(1), 59–63.

Dr Cathy Jaynes is an experienced flight nurse, educator, and researcher. She currently works with Monarch Medical Technologies as a clinical specialist coaching hospitals in the use of software developed to improve safety and efficacy in the dosing of dangerous medications. She remains involved in storytelling through Safety Story workshops and by serving on the Boards of Patient Voices and Nurstory.

8

Working with Dignity and Respect: Improving Mental Health Services with Digital Stories

Patrick Cahoon, Carol Haigh, and Tony Sumner

Introduction: Human Rights in Health and Social Care

In 2004, a MORI poll conducted by Ben Page found that the issue that ranked most highly in service users' concerns was being treated with respect (Page 2004), reflecting—in the views of service users—the recognition by legislators of a need to define human rights more widely.

Article 8 of the Human Rights Act (HMSO 1998) gives the right to respect for private and family life, home and correspondence. Privacy and

P. Cahoon (✉)
Greater Manchester Mental Health NHS Foundation Trust, Prestwich, Manchester, UK

C. Haigh
Faculty of Health, Psychology and Social Care, Manchester Metropolitan University, Manchester, UK

T. Sumner
Patient Voices Programme, Pilgrim Projects Limited, Landbeach, Cambridgeshire, UK

© The Author(s) 2018
P. Hardy, T. Sumner (eds.), *Cultivating Compassion*,
https://doi.org/10.1007/978-3-319-64146-1_8

dignity are fundamental to the well-being of individuals within the healthcare system, and every member of the nursing workforce should prioritise dignity in care, placing it at the heart of everything they do. When dignity is absent from care, people feel devalued, lacking control and comfort. They may also lack confidence, be unable to make decisions for themselves and feel humiliated, embarrassed and ashamed. Three integral aspects—respect, compassion and sensitivity—are central to providing dignity in care. In practice, this means:

- Respecting patients' and clients' diversity and cultural needs; their privacy, including protecting it as much as possible in large, open-plan hospital wards; and the decisions they make
- Being compassionate when a patient or client and/or their relatives need emotional support, rather than just delivering technical nursing care
- Demonstrating sensitivity to patients' and clients' needs, ensuring their comfort

The importance of healthcare staff's focus upon, and commitment to, the issues of dignity, respect and privacy when caring for older people or those with mental health needs is well documented (see, e.g. Levinson 2007).

The focus of this chapter is to explore how Patient Voices reflective digital stories were created at, and used by, the former Manchester Mental Health and Social Care NHS Trust (Manchester MHSCT) to enhance training and awareness of dignity, privacy and respect amongst service users and service providers.

Background and Aims of the Project

The Trust was an NHS organisation responsible for providing mental health and social care services in the Manchester area until January 2017, when it became a part of the Greater Manchester Mental Health NHS Foundation Trust, (GMMH), a new organisation that employs over 5000 staff, across 140 different locations. GMMH supports around 53,000 service users and has 832 inpatient beds and an annual income of around approximately £280 million. As a Foundation Trust GMMH has 22 elected governors and 10,600 members.

The original aim of the project was to use the medium of digital stories as the basis for developing educational resources. However, it quickly became much more than that. Since the inception of the programme, we at Patient Voices had argued that the stories provided a resource that could:

> ...redress the balance of power between healthcare clinicians and managers and the people they serve, and provide decision makers with a different kind of opportunity to understand the needs of patients—other than the dry results of surveys and statistics. If patients are really to be 'at the heart of health care', then their views and their stories are of paramount importance in any attempt to reform healthcare services. (Hardy 2004)

Following the disastrous patient experiences at Mid Staffordshire NHS Trust, this aspiration from Patient Voices was reflected in the Francis report into the events:

> If there is one lesson to be learnt, I suggest it is that people must always come before numbers. It is the individual experiences that lie behind statistics and benchmarks and action plans that really matter, and that is what must never be forgotten when policies are being made and implemented. (Francis 2010)

Patient stories have been recognised as making a significant contribution to understanding the patient experience; they acknowledge the patient's own areas of expertise, that is, his or her own life and unique experience of illness (Hardy 2007). When this project began, we had no idea how the application of these stories would flourish and evolve.

Meeting the Storytellers

The original impetus behind the storytelling workshops was to collect stories of service-user experiences. Since the emotional investment required from storytellers is immense, and understanding the importance of both informed consent and participant engagement, we recruited our first brave storytellers from a patient involvement conference/study day that was organised by Manchester mental health services. We were given a slot in which to introduce the concept of digital stories and to demonstrate their visceral emotional appeal. As always, the easiest way to explain what digital stories are was to show people a digital story, which is what we did.

There is an argument promulgated by some people that careful selection of exemplar stories is crucial, and there is some truth to that. However, since the stories reflect the 'real-life' experiences of storytellers, it is not unreasonable to suppose that, in any audience, there will be at least one or two people who will be emotionally affected by any story. We took comfort from the fact that our session was the one before lunch, which allowed anybody who was overly distressed to seek some quiet time to collect themselves. The nature of the day also meant that a number of mental health professionals who were known to the service users were in attendance and could provide specialist input should it be required.

As it turned out, our concerns were groundless. Yes, a number of people became tearful at the stories shown but any distress was immediately overshadowed by enthusiasm to take part in the project. Several people who volunteered wanted to share their stories there and then. This was an illuminating moment for us, since it showed us that these individuals had held their stories inside, sometimes for decades, and had been waiting patiently for a platform that would enable them to share them and people who were willing to hear them.

Creating the Stories

Since that first meeting in early 2011, there have been 12 workshops and 81 stories, created by 74 storytellers. The original focus of the project was to explore service provision through the stories of service users like Catherine—*The child within my bipolar* (Skelton 2012)—but an acknowledgement of the interdependency between the stories of service users and carers lead to the widening of the programme's catchment, resulting in the stories of carers, such as Lindsey's *Rites of passage* (Cree 2012).

The stories were shown in Board meetings and even, with consent from storytellers, by the BBC in the Triangle Shopping Centre in

Manchester. As the effects of the stories and experiences of storytelling spread through the Trust and the wider community, it became clearer that, as Mitch Albom said:

Each affects the other and the other affects the next, and the world is full of stories, but the stories are all one. (Albom 2003)

With this in mind, the project has broadened its approach in Manchester still further.

First, staff members were invited to tell and contribute their stories, to add another valuable perspective to the evidence of experience that the project was building, with contributions such as *I love my job!* (Mykoo 2013). Just as patient and carer stories have driven change and innovation in care, this particular story has prompted reconsideration of staffing rosters and the introduction of 'protected time' for some job roles/wards.

Second, a workshop with leaders from the diverse cultural communities within the city of Manchester was run. This workshop had both tactical and strategic objectives:

- To gather stories of diverse cultural experiences of mental and social care
- To introduce members of diverse community groups to the process and programme with the aim of exploring the wider diffusion of the Patient Voices storytelling approach through the communities the Trust serves

Despite the wide and varied experiences of the storytellers, whether carers or service users, what has been interesting is the courage and bravery with which they share their stories. The creation of the stories within the safe and secure environment that is created in a Patient Voices workshop allows for the blossoming of a social altruism. By this we mean that storytellers often state that they want to share their story so that other people (whom they are unlikely ever to meet) will be helped or reassured that their situation is not unique and that there is someone else who understands what they have experienced.

How Was It for the Storytellers?

Post-workshop feedback sessions reported very favourable responses from storytellers, describing the process as 'very supportive—we all helped each other', 'calm and relaxing', 'very enriching' or 'providing the ability to reflect and look at my issues in totality'.

These responses, made in the immediate aftermath of the workshop, are validated by the fact that several storytellers have returned to make second stories in later workshops, sometimes commenting within their stories on how the opportunity to be heard through the process has itself been important to them, as in *Butterfly* (Mahmood 2013).

After making his first story *Labour of Love* (Rahman 2012), one storyteller has now been to three further Patient Voices workshops, telling a sequence of stories that powerfully illuminate his experiences as a carer over a 3-year timeframe.

Using the Stories: A Flexible Resource

The original impetus for the Manchester mental health stories was a perceived need for educational and reflective prompts for staff. The first use of the stories was actually in a reflective session with service users, storytellers and staff after the first workshop in November 2011 and they have subsequently been used to trigger discussion and dialogue during training sessions. However, one of the strengths of the stories is their flexibility (Hardy 2007) and they have also been used in innovative and imaginative ways, for example:

- As part of the interviewing process for new staff (including the Chief Executive of the former Manchester Mental Health and Social Care Trust)
- To educate and inform the public
- At the start of all Board meetings

In healthcare research, it is widely held to be important to involve service users and members of the public in the planning and running of a research project, but healthcare services are only now beginning to make a link between increased user involvement and enhanced service provision (Dalton et al. 2016).

Recruiting for Compassion

In England, the Department of Health (DH) produced a document focusing upon the role that service users could play in the development of patient-centred services, highlighting that it was important that the providers of healthcare services recognised that patients had an expertise that had hitherto been ignored. In addition, the challenges facing the often lone Trust Board patient representative were highlighted (Haigh 2008); the same concerns exist around inviting service users onto interview panels, especially for senior posts.

To obviate this situation, Manchester mental health services had been incorporating the viewing of one or more of the patient stories into the interview process for new recruits up to and including the former Chief Executive. Service-user representatives on the interview panel are then able to use these Patient Voices as a foundation for discussion and a stimulus against which they can assess the values and emotional responses of candidates, thus ensuring that the voices of patients, service users and carers are central to the recruitment process and that the attitudes of new staff are in line with the values, mission and expectations of the Trust (Sumner 2013).

Raising Awareness of Mental Health Issues

Education and raising public awareness and concern around mental health issues are of key importance for the Trust. The stories were shown in various public arenas on World Mental Health Day 2013 in order to highlight the patient voice and show real people explaining their real experiences in their real voices. Helping to emphasise the message that mental health is everyone's concern is seen as a powerful benefit of the stories.

Bringing Insights into Service-User Experience to the Board

At the height of the programme, every Trust Board meeting at the former MMHSCT started with the showing of a Patient Voices story. The aim of this strategy was to focus the attention of the Board members on the reasons for their meeting (to run a Trust that provides care for service users) and to place the voice of the patient at the heart of the decision-making process. When one story *'Listen! Believe! Act!'* (Larkin 2013) was presented at Board, the former Trust CEO was prompted to write in her blog that:

> *I was genuinely humbled by the courage of one of our digital patient stories at Board this month. 'Listen, Believe, Act' told the story of someone who had felt unheard, disbelieved and untreated as she travelled through mental health services from her early teenage years to young adulthood. It was a really moving illustration of just how critical it can be to really listen, to believe what we hear and then to act upon it in good faith.*
>
> *I recognise that, as a Board, we will need to listen more carefully and more often to our staff. We need to trust and believe the feedback we receive from those on the frontline. And we need to act on that feedback as vital intelligence which will help us all to do a better job, whatever our role in the organisation. We are all in it together, after all.* (Moran 2014)

The Care Quality Commission (CQC) inspected the former Trust in 2015 and, in its report on the Trust, wrote that:

> *The trust was one of the first mental health trusts in the country to introduce the patient stories initiative which involved a range of patient stories being used at the trust board meetings for learning and sharing purposes. Patient stories highlighted how services had responded to people's care and treatment needs. We observed a trust board meeting and saw the powerful nature of starting the formal board meeting with one of these stories.* (Care Quality Commission 2015)

Co-producing Improvement Goals and Activities

The stories have provided both highly qualitative data from which themes and issues that concern and affect service users may be drawn and effective calls to action for management within the former Trust. For example, when the stories are shown to the Board, members were tasked with articulating the top three actions that would be taken to assure themselves that issues highlighted by the stories are less likely to happen in the future. Themes raised in a number of stories that went to the former Board resulted in a range of actions taken or assurances provided.

These have included the introduction of patient-led 'dignity walks' and of improved welcome packs for all new admissions on in-patient units; the use of QR codes and smartphones; the agreement to standardise approaches to ward activities on all Manchester inpatient sites; and to sign up to the 'Star Wards' initiative. In addition, the former Trust obtained a £1.1 million grant to increase involvement of service users in Care Programme Approach (CPA) processes and seen increased patient use of the 'Choice and Medication' website.

Community Awareness

Research conducted by the Royal College of Psychiatrists (Bailey et al. 2013) has identified an 'esteem gap' that prevents the achievement of parity between physical and mental health. The stories created by service users and staff in Manchester have been used to help address this 'esteem gap' by creating greater awareness in the community of the nature of the Trust's work, the challenges it faces and the successes it has achieved. In addition to released stories being available to view on the Patient Voices website, this has been done through the use of the stories in public events and screenings and in local and national media:

- The experiences of its service users and staff were covered on the BBC Radio 4 'Today' programme (Stanbridge 2013).
- The Trust delivered a project in the build-up to World Mental Health Day where the stories where shown on the BBC Big Screen located in Manchester's busy Triangle shopping district.
- The Head of Quality Improvement, along with one of the service users who participated in the programme, took part in a live radio interview on the BBC Radio Manchester mid-morning show on Monday, 8 October 2012.

- The programme received coverage in the *Manchester Evening News*, *Mental Health Today* and *Breakthrough* magazine.

Improvement in Performance Metrics

Health and social care organisations in England, as in other health economies, are increasingly challenged by efficiency or performance targets underpinned by appropriate metrics.

One of the key findings from the Trust's work with digital storytelling and digital stories has been significant improvements in the Trust's performance against key performance indicators.

These have included reductions in the level of complaints received by the Trust. After 2 years, there was a 45 per cent reduction in complaints related to care, a 9 per cent reduction in complaints related to staff issues and a 22 per cent reduction in complaints related to communication. Associated with these reductions in complaint levels has been a 50 per cent reduction in clinical negligence (CNST) claims.

These changes saw the former Trust achieve the highest CQC 'respect and dignity' scores in England for two consecutive years, with an overall quality of care that is good or excellent. In assessments of patient satisfaction, 91 per cent of respondents say staff listen and care, and 95 per cent of a sample of 2018 patients would recommend the Trust.

Conclusion

It may seem odd, or ironic, to end a description of the nature, progress and success of a digital storytelling project—in itself an overtly qualitative form of data-gathering—in such a quantitative manner, but in the real world of cost and improvement targets, these numbers are key to getting funding and authorisation, and they have an undoubted influence on how projects are received, such as when the project became a finalist in the 2013 *Health Service Journal*'s 'Innovation in Mental Health' Awards (HSJ 2013).

Service users, carers and staff all have valuable insights that can contribute to the improvement of existing services, identify gaps in provision and point towards innovative developments in service provision and commissioning.

Ensuring that storytellers have agency in the construction and sense-making in the process of storytelling creates stories with ownership, veracity and power that are close to the issues as seen and experienced by storytellers, rather than the care organisation.

Finally, the stories have helped create a 'patient-powered' culture. In 2013, the former Trust secured in excess of 10,500 separate counts of service-user feedback, from a patient population of around 13,800 (at the time). As a result, they were better able than ever to aggregate feedback and identify specific thematic issues or concerns.

Key Points

- Staff, carers and service users all benefitted from the experience of participating in a reflective storytelling process.
- In addition to identifying opportunities for change in service provision and development, reflective digital stories created by staff, carers and service users can act as powerful catalysts for, or promoters of, change.
- The stories can be used to get under the skin of the statistics, bring issues to life and co-produce simple locally owned actions that benefit staff and patients alike.
- The stories have strengthened the patient voice and inspired a real confidence that feedback can truly influence service improvement.
- Stories are an effective way of linking one patient's experiences to Board debate and decision-making and the introduction of organisation-wide improvements that affect many thousands of people.
- Care that is dignified, respectful and compassionate is not only better for service users but results in significant savings in time and money for the organisation.

References

Albom, M. (2003). *The five people you meet in heaven* (1st ed.). New York: Hyperion.

Bailey, S., Thorpe, L., & Smith, G. (2013). *Whole-person care: From rhetoric to reality achieving parity between mental and physical health (summary)*. London: Royal College of Psychiatrists.

Care Quality Commission. (2015). *Manchester Mental Health and Social Care Trust Quality Report.*

Cree, L. (2012). *Rites of passage.* Pilgrim Projects. Retrieved March 2014, from http://www.patientvoices.org.uk/flv/0647pv384.htm

Dalton, J., Chambers, D., Harden, M., Street, A., Parker, G., & Eastwood, A. (2016). Service user engagement in health service reconfiguration: A rapid evidence synthesis. *Journal of Health Services Research & Policy, 21*(3), 195–205.

Francis, R. (2010). *Independent inquiry into care provided by Mid Staffordshire NHS Foundation Trust January 2005–March 2009* (Vol. 1). London: The Stationery Office.

Haigh, C. (2008). Exploring the evidence base of patient involvement in the management of health care services. *Journal of Nursing Management, 16*, 452–462.

Hardy, P. (2004). *Patient Voices: The rationale.* Pilgrim Projects. Retrieved from http://www.patientvoices.org.uk/about.htm

Hardy, P. (2007). *An investigation into the application of the Patient Voices digital stories in healthcare education: Quality of learning, policy impact and practice-based value.* MSc dissertation, University of Ulster, Belfast.

HMSO. (1998). *The Human Rights Act.* London: HMSO.

HSJ. (2013). Health Service Journal Awards shortlist announced. *HSJ.* Retrieved from http://www.hsj.co.uk/news/hsj-awards-shortlist-announced/5062539.article#.U33yWk1OX_U

Larkin, F. (2013). *Listen! Believe! Act!* Pilgrim Projects. Retrieved March 2014, from http://www.patientvoices.org.uk/flv/0745pv384.htm

Levinson, R. (2007). *The challenge of dignity in care: Upholding the rights of the individual: A report for help the aged.* Help the Aged.

Mahmood, N. (2013). *Butterfly.* Pilgrim Projects. Retrieved May 2017, from http://www.patientvoices.org.uk/flv/0718pv384.htm

Moran, M. (2014). *CEO Blog—Listen, believe, act.* Chief Executive's Blog, Vol. 2014. Manchester Mental Health and Social Care Trust, Manchester.

Mykoo, J. (2013). *I love my job!* Pilgrim Projects. Retrieved March 2014, from http://www.patientvoices.org.uk/flv/0661pv384.htm

Page, B. (2004). What they really really want. *Health Service Journal, 114*(5900), 16–19.

Rahman, H. (2012). *Labour of love.* Pilgrim Projects. Retrieved May 2017, from http://www.patientvoices.org.uk/flv/0596pv384.htm

Skelton, C. (2012). *The child within my bi-polar.* Pilgrim Projects. Retrieved May 2017, from http://www.patientvoices.org.uk/flv/0576pv384.htm

Stanbridge, N. (2013). *PND mother: "I wanted to kill myself"*. BBC Radio 4 Today Programme. BBC, London.

Sumner, T. (2013, December 4). Retrieved from https://www.hsj.co.uk/topics/technology-and-innovation/how-we-can-recruitfor-compassion/5065601. article

Patrick Cahoon is Head of Quality Improvement at Greater Manchester Mental Health NHS Foundation Trust. Previously, as Head of Patient Experience, Patrick had the responsibility for capturing and reporting on patient experience and putting in place systems and processes that help the organisation listen to people and act on their feedback, ensuring centrality of the patient experience in the design, delivery and improvement of services.

Dr Carol Haigh is Professor of Nursing at Manchester Metropolitan University and has over 30 years' experience of working in healthcare settings and. She maintains strong links with the wider clinical disciplines, facilitating improvements in patient engagement and experience using social media. Her research interests centre on ethics, social media and technology in relation to health.

Tony Sumner is a co-founder of the Patient Voices Programme and a director of Pilgrim Projects. With degrees in physics and astronomy and astrophysics, and many years' experience working in the software industry, he is particularly interested in how technology and storytelling can intersect to promote deep reflection.

9

Breathe Easy: Digital Stories About COPD

Matthew Hodson

Introduction and Background

With the recent and current rapid changes within the National Health Service, there has been a growing energy and commitment to support patients with long-term conditions in their own homes. Providing high-quality care closer to where patients live makes them less reliant on hospital services and there is now an increased emphasis on ensuring that patients are at the heart of decision-making.

This chapter looks at a project undertaken with Patient Voices to work with a group of patients with a long-term respiratory condition called Chronic Obstructive Pulmonary Disease (COPD). COPD is a life-limiting condition for which there is no cure although there are, of course, guidelines for its management (NICE 2010). Of those patients diagnosed with COPD, 80 per cent are smokers. The most commonly reported symptoms are breathlessness, cough and sputum production. The severity of these symptoms varies between individuals but tends to worsen

M. Hodson (✉)
Homerton Hospital, London, UK

© The Author(s) 2018
P. Hardy, T. Sumner (eds.), *Cultivating Compassion*,
https://doi.org/10.1007/978-3-319-64146-1_9

141

over time, with some patients with very severe disease reporting worse symptoms than those with lung cancer. Many patients experience anxiety and depression because of their poor quality of life.

As the clinical lead for the Acute COPD Early Response Service (ACERS) team, I was undertaking a service review and felt that capturing the patient experience was fundamental and at the centre of ACERS' healthcare delivery. Previous attempts had been varied and had included attempts at focus groups, but the majority of patient feedback captured was more concerned with patient satisfaction:

> *Was the hospital outpatients department good or bad?' 'Did the nurse explain enough to you—yes or no?*

I felt this didn't truly capture the essence of patient experience. The untold patient story is one that reflects their lived experience and this is an idea still not fully understood in the NHS. Even though much has been written about the ethos of capturing patients' experience, many confuse the terminology and interpret patient experience as a level of satisfaction or report it as a patient outcome. The NHS does not currently give us the right tools to measure patient experience in COPD.

The Journey Towards Patient Voices

I was first introduced to the concept of digital stories and the Patient Voices programme following a discussion with a colleague from the communications department at my local Primary Care Trust. I have always loved a good story and what really drew me to compassionate care in COPD was the fact that many people who live with this terrible condition have an important story to tell about their life or a journey or pathway taken in life. The patient's journey to diagnosis with COPD is one of the things I always ask about when meeting them for the first time. *'Tell me, what do I need to know about you?'* is a phrase I learnt from an excellent palliative care consultant. Patients who have spoken about their experience of COPD say:

'It's a disease of which there is no beginning.'
'It has just crept up on me like old age.'
'I was so relieved to hear I didn't have cancer, but then I was told I had COPD.'
'What's that?' I asked the doctor. 'It's like asthma. I was told.'

Often patients felt their symptoms were age-related or due to smoking, not because of an underlying respiratory disease. Misdiagnosis is common, as many patients are told they have asthma when in fact they have COPD. Some patients say that a hospital admission was a significant event in their eventual diagnosis, where for many years they had had the early signs of COPD but it had never been picked up by a healthcare professional despite the patient reporting symptoms.

At the time of the service review it was clear we had statistics for reduction in bed days and hospital re-admissions but what was missing for me, as a nurse and head of the service, was the qualitative narrative to support this. What must it be like to be given a diagnosis of COPD or to be told that you need a referral to a hospice for palliative care, as medically there are no other options? These are powerful words we use daily but do we really reflect on how these phrases impact on the patient's experience of health services?

My previous attempts at collecting patient experience had either been through a questionnaire or a patient focus group for people with COPD and users of the ACERS service. Feedback on what it feels like to have COPD was then presented at meetings with informed commissioners and managers, for example:

Frightening, the feeling that you can't breathe and this may be your last breath, but knowing the ACERS team are there reassures me.

I was never told anything about COPD, until I met the COPD nurse from ACERS years later.

Breathlessness is a silent symptom and a diagnosis of COPD is a shock for some people, especially when the person is told there is no cure and no medication can be prescribed. I wanted to convey the compassion the team and I felt for our service users and to capture the essence of what it is the team achieves for its service users.

Viewing the digital stories on the Patient Voices website provided me with an everlasting memory of the moving, compassionate and inspiring stories made by people living with COPD and other diseases. I was certain that digital stories would enable me to capture patient experience in a powerful way that for the first time would convey the true experience of our patients and enable us to build on their experience of engagement with healthcare professionals and the ACERS service.

Preparing for the Workshop

We used posters and an awareness event to publicise the workshop and, eventually, after much discussion about the logistics and operational issues of commissioning Patient Voices to undertake the workshop, the participants began their journey.

Unfortunately, due to the chronic nature of COPD, many patients who were invited to take part in the digital storytelling process felt that a commitment of 3 full days was too much of an obligation. Some were put off by the thought of using computers and video editing software; others felt that they didn't have a story to tell in spite of us having listened to them and received compliments from them about the ACERS service.

We arranged for the storytelling workshop to be held at a local hospice, St Joseph's in Hackney. The workshop venue is critical to success because space and quiet time to think and reflect are paramount. The hospice was an ideal location because it offered open space and was familiar to many of our patients as the venue for the local 'Breathe Easy' group. The venue is light and airy, and tea, coffee and biscuits were available all day—all essential to ensure a manageable day for our particular patient group.

On the first day of the workshop we had a small, mixed group of elderly patients, plus myself and Laura Graham, an experienced physiotherapist who leads on the pulmonary rehabilitation group for the team and who is a familiar face for all our patients.

Pip and Tony began the day with introductions and, as we went around the room, the patients introduced themselves, often followed by 'I've never used a computer in my life, but I'm willing to give it a try.' The first full day focused on the patients who attended the COPD group run by Laura and me, although we both agreed that we would also make and tell a story about our profession and why we decided to specialise in respiratory/COPD care.

Introducing the Project to Storytellers

We explained the reasons for the workshop to the patients and told them the main theme of the stories would be their journey through COPD and interactions with healthcare services (especially contact with the ACERS service), or a specific aspect of the ACERS service, such as attendance at the hospice or the pulmonary rehabilitation group. By this time an air of confusion surrounded the group and clarity was needed on what was expected from us all. Details of the workshop and of the Patient Voices website had been given to the participants before the workshop but it turned out that I was the only one who had viewed some of the stories.

In view of this, it was felt this was the ideal time to show a completed COPD Patient Voices story to the group—one that had been made by a similar COPD team about their patients' experiences of using telehealth (another area where 'data' doesn't support patient experience in the difference it makes to the quality of people's lives). We watched *Breathless* (Simons 2010) and I was very moved by James's story. However, I wasn't ready for what came next, when Pip asked us how we felt about the story. There was silence in the room as we all paused to reflect on the images we had seen, accompanied by the deep voice of James telling his story, a man we had never met but whose words were instantly recognisable to me from listening to people describe their symptoms of COPD. James's words spoke an emotional language that was so powerful in its delivery and his message was understood and shared by many in the group.

Creating the Stories

I hoped that we might be able to create something similar but was apprehensive, given that our patients had no IT experience. Little did I know that the participants around me would produce some outstanding patient stories.

A key aspect of the workshop was that both patients and clinicians took part. This was important because it gave a greater sense of partnership—we were *all* storytellers and we were *all* able to talk through our concerns and benefit from feedback. The fact that some of us were clinicians and some were patients became almost invisible during the workshop itself, as we worked together so well. This ability to work together led to a high degree of transparency and openness when talking about very personal aspects of our stories.

Pip and Tony facilitated during the workshop and they were invaluable in helping participants to think about the particular story they might wish to tell. At no time did they try to steer participants towards a particular story—it was clear from the outset that ownership of the story always remains with the participant.

The next few days were action packed as we spent time refining and editing our scripts, sorting images, choosing music and pulling together our stories. During this time there was a lot of laughter, quite a few tears and some frustration but also a sense of camaraderie. Each picture had its own story and I felt so privileged to have an opportunity to share these with my patients. Anne's story, *Coming out* (Hamblin 2012), describes a woman of almost 80 years, who had enjoyed gardening, photography and walking the dog. The story captures her life in pictures whilst describing her encounter with the ACERS team that leads to her learning to exercise again and to manage her condition more effectively. Mary's story, *The eleventh hour* (Durkin 2012), describes the benefits of pulmonary rehabilitation but also highlights the need for earlier diagnosis and treatment and is an excellent example of patient experience in COPD care.

Finally, on the last afternoon of the workshop we previewed the stories, with Tony showcasing each storyteller's story. The pictures, music and words in each story were amazing—so compassionate in their delivery and so believable to the audience. Our participants will truly inspire others living with COPD.

Core Values of Nursing

A lack of compassion in the nursing profession had been very much in the media spotlight at the time of the workshop. Shocking stories of poor-quality nursing care throughout all aspects of service delivery were highlighted in the Francis report into the appalling care at Mid Staffordshire Hospital (Francis 2010). As a result, I felt that truly understanding the patient experience had never been more critical. Alongside the national responses to the Francis report was a document called *Compassion in practice: nursing, midwifery and care staff, our vision and strategy* (Cummings 2012), intended to put six core values at the forefront of all nursing care to ensure high-quality care is delivered at every patient contact. The core values are also known as the 6Cs: care, compassion, competence, communication, courage and commitment.

As a nurse consultant, I wanted to use these core values to enhance the care delivered to patients, alongside a seventh C—COPD—which is at the heart of the ACERS team, to ensure nurses provide coordinated, effectively communicated and compassionate quality care, through a competent and courageous workforce for the safety of our COPD patients. Therefore, a secondary aim of the project was that the stories would also provide insights into whether the 7Cs were embedded in the ACERS service. This was demonstrated by Patricia's story, *Just around the corner* (Alexander 2012). Her story unfolds from an acute admission to the hospital and powerfully reveals how the COPD care and support she received from the local hospice enabled her to live with her condition.

How the Stories Are Used

We have used the stories in several different ways but one of the most powerful ways has been during presentations about the Breathing Space clinic, for which the ACERS team won a national award. By showing one of these stories, I can demonstrate the storyteller's real-life experience, enabling viewers to walk in someone else's shoes for a few minutes and try to understand what it is like to live with COPD.

I also believe that the stories have led to a greater sense of compassion in COPD care. Though difficult to quantify, healthcare professionals who have listened to and watched the stories have talked about the empathy, care and respect shown, which has fuelled them to reflect on their own practice. I plan to take the 7Cs further and utilise these stories so nurses are able to reflect on the positive and negative experiences shown.

Learning from the Workshop

During the workshop, we spent a lot of time reflecting and it was during this time that I thought of some learning points that I had not really considered before. One of the most unforgettable ones for me was the memory of my mum telling me I had asthma when I was a child and taking my blue inhalers regularly. I found myself wondering whether my career choice later in life—specialising in respiratory disease—was just a coincidence or whether it was a result of my childhood experience. My own story, *Small impact, big difference* (Hodson 2012), is an example of my commitment to providing quality care for patients, inspired by my own experience of breathlessness. My colleague Laura recounted a personal view of her late grandfather in her story, *Making a difference* (Graham 2012), and we both spent a long time reflecting on childhood experiences and what prompted us to go into healthcare.

We all have a good story to tell—some love to shout about theirs, others do not—but what is really important is what we can learn from a Patient Voices workshop and the digital storytelling process. Following this workshop, in 2013 I was honoured with the title 'Nurse of the Year' and, as a result, have heard from a number of nurses and clinicians who would like to organise a similar workshop. People often tell me that the patient voice is the most powerful form of feedback. For me, the idea of stepping into the shoes of a patient and the real-life experience of their interaction with healthcare and healthcare professionals can tick a thousand boxes. As a clinician, this is what I want to hear and I hope it is what a chief executive would want to hear. There is value in collecting both patients' and clinicians' stories as long as there is a purpose and clear understanding of the reasons why this is being done and the journey the stories will take after they have been made.

Conclusion

This was a workshop that I will never forget. I feel fortunate to have worked with the participants who discussed, edited and re-evaluated their personal experience to produce Patient Voices stories that they wanted to share.

Patient experience is just that: it's their experience, not ours. We must listen and take action if we in the NHS want to make changes. The biggest change makers are not politicians, clinicians or managers; they are the patients themselves—those who live with long-term conditions know what they want from care—and we must begin by listening to them. The Patient Voices programme provides powerful opportunities to enable us to do just that.

The 6Cs are everyone's responsibility. Individual nurses (and other clinicians), as well as patients and those who care for them, can provide important feedback that can result in changing the culture of an organisation. To deliver a modern NHS and provide high-quality, compassionate care for patients with COPD, we must act upon local needs and take time to listen to patients (and invest sufficient money to enable us to do this). Only then can we ensure sustainability for the future of respiratory services and the wider NHS.

The value of Patient Voices is that they recognise each voice as an individual and ensure that compassion is maintained throughout the patient's journey—I feel privileged to have been on one of those journeys with them.

Key Points

- Pre-course information and recruitment of storytellers is key, but it is important to be clear about the aims of a digital storytelling project. Ask yourself: *What are these stories for? What am I going to do with them once they are finished?*
- Generic advertising is fine but targeted recruitment is better and this can sometimes pose a challenge.
- Adequate briefing for storytellers and workshop sponsors/commissioners is important and it can be helpful to speak to someone who has already organised a workshop. For example, it's useful to think about things such as this for patients and the need for frequent refreshments and so on.
- Patients and clinicians can work in partnership to deliver and understand what quality patient experience is.
- Digital stories can lead to a greater understanding of patients as it is possible to really appreciate their lived experience.

References

Alexander, P. (2012). *Just around the corner*. Pilgrim Projects. Retrieved May 2017, from http://www.patientvoices.org.uk/flv/0606pv384.htm

Cummings, J. (2012). *Compassion in practice. Nursing, midwifery and care staff, our vision and strategy*. London: Department of Health.

Durkin, M. (2012). *The eleventh hour*. Pilgrim Projects. Retrieved May 2017, from http://www.patientvoices.org.uk/flv/0605pv384.htm

Francis, R. (2010). *Independent inquiry into care provided by Mid Staffordshire NHS Foundation Trust January 2005–March 2009* (Vol. 1). London: The Stationery Office.

Graham, L. (2012). *Making a difference*. Pilgrim Projects. Retrieved May 2017, from http://www.patientvoices.org.uk/flv/0602pv384.htm

Hamblin, A. (2012). *Coming out*. Pilgrim Projects. Retrieved May 2017, from http://www.patientvoices.org.uk/flv/0603pv384.htm

Hodson, M. (2012). *Small impact, big difference*. Pilgrim Projects. Retrieved May 2017, from http://www.patientvoices.org.uk/flv/0601pv384.htm

NICE. (2010). *Chronic obstructive pulmonary disease: Management of chronic obstructive pulmonary disease in adults in primary and secondary care* (partial update). NICE guidelines. National Institute for Health and Care Excellence, London.

Simons, J. (2010). *Breathless*. Pilgrim Projects. Retrieved May 2017, from http://www.patientvoices.org.uk/flv/0447pv384.htm

Dr Matthew Hodson MBE is a Chief Nurse, an Honorary Respiratory Nurse Consultant at Homerton University Hospital in London and Chair of the Association of Respiratory Nurse Specialists. He was the 2013 *Nursing Standard/* RCN 'Nurse of the Year' for work around end-of-life care for people with advanced COPD.

Part III

Transformational Learning

Pip Hardy and Tony Sumner

Education is the kindling of a flame, not the filling of a vessel. Socrates

It was never the intention of the Patient Voices Programme to encourage the acquisition of facts, provide solutions or, indeed, offer training. Many years' experience of designing open learning materials had taught us that inspiration and motivation are the prompts to reflection that will, in turn, shape new understandings, adjust beliefs and alter behaviour—in short, to transform the learner in some way. It was precisely this kind of inspiration and learning that we hoped the Patient Voices stories themselves would evoke; it was to be some time before we realised the transformative potential of the digital storytelling process, particularly with respect to the development of the skills of critical reflection.

It is our view, and one that is shared by many other educators, that the ability to reflect on experience is the cornerstone of education. We have been inspired, in particular, by the work of John Dewey (Dewey 1938) and Donald Schön (Schön 1987) both transformational educators who regarded reflection as central to individual learning. Going one step beyond personal change, Parker Palmer viewed learning and knowing as communal acts, carried out with the heart as much as the head (Palmer 1983), and of course, digital storytelling might not exist if not for the inspirational work of Paulo Freire and his recognition of the need for critical consciousness in order to bring about transformation

(Freire 1973). The theory of transformational (or transformative) learning has been discussed at length by Jack Mezirow (Mezirow 1991) drawing on humanistic and psychological theories such as those expounded by Carl Rogers (Rogers and Freiberg 1969). These educators and others acknowledged the importance of emotion in the experience of learning (Salzberger-Wittenberg et al. 1999); it was precisely this alliance of heart and head that we observed in digital storytelling workshops, leading to new insights and, often, changes in behaviour. We, therefore, thought that digital storytelling could fruitfully be used as way of teaching reflection at undergraduate and post-graduate levels, and of deepening the reflective capacity of qualified health professionals.

The chapters in this part illustrate just how transformational a process the Patient Voices workshops can be, focusing initially on the experience of five, originally sceptical, medical students, from the perspective of their educators and the students themselves, and then looking at the preparation of mental health student nurses for the actuality of clinical practice. Their experiences provide a strong case for the use of digital stories in the ongoing professional development of health professionals.

Chap. 10 "Reflection: They Just Don't Get It! Digital Stories with Junior Doctors" details how five final year medical students created digital stories as a component of their training. Analysing the process offers insight into the power and potential of digital storytelling to enable deep reflection on clinical experience, in particular its emotional impact, suggesting that this might be a means to develop a more compassionate reflective framework for personal, professional and inter-professional development.

In Chap. 11 "Reflection: Now We Get It!" the medical students themselves reflect on the transformative nature of their experiences of the 'Student Voices' project and the opportunity it gave them to develop their professional identities and as individuals. They acknowledge the importance of time to question themselves and find their significant stories; mindfulness and a person-centred approach; reflection as a tool for learning rather than assessment; tapping into emotions and the ability to challenge and learn from past actions.

In Chap. 12 "The Shock of Reality: Digital Storytelling with Newly Qualified Nurses", Gemma Stacey finds digital storytelling a way to help stop the cycle of repeating past mistakes with generations of newly qualified mental health nurses. Conflict between expectations and the actuality of clinical experience produces negative effects on nurses themselves, attrition rates and quality of care. Gemma considers hurdles to hosting the workshops, such as funding, and more complex personal factors such as disclosure, vulnerability and feelings of disloyalty, but also the benefits to the students of validation and sensitivity to their needs, and of creating a valuable teaching tool for transformative reflection.

References

Dewey, J. (1938). *Experience and education*. New York: Collier.

Freire, P. (1973). *Education for critical consciousness* (Vol. 1). London: Continuum.

Mezirow, J. (1991). *Transformative dimensions of adult learning*. San Francisco: Jossey-Bass.

Palmer, P. J. (1983). *To know as we are known*. New York: Harper & Row.

Rogers, C. R., & Freiberg, H. J. (1969). *Freedom to learn*. Columbus, OH: C. E. Merrill.

Salzberger-Wittenberg, I., Williams, G., & Osborne, E. (1999). *The emotional experience of learning and teaching*. London: Karnac.

Schön, D. (1987). *Educating the reflective practitioner: Toward a new design for teaching and learning in the professions*. Higher Education Series. San Francisco: Jossey-Bass.

10

Reflection: They Just Don't Get It!— Digital Stories from Junior Doctors

Liz Anderson and Dan Kinnair

Introduction and Background

Patient experience is central to developing effective interprofessional education (IPE), that is, learning for health and social care students that brings together practitioners or learners from different professions. IPE *occurs when two or more professions learn about, from and with each other to enable effective collaboration and improve health outcomes* (WHO 2010).

Internationally, those who forward the IPE agenda meet every two years within a conference series entitled 'All Together Better Heath' (ATBH). In 2006, the Patient Voices programme was showcased as a valuable resource for IPE educators at ATBH III, in London. The project leads, Pip Hardy and Tony Sumner, ran interactive workshops on digital

L. Anderson (✉)
Centre for Medicine, University of Leicester, Leicester, UK

D. Kinnair
Bradgate Mental Health Unit, Glenfield Hospital, University of Leicester, Leicester, UK

© The Author(s) 2018
P. Hardy, T. Sumner (eds.), *Cultivating Compassion*,
https://doi.org/10.1007/978-3-319-64146-1_10

155

storytelling with delegates from around the world. The workshop was endorsed by the UK Centre for the Advancement of Interprofessional Education (CAIPE), an organisation of which both authors have been active board members. From here we attended several Patient Voices workshops and gained greater insight into the power and potential of digital storytelling.

Making our own stories about critical moments in our lives helped to highlight the power of personal reflection, and we developed and produced several stories, such as *Empty Chairs* (Anderson 2008), about midlife changes for women, and *Climbing Mountains* (Kinnair 2008), contrasting experiences of healthcare in Africa and those in the UK. Our experiences prompted us to consider their value for student learning within the medical school, and so we contacted Patient Voices to consider how digital storytelling might be adapted for medical students, and a project team consisting of the authors and the Patient Voices team was born.

As educators we were very aware that students found reflection on their learning difficult, despite numerous opportunities and approaches on learning how to reflect within the curriculum. We recognised that students have long periods of clinical exposure with direct patient involvement and experience many emotionally challenging situations, such as a patient dying. Sadly, there is limited time for students to fully understand the impact of these clinical experiences, which in the main go unrecorded, especially their emotional impact. Such experiences are commonplace for many people training in healthcare, who are expected to build resilience for future professional responsibilities. While completing their learning placements, medical students reflect using short written pieces or reflective diaries prepared and read by placement educational leads, and they can share personal concerns with tutors. Our exposure to digital stories had made us wonder if there was a place for using this methodology to help students retell and unpack their raw emotions in a rather different way.

Reflection Is Vital

Following the events in the Mid Staffordshire Foundation Trust (Francis 2013), it is even more pressing that all healthcare staff have time to stop, think and reflect on their individual and team practices. At times it is too easy to get stuck in following an existing process for patient care that has long since ceased to be effective and which may even sometimes be identified as being unkind. Reflection should not simply be done as a mandatory requirement for appraisal and revalidation or as a response to a complaint. Instead, it should be done in a thinking, intelligent way to develop better services and more responsive patient care. Reflection can be individual and personal and should also be used to examine behaviours and attitudes seen within and between teams. All too often, postqualified staff complain of a lack of time for thought and reflection when managing the most challenging emotional situations in their day-to-day working lives. For the project team, the opportunity to offer students a meaningful reflective experience early in their careers may have longlasting benefits for patients and may help to develop compassionate, mindful professionals of the future.

Our Project: Digital Storytelling as Reflection

Our project aimed to analyse how medical students might reflect on their clinical experiences using the Patient Voices digital storytelling process. Medical students, unlike other students, have an elongated programme that enables a period of uninterrupted study during a Student Selected Component (SSC). We chose a 3-week period within the SSC programme, in the late summer, for students in the last year of their training.

We submitted a study brief in the summer of 2008, in partnership with Pilgrim Projects/Patient Voices, for students to select this SSC, entitled 'Student Voices: Digital Storytelling in Healthcare.' The traditional format for making stories was adjusted. The team produced a student workbook containing further reading and activities related to reflection and including elements of digital storytelling, with the whole process elongated over 3 weeks. As this was a pilot, we had placed a ceiling of ten students. However, when we started we had only five male students who all stated that this was not their first choice.

The workshop began by exploring reflection for medical students and why this is so important. The General Medical Council expects that qualifying doctors should be able to reflect, learn and teach others and maintain a portfolio of reflections and learning needs. The outcomes expected of medical students are to 'continually and systematically reflect on practice and whenever necessary, translate that reflection into action' (GMC 2015a).

> Learners must receive regular, constructive and meaningful feedback on their performance, development and progress at appropriate points in their medical course or training programme and be encouraged to take action on it. Feedback should come from educators, other doctors, health and social care professionals and where possible patients, families and carers. (GMC 2015b R3.13 p. 26)

As a result, 'Portfolios' have had a recent surge in importance for undergraduate professional development, propelled by the General Medical Council directive that medical students should be able to: Establish the foundations for lifelong learning and continuing professional development, including a professional development portfolio containing reflections, achievements and learning needs (GMC 2015a, 21(b) p. 8).

This is in preparation for the requirements for Foundation training which over 95% of our graduates would undertake using e-portfolio-based learning.

Reflection has always been an essential attribute of health and social care professionals, especially doctors, who are often the first point of contact for patients (Sandars et al. 2008). It is seen as central to assessing personal competence and is now integral to remaining on the register of practising doctors held by the General Medical Council. All doctors have to be appraised every year and must bring reflective accounts of clinical practice as evidence of learning and progression (GMC 2012).

The introductory session analysed reflection by considering a number of theorists, mainly John Dewey (1938), whose words were placed in the student workbook, 'learning comes not from experience but from reflecting on experience,' as well as the work of Vygotsky and Rieber (1997), Moon (2004) and Kolb (1984).

Students were then directed to watch several Patient Voices stories from the website, to analyse the impact of the stories on them personally and to consider the extent to which each of the seven elements of digital storytelling (Lambert 2006) contributed to the meaning of the story. The main aspects they considered were the simplicity of the story and how the author used visual pictures and music to enhance the message. This energised the students to start to consider what story they wished to tell from their clinical learning. They were not given any directions as to what story to tell but were encouraged to choose their own critical moments. All students could bring to memory meaningful clinical experiences and they began to write down their recollections using a story board.

The group was typical of students completing reflective writing exercises in that they failed to get to the heart of the story. They produced copious notes, but the story board helped them to work towards a concise account with only the salient points, told in the manner of a story, rather than a report. Some students had two stories. This period of exploration of the Patient Voices website and time to write their own story took most of week 1. The students' story notes and first drafts were emailed to all the team. Finally, a story circle helped to focus down on the core elements of the narrative. Each student had two stories which could be clearly retold within a 2-minute window. In preparation for the following week, they spent time searching for images to enhance the story. This meant returning to clinical units and seeking permission to take photographs of clinical areas. Collecting the elements (photos, voiceover, music, etc.) they would need to pull together, their digital story was work they all enjoyed.

There is no doubt that when it came to learning about the technology behind mixing a digital story, these IT-literate students were a pleasure to work with. They enjoyed taking and editing photos, capably using Photoshop to enhance the images and quickly learning how to add action by zooming in on part of an image and exploring different filters and effects to support the mood of their story. In fact there was no length of time they could not sit and practise these skills, often working until well after 5 p.m. The students were eager to see a worthy final product and were completely enthralled by the whole process. We, meanwhile, were quietly delighted that students who had come to a workshop with such scepticism were so engaged.

Presenting the Stories

The students' sheer delight in showing their final stories was wonderful to observe. A presentation session was organised to share their experiences with the head of clinical practice and the head of the medical school and several teaching consultants and senior academics attended. The workshop therefore concluded at the end of 3 weeks, with the students consenting to share all of their stories on the Patient Voices website and with a final feedback session in which the heads of the medical school were both amazed and delighted at the outputs. Table 10.1 outlines details of the stories posted on the Patient Voices website as 'Stories from the University of Leicester Medical School SSC workshop for junior doctors in training' (www.patientvoices.org.uk/lssc.htm).

Student Evaluations

Any solid piece of learning requires the educator to evaluate the student experience. Throughout the project the students completed a weekly diary and, in addition, they filled in a post-course evaluation questionnaire and spoke with a researcher about their experiences. These findings have already been shared elsewhere (Anderson et al. 2012) but the value of the digital storytelling process for the students is described below.

The Emotional Content of the Stories

Each student chose a highly emotional theme, including patient care prior to death (*Yeah, I'll go*; *Can I have a hand please?*); what it means to remain calm and professional when working with the public (*Be patient with us*; *Are you happy in your profession?*); the complexity of emotions within clinical uncertainty (*Heart of stone*); and care of the dying and environments for hospice care (*Care of the dying?*; *Your type*). Many of the stories offered insights into the pressures on frontline staff in modern healthcare. We were not surprised about the content, which confirmed our project aims to explore further student emotional challenges when in

Table 10.1 Digital stories and summaries

Digital story	Summary
Heart of stone (Al-Alousi 2008)	Salam is shocked and angered when an emergency operation doesn't go according to plan, but he comes to realise that things are not always what they may seem and even consultants have feelings
Be patient with us (Pang 2008a)	Weehaan became acutely aware of the tensions between caring for the patient and caring for the family—and pleads for tolerance while he learns to find the right balance
Are you happy in your profession? (Tangri 2008)	Abs had a successful career as an accountant in London before deciding to go to medical school. Despite the ups and downs, his chosen path seems to be the right one
Yeah, I'll go (Critchfield 2008)	Matthew is keen and enthusiastic to successfully perform a 'by-the-book' catheterisation, but the discovery that there is more to his vocation than technical know-how leads him to reflect on the true nature of caring for patients
Can I have a hand please? (Pang 2008b)	Patients in the last days and hours of life can sometimes be challenging and even unreasonable. As the only male professional on the ward, Weehaan was at first frustrated, but then patiently responds to the final requests of a dying man
Your type (Corry-Bass 2008b)	When Steve chooses a placement at a hospice in order to learn some of the 'softer' skills that he thinks will help him in the practice of emergency medicine, a casual remark causes him to reflect on what 'type' he needs to be to care for people facing death
Care of the dying? (Corry-Bass 2008a)	There are many preconceptions and stereotypes surrounding hospice care. When Steve chooses a hospice for his clinical placement, he is pleasantly surprised to find that care of the dying is not at all what he had anticipated

clinical placements, and many of the stories identify kindness and compassion as a key theme. In the stories, the students identified what they would do differently in the future and how they have developed as a result of the storytelling.

All of the students repeatedly stated what a great time they had on the SSC. They had made new friends and enjoyed learning new techniques in a relaxed atmosphere.

Reflection

All the students stated that, for the first time, they had really completed a process that had shown them the true meaning of reflection: 'really pleased to be able to reflect on my experiences in a meaningful and constructive way' (Student 1); 'nice to be able to reflect on something of my choosing and not something the Medical School told us to reflect on' (Student 2).

Several years later, in 2016, one of the now-qualified students returned to the medical school to endorse the value of this method of reflection, again confirming that this was the only time in his training that he actually understood what reflection really meant and its ongoing value to help shape future practice.

The Value of Stories

The production of their stories helped the students to think more deeply about their clinical learning: 'the small details in everyday practice that could improve aspects of clinical care' (Student 5).

Listening

The group had not only worked as individuals on their own stories, but they had supported and become engaged through the story circle in each other's story. This and analysis of both the groups and their own story had made them consider the valuable role of listening in medicine, not just to the spoken word but to the awareness of situations and everything around them when in clinical areas.

Organisation and Self-Management

The process had been time-limited and many wanted more time and worried that they would not meet the deadline and be ready to share their story on the last day. In fact, what they could see was the process had helped them to consider self- and time management.

Value of Digital Stories

All the students stated that they would consider using this approach when in clinical practice. They could see that they might work with patients to create stories to help them in their practice of medicine or that they might use critical learning moments and turn them into digital stories for appraisal. They therefore perceived the process as:

- a means to capture critical incidents in clinical care and their impacts
- a way of using visual material for learning
- a process to help them fully listen to patient experiences
- a tool for reflection on learning
- a tool for presenting their reflections-on-actions taken in clinical work.

These views are summarised by these extracts from the students' evaluations:

Benefit to Themselves and Others

I enjoyed the course. I produced a digital story that I am pleased with. I have improved my reflective abilities and I found that I had many stories I could have used from clinical practice. (Student 3)

I expect my video to be used—this is particularly pleasing as I feel others will strongly benefit from my experiences. (Student 4)

I produced two powerful stories that can benefit other people—patients and healthcare professionals. Two important reminders … to say have patience with patients all the time—the main theme of my stories is also an important aspect of being a [professional] doctor. (Student 5)

The benefits for others included those who attended the final presentation session, the authors and medical school leads. At the presentation session, one consultant working in a clinical area that resonated with one of the stories commented that she would return to her team and share the impact and personal learning. A general practitioner attending the presentation aligned the process to his educational work in medical humanities. The presentation reopened clinical memories for all who attended, including the authors.

The stories highlighted the emotional power of the day-to-day experiences that all health and social care professionals must manage. It is clear that these early clinical experiences stay with us for the rest of our working practice. Digital storytelling allows these memories to be distilled and meaningfully reflected upon, even many years later. There was much debate and discussion over coffee after the stories were shown.

How the Stories Have Been Used

The stories were developed by medical students to offer them a transformative moment in time to appreciate reflection in action. Our evaluation of these students led us to believe that this really was the case and that the power of making a digital story was something we would like many students to appreciate. We anticipate repeating this process in the future, and the medical school continues to work with Patient Voices in patient involvement and the process of digital storytelling. A similar process has been endorsed elsewhere for medical education as a method for reflection (Sandars 2009).

Use of the Stories Today

The final outcomes (seven stories were placed on the Patient Voices website) have been used for teaching in a number of ways. They have been used to prepare students for their clinical practice and are shown by the head of the clinical curriculum in a lecture for all medical students about to go on clinical placements. Although increasingly medical students access clinical opportunities in their early training, it is not until their later training that they are fully exposed to day-to-day healthcare delivery. At this later stage, students' clinical placements expose them to what it feels like to work in hospitals and in the community. Much of this practice is about professional responsibility, dealing with emotional engagement in clinical situations and learning with and from patients and other members of the clinical team, all while preparing for finals.

The stories help to highlight some of the emotional, ethical and professional issues medical students may face. In addition, during their clinical blocks, they return to the medical school for several sessions on professionalism. These stories have been used in small-group work as a trigger to unpack their own clinical insights and to ensure that our students adhere to the highest possible standards of practice recently endorsed by Francis, namely, patient-centred practice based on advocacy, accountability, transparency and responsibility (2013). An example of the way one of the stories is used in small-group teaching is described in the case study below.

Case Study: Use of Medical Students' Stories in Professionalism Teaching—Annual Workshop on Professional Practice

Matthew's story: *Yeah, I'll go* (Critchfield 2008)

This story was used to generate debate and discussion on the theme of 'professional responsibility.' Many medical students, just like Matthew, find themselves in situations that cause them a dilemma. Matthew needed to have completed a procedure (here catheterisation) and wanted to appear willing and eager both to gain his competence and also to help more senior colleagues. However, in stepping forward to complete any patient-centred procedure, certain steps must be followed: first, to ascertain whether the procedure is actually required and, second, to seek consent from the patient themselves. Neither of these steps was fully explored to a satisfactory level in this scenario. Matthew was left feeling uncomfortable about actions for which he was accountable, even as a student, because he conducted the procedure in the belief that requests from senior staff automatically warranted his compliance.

Today's NHS is being asked to challenge a culture in which there is a lack of 'candour,' 'accountability' and 'responsibility' (Francis 2013). Should Matthew's actions have been scrutinised, the whole team, including Matthew, would have had to account for their actions. Matthew would have been found wanting as he could not justify what he did as simply responding to the requests of senior staff. All NHS staff, including students, must think for themselves.

Conclusion

Sceptical male medical students towards the end of their training engaged and benefitted from making digital stories using critical learning moments from practice. They highlight to educators some of the challenges our students face when working in frontline clinical care. The medical school can now draw upon these stories to prepare students for clinical practice. Digital stories can highlight current issues within clinical areas as seen here through the eyes of observant and often manipulated students. This is extremely relevant today in light of the concerns raised in the Francis report (2013). We continue to use these stories in lectures and small-group teaching, and Patient Voices have shown them at many national and international meetings around the world; the stories can also be viewed on the Patient Voices website.

We end with an extract from the focus group:

> *Those medical students that do not want to do this should be made to do it as it is probably these to whom it would have the greatest effect—it has on us.*

Key Points

- Medical students valued making digital stories to learn how to reflect upon critical moments from clinical practice.
- The process of producing a Patient Voices digital story helped medical students to learn how to reflect in a more meaningful way.
- The power of the stories belongs to the individuals who produce them in a snapshot of time, but have long-term capacity to influence because they resonate with others who share similar experiences.
- Patient Voices bring a mixture of IT expertise, educational design and development experience, writing and editing skills, understanding of storytelling and recognition of the support necessary for people to tell

difficult stories. They are pivotal for making reflective digital stories from within the context of the lived experiences of health and social care.

- Making a personal digital story has high emotional gain if the stories are based on key life moments. The process can be cathartic and emotional and any personal story can only emerge from within a supportive framework such as that offered by Patient Voices.
- Digital storytelling might be a means to develop a more compassionate reflective framework for personal and team developments. This has never been more important given the pressures on healthcare nationally and internationally and the reports in the media, which often have as a theme the lack of compassion in healthcare.

References

Al-Alousi, S. (2008). *A heart of stone?* Pilgrim Projects. Retrieved May 2017, from http://www.patientvoices.org.uk/flv/0258pv384.htm

Anderson, L. (2008). *Empty chairs*. Pilgrim Projects. Retrieved May 2017, from http://www.patientvoices.org.uk/flv/0184pv384.htm

Anderson, L., Kinnair, D., Hardy, P., & Sumner, T. (2012). They just don't get it: Using digital stories to promote meaningful undergraduate reflection. *Medical Teacher, 34*(7), 597–598.

Corry-Bass, S. (2008a). *Care of the dying*. Pilgrim Projects. Retrieved May 2017, from http://www.patientvoices.org.uk/flv/0259pv384.htm

Corry-Bass, S. (2008b). *Your type*. Pilgrim Projects. Retrieved May 2017, from http://www.patientvoices.org.uk/flv/0260pv384.htm

Critchfield, M. (2008). *Yeah, I'll go*. Pilgrim Projects Limited. Retrieved May 2017, from http://www.patientvoices.org.uk/flv/0257pv384.htm

Dewey, J. (1938). *Experience and education*. New York: Collier.

Francis, R. (2013). The final report of the Mid Staffordshire NHS Foundation Trust Public Inquiry.

GMC. (2012). *Ready for revalidation: The good medical practice framework for appraisal and revalidation*. London: General Medical Council.

GMC. (2015a). *Outcomes for graduates (Tomorrow's doctors)*. Manchester: General Medical Council.

GMC. (2015b). *Promoting excellence: Standards for medical education and training*. Manchester: General Medical Council.

Kinnair, D. (2008). *Climbing mountains.* Pilgrim Projects. Retrieved May 2017, from http://www.patientvoices.org.uk/flv/0183pv384.htm

Kolb, D. A. (1984). *Experiential learning: Experience as the source of learning and development* (Vol. 1). Englewood Cliffs, NJ: Prentice-Hall.

Lambert, J. (2006). *Digital storytelling: Capturing lives creating community* (2nd ed.). Berkeley, CA: Digital Diner Press.

Moon, J. (2004). *Handbook of reflective and experiential learning: Theory and Practice.* Abingdon: Routledge and Falmer.

Pang, W. (2008a). *Be patient with us.* Pilgrim Projects Limited. Retrieved May 2017, from http://www.patientvoices.org.uk/flv/0261pv384.htm

Pang, W. (2008b). *Can I have a hand, please?* Pilgrim Projects Limited. Retrieved May 2017, from http://www.patientvoices.org.uk/flv/0262pv384.htm

Sandars, J. (2009). The use of reflection in medical education: AMEE Guide No. 44. *Medical Teacher, 31*(8), 685–695. doi:10.1080/01421590903050374.

Sandars, J., Murray, C., & Pellow, A. (2008). Twelve tips for using digital storytelling to promote reflective learning by medical students. *Medical Teacher, 30*(8), 774–777.

Tangri, A. (2008). *Are you happy in your profession?* Pilgrim Projects. Retrieved May 2017, from http://www.patientvoices.org.uk/flv/0256pv384.htm

Vygotsky, L. S., & Rieber, R. (1997). *The collected works of LS Vygotsky: Problems of the theory and history of psychology* (Vol. 3). New York: Plenum Press.

WHO. (2010). *Framework for action on interprofessional education and collaborative practice.* Geneva: World Health Organization.

Dr Liz Anderson trained as a Nurse and worked as a Midwife and Health Visitor. She is Professor of interprofessional education at Leicester Medical School where she also leads on patient safety. She works in partnership with patients in delivering education and leads the local patient and carer group. She is a CAIPE Fellow and a National Teaching Fellow.

Dr Dan Kinnair is a Consultant Psychiatrist, Honorary Associate Professor at the University of Leicester Medical School and Associate Postgraduate Dean at Health Education England in the East Midlands. He is responsible for the mental health training of undergraduate medical students and has a particular interest in interprofessional education.

11

Reflection: Now We Get It!

Steve Corry-Bass, Matthew Critchfield,
and Weehaan Pang

Editors' Note

Elsewhere in this book, contributors have spoken of how the Patient Voices projects and workshops that they have sponsored have provided opportunities for storytellers to reflect upon their experiences.

For junior doctors in training, *Outcomes for Graduates* (*Tomorrow's Doctors*) (GMC 2015) formally puts in place reflection as a key aspect of professional practice and development. Several of the storytellers who took part in the Patient Voices project described in the previous chapter

S. Corry-Bass (✉)
Northampton General Hospital, Cliftonville, Northampton, UK

M. Critchfield
Neville Centre, Leicester General Hospital,
Leicester, UK

W. Pang
Royal Wolverhampton NHS Trust, New Cross Hospital,
Wolverhampton, UK

© The Author(s) 2018
P. Hardy, T. Sumner (eds.), *Cultivating Compassion*,
https://doi.org/10.1007/978-3-319-64146-1_11

wanted to contribute something about how that reflective process has played an important role in their developing professional identity.

This chapter consists of three distinct but related—and invaluable—reflections on that process.

Reflection: Now I Get It!

Steve Corry-Bass

It's fair to say that I never planned on attending the 'Student Voices: Digital Storytelling in Healthcare' workshop, led by the Patient Voices Programme, in summer 2008. In fact, none of us had chosen Student Voices as our first option for that summer's Student Selected Component (SSC) of our medical degree. My summer was originally going to involve a tonsillectomy, but that is, as they say, another story. It's also fair to say that given my previous experiences of reflection and reflective learning, I did approach the first session with some trepidation and cynicism. Three weeks of reflection, well…

However, all preconceptions were gone as soon as I entered the room and saw chairs in a circle with scatter cushions, and no desks or notebooks in sight.

Not only was the module a transformation for me in my appreciation of reflection as a process, it also served as an opportunity for me to develop as an individual, and as a reflective practitioner in my own right, building on my own professional identity.

Through this chapter I hope to be able to bring to you, the reader, something of the transformation that this sceptic had after meeting Pip and Tony and taking part in the 'Student Voices: Digital Storytelling in Healthcare' workshop.

Reflection

From the moment you start medical school, there is a requirement placed on you as a student to 'continually and systematically reflect on practice and … translate that reflection into action' (GMC 2015), and this continues once working as a qualified practitioner. My school strove to ensure you had ample opportunity to achieve this, through provision of numerous occasions to reflect on experiences. However, prior to attending Student Voices in my final year, reflection had become just another form of assessment, another box to tick, another hoop to jump through. Reflection had been about writing 1000 words on an experience, ensuring that I utilised the approved headings/technique. It was no longer deep or transformative; it was correct and appropriate to ensure that I could evidence achieving the competencies, and would be signed off at the end of the module. It had been a record of what I had learnt and what I would do differently in the future, not *how* I had learnt or *how* my future practice and actions would be influenced by it.

Student Voices was, therefore, a revelation for me. I was given the opportunity to spend time with Pip and Tony considering what had happened over the past 5 years of medical school and what I wanted to talk about. I was given time to think about what I had done, what I hadn't done, and what I hoped to do in the future; where I hoped my career would take me, my dreams and aspirations. I was given time to challenge my thoughts, time to challenge the actions of my past, and time to consider how events had made me the student I was today. All this I was able to do, without the feeling of time or pressure, without the sense that I had an impending deadline. I could explore my thoughts and feelings at my own pace and reflect properly on what had been a whirlwind journey and only the start of a much greater adventure.

It was through this process that I came to appreciate the number of transformative moments that had occurred during my time at medical school, the number of life-changing events I had been witness to, the interactions I had had with patients and with others. But what had had most meaning for me and what could I then take forward and turn into a digital story?

I thought about the first time I had met a patient on a ward, the first operation I had seen, outpatients' clinics, different hospitals and community teams, treatments and (inevitably) death. All these experiences had been so rich, and looking back at them, I could appreciate how they had impacted future decisions, even if at the time I didn't realise their significance. I could see that I had learnt from my experiences and through Student Voices giving me time to reflect, I could see how I had grown as a person.

Equally, however, I was struck with a sense of fear; there had been so many moments in the last few years that had been so deep and profound in their effects on me: how could I pick just one to create a story about? Which was the most meaningful for me, and, once transformed into a digital story, which experience would be the most useful and interesting to others?

I had become so focused on final exams, which were only 7 months away, and ensuring that I would pass them that I had lost sight of the bigger picture: I had lost sight of why I wanted to become a doctor. Having time to think and reflect on what had happened, with no pressure to write X words or to use Y headings was refreshing and much needed. The chance to sit and talk with Pip, Tony and the others about my experiences allowed me to realise how much I had changed, how much I had learnt and how much there was still left to learn.

Distillation

As I thought about events and occurrences, and began to distil one experience down to its essence, I realised that I had two stories to tell: how I had found a hospice, and how the hospice had found me. I found myself writing about my preconceptions of hospice care and care of the dying, and another story about the type of student you had to be to attend a hospice placement, after a consultant quipped, 'We don't usually get your type here'. The entire placement at the hospice had been fulfilling and rewarding, but with the assistance of Pip and Tony, I was able to turn this experience into two digital stories, reflecting on some of my experiences: *Care of the dying?* (Corry-Bass 2008a) and *Your type* (Corry-Bass 2008b).

Through the process of finding images and music to use with my digital story I was afforded further opportunity to think and reflect. 'A picture is worth a thousand words' is a phrase often quoted, and we also know that music can prompt a reflective attitude; it can aid in the creation of space and can encourage powerful emotions and reflections

(Blasco et al. 2006; Janaudis et al. 2011). Looking for media to accompany my stories was perhaps the most challenging part: how to complement the spoken word, how to enhance my message and how to bring the viewer into my story, to be a part of something that was both personal and something I wanted to share.

Following the workshop, reflection has become a deeper and more meaningful process. I have found myself asking my own tutees to reflect on things that make them 'take a breath'—the things that they tell their friends about at home, the things that they think about days and maybe weeks later. These are the experiences that are significant; these are the experiences that have a profound effect on who they are; and these are the experiences that will shape the practitioner they become in the future.

Professional Identity

The Student Voices SSC allowed me to consider how the 18-year-old A-level student had become a medical student and was (soon) to become a doctor. It allowed me to consider more deeply what it meant to be a doctor and the 'type' of person who became an emergency medicine physician. Here, I am not just referring to knowledge, dexterity, time management and technical abilities—which are all, of course, important traits for anyone who is looking to work in the busy and ever-changing environment of an emergency department. I am referring to the ability of the doctor as a communicator, the doctor as a healer and the doctor as a person. Student Voices allowed me to realise that I had already begun the process of exploring this side of my identity—how I had developed as an individual from a generic curriculum; how to communicate with people; and how to maintain that person-centred approach which is so important, without losing the technical knowledge and know-how.

If it hadn't been for the opportunity that Student Voices afforded me then, I am not sure I would have spent time appreciating the depth and the richness of my experiences. Since the workshop, I have been more mindful of what is happening, analysing situations and afterwards considering how they might have played out differently had I acted differently.

Within this, I am also mindful of not only how I conduct myself with other staff but also with patients and their relatives.

Moving forwards, I would encourage everyone, regardless of professional or social status to consider, 'Who am I?', 'What am I doing?' and 'Where am I going', as a means to reflect on their own identity and that of those around them.

Conclusion

Student Voices turned me into somewhat of a reflective practice convert. Initially sceptical of the term through its overuse, it allowed me the chance to realise what reflective practice was, what it wasn't and how it could be used for learning and development.

Reflecting on Reflection: Experiences of a Patient Voices Workshop

Matthew Critchfield

In the last few months of medical school, we had the opportunity to choose our final Student Selected Component (SSC). While many of my colleagues chose to spend clinical time in areas that they were likely to pursue as careers, I was drawn to an alternative option with the title 'Student Voices: Digital Storytelling in Healthcare'. I read a little about it and thought it sounded like something a bit different and put it down as an option, although I'll admit it was not my first choice. When I was told some weeks later that I had been allocated this SSC, I was a bit sceptical as to what it might involve, and half wished that I was going off to the wards again where I felt comfortable. I recall the first few days of the workshop and doing the story circle and thinking—am I wasting my time here?

Although it is now 5 years since I did that workshop, it has turned out to be one of the most memorable experiences I had at Leicester Medical School and has heavily influenced my attitude and approach to reflective practice. I am now working in psychiatry where being reflective is as much a part of treatment as it is about consolidating, processing and unpicking one's own experience and learning.

Reflective Practice

'Reflective practice' is a term that gets used a lot at medical school. We are told, for example, that it is 'an essential characteristic for professional competence' (Mann et al. 2009). It is drummed into us that the General Medical Council states that we must be able to provide evidence of reflective practice throughout our careers. As I recall, most of us were sick to the back teeth of the phrase, and many felt that time spent formally reflecting was a 'wishy-washy' part of the course and far less valuable than spending time in the operating theatre or the wards. We were issued workbooks to guide and assess our learning through the various clinical placements, and many of the workbooks called for written 'reflections' of our experiences during the placement. For many of us, these sections ended up being hurriedly filled in before handing in the book at the end of the placement.

The story I produced at the Patient Voices workshop, *Yeah—I'll go* (Critchfield 2008), tells of how, when I jumped at the chance to practise a clinical procedure, what I actually learnt about was compassion and what it really means to provide medical 'care'. I am certain that this is the most considered and thought out piece of formal reflection that I have produced to date.

The workshop was run over 3 weeks, and much of that time was spent practising storytelling, writing and producing, with the goal being to produce a tangible piece of reflection in the form of a digital story. In order to achieve this, I had to really think about, dissect and unpick my thoughts about how I had experienced the events I had chosen for my digital story. I wanted to capture the event itself, the emotions attached to it, the learning and how my approach to practice had altered as a result. Getting all this down to just a few minutes was not an easy task. In my opinion, the process of producing this digital story encapsulates what is meant by reflective learning. Considering which images to use and whether to include music to accompany the narrative adds a dimension that is not present in traditional written reflection. It is possible that these processes tap into emotions and feelings in a deeper sense.

In my postgraduate training as a junior doctor and psychiatrist, I have attended other formal courses on reflective practice, and I have been struck by the huge variation in understanding amongst my peers about what reflection in practice is. I was also fortunate enough to attend a weekly Balint group for a year with my psychiatry trainee colleagues. This has provided a rich source of discussion and a chance to reflect, both on an individual level and as a group, on our experience of patients' stories encountered in psychiatric practice. Collecting written evidence of reflective practice forms a significant part of the 'ePortfolio', an online log of what can sometimes feel like a sea of assessments, learning objectives, outcomes and reports that we as junior doctors have to undergo and record as evidence of our competence. I'll admit that at times the 'reflection' I do for the purpose of this portfolio is reminiscent of those workbooks at medical school.

Conclusion

Yeah, I'll remains my only digital story. I have not made any more since doing the workshop in 2008. For me, balancing the busy life of being a junior doctor with my young family leaves little time, and there is no doubt that the time needed to make digital stories is more than I can afford. However, I am certain that the time spent making my story as a medical student helped me to realise how powerful reflection is as a learning tool. It has shaped the way that I approach my reflective practice more than any other teaching.

I think it is the sheer depth to which one needs to think about an experience in order to make a digital story that forces you to understand the reflective process. I would strongly encourage all medical students to consider and develop their reflective abilities as early in their career as possible. It remains an essential component of professional practice and must not be side-lined in the minds of students as 'wishy-washy'. There is considerable evidence outlining the benefits of reflection in healthcare education (Mann et al. 2009), and I think it would be wonderful if all medical students were given the time and opportunity to make at least one reflective digital story.

When You Reflect Out Loud: Digital Storytelling for Learning and Understanding

Weehaan Pang

I attended the digital storytelling workshop as a final-year medical student as part of my special study module. I wanted to do something not entirely academically related, to have a different 'end product' out of it. It was a great decision, as I learned a lot about effective reflection and also mastered the art of 'digital storytelling' to voice out my reflection, to share with many others. I am glad that the video clips I made during the workshop have been featured in several teaching programmes and conferences.

Reflecting in the storytelling workshop was done very differently from all the 'reflections' we were taught to produce as part of our assessment in medical school, where there is a fixed structure to follow, often done half-heartedly as tick-box exercises. In the workshop, we were encouraged to reflect on all aspects of our experience in clinical setting as medical students, and to pick one or two stories that we thought were worth sharing. There was no fixed structure to follow or a marking scheme to grade our work. The idea was to produce something that was personally meaningful and potentially influential in our future career.

The workshop went through the process of reflection, brainstorming ideas, materials preparation, structuring the digital story, preparing and recording a voiceover and editing the final video. Selecting photos that fit the storyline was the most challenging part. Since it was an audiovisual project, I tried to include images that would serve to paint a mind picture of the actual setting, to lead the audience to engage in a similar thinking process to mine. The voiceover process added emotions to it, to maximise engagement. The step-by-step approach was very learner friendly. At the end of the workshop, each of us walked away with a successful piece of work and an important life-long skill that continued to benefit us on many occasions.

Reflecting on Experience: *Can I Have a Hand, Please?*

My first story, *Can I have a hand, please?* (Pang 2008b), reflects on my experience as a part-time healthcare assistant on an elderly care ward. I was on night duty with a patient who became agitated and delirious in the middle of the night. I repeatedly attended this elderly gentleman, Mr. A, who pressed the buzzer for help to get comfortable. On a busy night with many unwell patients, even with efficient time management, the goodwill to spend more time with the patients who needed most attention may not be fulfilled. Mr. A had been deteriorating on the ward for the last few days and was known to be terminally ill. I was a little frustrated to be called so often, when there was a long list of jobs awaiting completion. He passed away in the morning.

Reflecting back immediately after the shift, I could have done much better. Instead of attending his calls repetitively, in an attempt to keep him settled, I should have identified his moribund state and proactively initiated to call for a proper palliative input to make him more comfortable at the end of life.

This particular piece of reflection has continued to influence my practice as a doctor. As a busy NHS worker who is expected to multitask and to achieve perfection at all times, the stress could be overwhelming. I aim to review and adjust my attitude regularly when dealing with tricky tasks to ensure provision of best care to my patients at all time. One key phrase I use to remind myself: 'it is not personal!' Besides, I also make a mental note to think outside the box, to understand the underlying reasons of particular behaviour in a patient and act upon it accordingly.

Reflecting on Experience: *Be Patient with Us*

My second story, *Be patient with us* (Pang 2008a), is a plea for the general public to understand NHS workers. The story highlighted my experience in dealing with impatience amongst patients and family members in the hospitals. It is understandable that when someone is ill they expect the best care from the healthcare professionals to help restore their health.

Dr Steve Corry-Bass is an Emergency Medicine registrar, undertaking sub-speciality training in Pre-Hospital Emergency Medicine. He also holds an MA (Education), volunteers his time as a University Personal Tutor, and is involved in the development of eLearning resources for St John Ambulance and the Royal College of Emergency Medicine.

Dr Matthew Critchfield studied medicine at Leicester Medical School as a mature student. Prior to commencing his studies, he spent several years working as a carer for the Leonard Cheshire Foundation and as a physiotherapy assistant. He graduated as a doctor in 2009 and became a member of the Royal College of Psychiatrists in 2013. He is currently a Higher Trainee in adult and old age psychiatry in Leicester.

Dr Weehaan Pang is a qualified doctor currently training to become a Specialist in Clinical Radiology. While at medical school, Weehaan worked as a part-time healthcare assistant. The time spent looking after patients at the bedside and listening to their stories continues to enhance his overall experience as a clinician.

12

The Shock of Reality: Digital Storytelling with Newly Qualified Nurses

Gemma Stacey

Introduction

This chapter describes a project that aimed to improve the experiences of newly qualified mental health nurses during their transition from student to qualified nurse. It represents a cycle of stories, with one influencing the next, and began with my own story and those of my friends making that same transition over 12 years ago. Our stories involved feeling overwhelmed by the weight of responsibility; unsupported by established healthcare professionals working around us but not with us; and in some cases frightened by incidences we had been involved in and felt underprepared to respond to or move on from. For me, the distressing experiences encountered had been dealt with, processed and dismissed as an overreaction due to my inexperience and lack of maturity. Some of my friends had done the same, but others had chosen to leave nursing and pursue alternative careers. I was enjoying a satisfying role as a community mental

G. Stacey (✉)
School of Health Sciences, Royal Derby Hospital, University of Nottingham, Derby, UK

© The Author(s) 2018
P. Hardy, T. Sumner (eds.), *Cultivating Compassion*,
https://doi.org/10.1007/978-3-319-64146-1_12

health nurse and thought little about my early experiences and the possible implications they could have had on my own mental health and how I perceived myself within the profession.

However, in my new position as a lecturer in mental health, the stories of my past re-emerged as I listened to the experiences of newly qualified nurses I had supported during their nurse education. They were encountering the same challenges as I and my friends had years before—it was obvious that the stories were repeating themselves. The people and contexts were different but the issues were the same and the consequences equally detrimental to some individuals. I learnt that some newly qualified nurses were already seeking alternative roles, and some were considering leaving nursing altogether. I met individuals who were showing signs of post-traumatic stress disorder and struggling to manage their anxiety when at work. Despite this, the support from within the service was non-existent, and there was a clear message that this was an inevitable reaction that was required in order for the newly qualified nurse to build resilience to the nature of the work.

I felt that this was an unacceptable resolution and began researching the literature that explored the transition process. I learnt that a significant body of literature existed and that it had originally been described by Kramer in 1974 as a:

> *'reality shock', defined as 'the reactions of new workers when they find themselves in a work situation for which they have spent several years preparing and for which they thought they were going to be prepared, and then suddenly find they are not. (Kramer 1974)*

The evidence suggests that this dissonance is due to the conflict between the expectations of the newly qualified nurse and the actuality of clinical practice.

This experience continues to be echoed throughout the recent literature exploring the lack of post-qualification support strategies, low job satisfaction and high attrition rates (Robinson et al. 2005; Forsyth and McKenzie 2006). The consequences are significant, as the coping strategies that newly qualified nurses employ to rectify this dissonance are shown to have negative effects on quality of care and maintenance of person-centred values (Mackintosh 2006). Despite this issue being reported first in 1974, the phenomenon of a 'reality shock' appears to remain and seems to have been accepted by education and practice as an inevitable aspect of professional socialisation.

I set out to explore educational approaches that could help students prepare for the challenges described by others and documented in the literature. It was at the International Nurse Education Conference in Dublin that I first encountered the work of the Patient Voices Programme and experienced the impact of a digital story (Hardy et al. 2008). I was instantly engaged and connected and felt the storytellers' struggles. It was a truly moving moment, and I felt compelled to talk to Pip Hardy about the newly qualified nurses and how digital stories might be the perfect fit for the educational innovation I had been looking for.

The Hurdles

After a number of discussions with Pip, it was evident that a synthesis of my vision had occurred, and after experiencing the digital storytelling process myself, I was assured that Patient Voices would work with the newly qualified nurses' stories in a sensitive and respectful way. However, gaining funding to support a workshop to create the stories was a challenge. Those within the technical world dismissed the complexity of the process as they were blind to the methodology that underpinned the creation of the short videos. Those within the educational world appreciated the value of the digital stories but were also at a loss to suggest options for funding as there were few avenues that supported the creation of educational resources.

Finally, funding was secured from the Centre for Integrative Learning and the Nottinghamshire Health Care Trust. A project was designed that would result in the stories being used within the pre-registration mental health nursing curriculum and in an online training website for established qualified nurses who were supporting newly qualified nurses during the transition process. This involved lengthy bid writing and presentations to funding boards. Some revisions had to be made to the project plan and the funding bodies were quite specific about the stories they wanted to be created. The usually flexible brief of a Patient Voices workshop had to become much more focused in order to satisfy the funders.

Recruiting the newly qualified nurses to attend the workshop was fairly straightforward due to the relationship I had with them and their shared desire to influence the experience of others. However, gaining permission for them to be released from their clinical roles to have 3 days' study leave was a challenge. It involved writing to and liaising with senior management and convincing them of the value of the workshop, both for the individual and the service as a whole. Permission was given for five newly qualified nurses to attend.

The final hurdle was one for the storytellers themselves. Having received the information on the digital storytelling process, they became concerned about their own vulnerability and how they would be perceived if those working with them discovered the struggles they had been experiencing. They became protective of the service and attempted to defend the lack of support or poor practice they had been exposed to. It appeared a process of self-censorship was occurring that could present a barrier to the digital storytelling process. One storyteller decided to limit the audience that she was comfortable with the story being shown to. She asked for it only to be used in presentations where students or professionals would be guided through a process of reflection to ensure judgements were not made of the service or individuals involved.

The Stories

Over the period of a 3-day workshop, the newly qualified nurses created digital stories that relayed an event or experience that was significant to them during their transition from student to qualified nurse. Whilst the digital stories that were created do not claim to be representative of all newly qualified nurses' experiences, the content of the stories is supported by events reported in the wider research literature exploring this transition process. These digital stories reiterated the overarching impact of a reality shock stemming from the gap between expectation and actuality. However, the cause of this shock appeared to be varied and resulted from different challenges.

The stories were grouped into themes, the first of which related to the conflict the newly qualified nurses experienced when their values where questioned or disregarded by established nurses, illustrated by Susanna's story, *Who Is an Expert?* (Morris 2009). This situation appeared to result in the newly qualified nurses questioning their personal beliefs and identity as nurses, due to lack of support and dismissal from those they were looking to for guidance. The stories present detailed reflections on the potential consequences of negative interactions with established nurses while offering powerful illustrations of bullying and hostility within a discipline known as 'horizontal violence' (McKenna et al. 2003).

The next theme was named 'The challenges of the therapeutic relationship,' illustrated by Rachel's story, *Are We There Yet?* (Hadland 2009). The content of these stories relates closely to the concept of emotional labour, which refers to the internal regulation of emotions required of nurses in order to adopt a 'work persona' that still enables them to express their (surface or deep) emotions during patient encounters. This concept has been discussed by Huynh and others (Huynh et al. 2008) who recognise that ignoring the impact of emotional labour can result in nurses employing defensive strategies to enable them to maintain emotional distance from their patients. The research on this issue in relation to professional socialisation implies that newly qualified nurses are encouraged by organisational culture to ignore this aspect of their work in order to prioritise practical tasks. These stories illustrate the personal impact on nurses of engaging on an emotional level with their patients and shed light on how this may become burdensome if ignored or unexplored.

The final theme relates to the emotional consequences of distressing events occurring in practice, illustrated by Vicky's story, *Maybe It Just Isn't the Right Job for You* (Baldwin 2009). In these stories, newly qualified nurses described significant incidents in their work and reflected on how these situations impacted upon them emotionally. These events represented extreme illustrations of emotional labour, and storytellers' reflections mirrored those typical of reactions to traumatic experiences. Despite this, there appeared to be a lack of recognition from within the service of the longer-term consequences of these experiences on individual nurses. As a result, the newly qualified nurses became embarrassed by their reactions and felt the need to present themselves to others as coping, a response that reflects Goffman's view about how people negotiate daily life and make conscious decisions about how they present themselves in the public arena (Goffman 2002). Goffman refers to creating a 'front' or image of oneself as an acceptable person and argues that such impression management is a fundamental component of all social interaction. These stories illustrate the ways in which students respond to expectations in order to evoke confirmatory feedback that may lead to the verification of conceptions about how they should behave as 'professionals' which, in turn, ultimately involves switching off emotions.

The Focus Group Discussion

The storytellers were invited to take part in a focus group discussion to consider their experiences of the digital storytelling process.

The group first considered their motivation to create a digital story and take part in the storytelling process. The most significant motivation appeared to be underpinned by a desire to take the opportunity to reflect on their experiences. One participant stated:

> *Just to take a breath and think about that [incident] intensively for a couple of days meant a lot. I could have just carried on and on and on and not really processed it, whereas I was able to get away from work and talk about it.*

For other storytellers, the opportunity to create a teaching resource which would communicate an important message was a motivating factor. These individuals felt dissatisfied with their own experiences and passionate about making a difference for others. They identified the digital story medium as a way of expressing their experiences in a manner which would command the attention of educators, service managers and even policymakers.

Despite these motivating factors, the storytellers found the process challenging for a number of reasons. First, some felt conflict with disclosure of their personal experiences into the public arena. They felt this placed them in a vulnerable position as they were allowing others to judge them, their feelings and their practice. It appeared they were attempting to maintain the meaning of the story whilst presenting themselves and others in the story in a way which was acceptable to them. For example:

I was worried about how people might judge my practice and what message they would take from the story. I was worried that potentially I could do more damage than good.

The storytellers also reflected on how surprised they were by the emotional consequence of the process. Whilst they identified this as a challenge, they also described it as a benefit of the process, as they felt this was due to the depth of reflection that they had engaged in. This was helped by them gaining validation on their reaction to events from sharing with others. One storyteller reflected:

When you speak about it you are quite detached—I speak about it but I'm not really thinking—it's just words. Whereas this made me stop and think for a longer period of time, away from work, with people who are nothing to do with my work, this was good, to validate my experience. It was really helpful.

The storytellers were also reminded of how difficult their experiences had been and realised how they had already become detached from certain emotional elements of their work through exposure and self-protection. They felt the storytelling process would maintain awareness of challenges and encourage others to offer support to future newly qualified nurses as they developed through their career.

How the Stories Have Been Used

The stories have now been integrated into a workshop that was designed by educationalists and counsellors for student nurses. The workshops aim to expose students to some of the challenges they may experience and engage them in small-group activities, which encourages them to empathise with the storyteller, consider how they might respond in similar circumstances, and identify personal development needs that they would like to be supported to explore outside of the workshop. The students who have taken part in these workshops have contributed to their evaluation and refinement. Below are some of the comments made by students to illustrate their perspective of the learning process. There were a number of comments relating to the authenticity of the stories, which appeared to enable students to relate to the storyteller:

> *It made my learning more meaningful and real.*
> *I felt many newly qualified nurses would feel the same way and it helps to hear first-hand from someone in a real-life situation.*
> *It made the session come to life.*

The students also acknowledged how the stories raised issues that were of concern to them. This presented a challenge to some members of the group:

> *It raised issues and problems which I had been thinking about in the back of my mind.*
> *I felt sympathy for the storyteller and fearful for my own progression to a qualified nurse in relation to the responsibility.*
> *It was a good way of discussing these issues and to identify your own that you perhaps hadn't realised you had until this.*
> *Highlights fears I have about qualifying.*

They commented on the reassurance they gained during the group discussions from sharing their concerns with others and realising that others had similar concerns. This suggests that the workshop also had a supportive function.

> *It helps you to realise the things you worry about are what others go through too, so you're not alone.*
> *I now realise that other people have the same worries as me and that most people are feeling the same as I am.*
> *It's good to know I am not alone when I feel my confidence is not as high as it could be.*

The authenticity of the stories and reflective discussions also appeared to enable the students to place themselves in the position of the newly qualified nurse and consider how they might respond to the challenges faced. This indicates that the students were starting to recognise their personal resources that would enable them to regain a feeling of control.

> *I recognised the fears, values and first expectations that the storyteller had as what I would have. It was encouraging to see how she dealt with them and that I am not on my own.*
>
> *I felt I could relate to the feelings she was experiencing. It made me look at how I would deal with that scenario.*
>
> *It was a situation any of us could relate to and put ourselves in when we qualify and made us think how we would behave/react to a similar situation.*
>
> *Makes you think about how you would act in this situation, which is good as it challenges your values and ideas.*
>
> *I appreciated thinking about strategies for conflict resolution and gaining a wider experience of seeing the points of view of others.*

The students were asked to compare this experience to other teaching approaches that aimed to encourage reflective learning. The students identified that the open structure of the workshop gave them space to reflect, as opposed to alternative approaches, which have been more focused on being taught reflective models. They also identified that the storytellers were modelling the reflective process, enabling them to observe reflection in action. Some students identified that this helped them to go on to reflect on their own experiences.

> *Normal reflection sessions are set out and structured. I felt able to explore more.*
>
> *I have always struggled with reflection but listening to someone else reflect made me also reflect.*
>
> *A lot better, more interactive and helped me to reflect in a deeper and more meaningful way.*
>
> *Probably the most I have reflected on anything as I was able to put myself in Susanna's shoes as she was the one telling the story, not just reading it.*

Additionally, the stories are integrated into an online learning tool for established nurses who are supporting newly qualified nurses during their transition. Early responses indicate that established nurses find the digital stories a powerful reminder of the difficulties experienced by newly qualified nurses and encourage them to be more aware of the nurses' emotional and support needs.

Note: A fuller evaluation of the educational intervention, including a model for using the stories to encourage newly qualified nurses to develop core strengths, has also been written up in a paper called 'Challenging the shock of reality through digital storytelling' (Stacey and Hardy 2011).

Conclusion

Whilst it is acknowledged that the digital stories themselves cannot address the wider issues around lack of support for newly qualified nurses or protect them from exposure to distressing or challenging incidents they might encounter, it is hoped that they provide a more authentic perspective that students can consider. This in itself will not rectify the problem, but it may give newly qualified nurses some tools to respond to these issues in a way that is less detrimental to their own mental health. Furthermore, by reminding established nurses of the challenges of newly qualified nurses, it is hoped that they may be more aware and sensitive to their support needs. In conclusion, it is anticipated that a different story might be told by future newly qualified nurses, one that incorporates a sense of control, expectation and positive adjustment as opposed to the reality shock that currently occurs.

Key Points

- The process of gaining funding to support projects involving digital stories should not be underestimated. It will often entail the project leader promoting the power of digital stories to a sceptical audience. However, the stories themselves are often the best way of convincing others of their value, so try to incorporate the opportunity to view them into the application process, either within a presentation or by providing a link within the paper application.
- Consider carefully your rationale for viewing digital stories as the best educational resource to promote the intended learning. Sceptics may need to be convinced of why digital stories as opposed to other approaches are justified.

- The storytellers will often need reassurance of how their stories will be utilised in the future. It is important to acknowledge that sharing their personal experiences may lead to a level of anxiety. This should be carefully responded to so that storytellers feel that they have control and do not lose ownership of the story when it becomes an educational resource.
- Remember the power of the stories even when you have seen them several times. When using the stories regularly within teaching, it is possible to become desensitised to the story and forget the potential impact it can have on an audience who is viewing it for the first time. Ensure that you respond to the reaction within the room and attend appropriately to how the audience receives the story.
- Remain open to the audience seeing something within the story that others have not. Although it is important to consider the educational framework the story fits within and the intended learning outcomes, you should also remain open to the possibility of unexpected learning to occur or discussions to be promoted that take you down an unexpected avenue.

References

Baldwin, V. (2009). Maybe it just isn't the right job for you? *Patient Voices: The shock of reality – Stories from newly qualified mental health nurses*. Retrieved from http://www.patientvoices.org.uk/flv/0367pv384.htm

Forsyth, S., & McKenzie, H. (2006). A comparative analysis of contemporary nurses' discontents. *Journal of Advanced Nursing, 56*(2), 209–216.

Goffman, E. (2002). The presentation of self in everyday life [1959]. In C. Calhoun et al. (Eds.), *Contemporary sociological theory* (pp. 46–61). Oxford: Blackwell.

Hadland, R. (2009). Are we there yet? *Patient Voices: The shock of reality – Stories from newly qualified mental health nurses*. Retrieved from www.patientvoices.org.uk/flv/0363pv384.htm

Hardy, P., Stanton, P., & Mangnall, J. (2008). *The potential of Patient Voices and digital storytelling to humanise health and social care (a symposium)*. Paper presented at the NETNEP, Dublin.

Huynh, T., Alderson, M., & Thompson, M. (2008). Emotional labour underlying caring: an evolutionary concept analysis. *Journal of Advanced Nursing, 64*(2), 195–208.

Kramer, M. (1974). Reality shock: Why nurses leave nursing. *AJN The American Journal of Nursing, 75*(5), 891.

Mackintosh, C. (2006). Caring, the socialisation of pre-registration student nurses, a longitudinal study. *International Journal of Nursing Studies, 43*(8), 953–962.

McKenna, B. G., Smith, N. A., Poole, S. J., & Coverdale, J. H. (2003). Horizontal violence: Experiences of registered nurses in their first year of practice. *Journal of Advanced Nursing, 42*(1), 90–96.

Morris, S. (2009). Who is an expert? *Patient Voices: The shock of reality – Stories from newly qualified mental health nurses.* Retrieved from www.patientvoices.org.uk/flv/0365pv384.htm

Robinson, S., Murrells, T., & Smith, E. M. (2005). Retaining the mental health nursing workforce: Early indicators of retention and attrition. *International Journal of Mental Health Nursing, 14*(4), 230–242.

Stacey, G., & Hardy, P. (2011). Challenging the shock of reality through digital storytelling. *Nurse Education* in *Practice, 11*(2), 159–164. doi:10.1016/j.nepr.2010.08.003; pii:S1471-5953(10)00107-1.

Dr Gemma Stacey is an Associate Professor in the School of Health Sciences at the University of Nottingham. She has published a number of papers and chapters reporting on educational approaches implemented in pre-registration nursing programmes which aim to promote transformational learning through in-depth reflection and critical dialogue within supportive educational forums.

Part IV

How Was That for You? The Healing Power of Digital Storytelling

Pip Hardy and Tony Sumner

To remember requires language, to heal requires story. (Baldwin 2005)

Since the very first workshop, described by Monica Clarke in her tenth anniversary tribute, it was clear that making digital stories could be beneficial for storytellers. Although the original intention of the Patient Voices Programme was to make available an accessible resource that people could watch and learn from, anecdotal and, increasingly, statistical and theoretical evidence is building up that strongly suggests that although the Patient Voices workshops are not offered as therapy, they are intensive healing and therapeutic experiences in their own right. An early influence on Patient Voices *Intoxicated by My Illness* (Broyard 1992). This, Anatole Broyard's final book, justified the need for more personalised care from health professionals while also enabling Broyard to face his own imminent death from cancer.

It wasn't until a little later, thanks to Mark Shea, that we came across the ground-breaking work of James Pennebaker, an American psychologist who conducted a series of experiments designed to discover whether regular writing about emotional subjects (such as childhood trauma) might have therapeutic benefits. The results of his work pointed overwhelmingly to the positive outcomes from this kind of regular writing and have been replicated over the years with many different groups, including patients affected by long-term chronic pain and students suffering from stress (Pennebaker 1997) (Pennebaker and Seagal 1999). His work has helped us to understand why people so often find the process of creating a digital story so therapeutic, even cathartic.

It is, perhaps, stating the obvious to mention the growing recognition of the value of the 'talking therapies', particularly during the twentieth century. All of the talking therapies rely on one person talking—often telling stories about their lives—to another person who, through attentive listening and mindful attention, with the help of a body of knowledge developed over more than a century, may be able to help the first person see things differently. The particular brand of therapy known as *narrative therapy* recognises the importance of the stories we tell ourselves and offers the potential to reframe these stories and, consequently, our perceptions of ourselves and the world in which we find ourselves. The work of Michael White and David Epstein (White and Epstein 1990) and Martin Payne (Payne 2005) is particularly relevant to this discussion.

The three chapters in this part examine this aspect of digital storytelling through first-hand experience, analytical psychological study and preparations for a team workshop.

In Chap. 13 'Healing Journeys: Digital Storytelling with Service User Educators', occupational therapist and senior lecturer Julie Walters explores the healing, therapeutic nature of digital stories as she experienced it herself and then, following up a workshop at Sheffield Hallam University, through her awareness of its potential as a healing tool for mental health service users and carers. She highlights the importance of active listening and careful facilitation of the workshops and the unique transformative and cathartic role that digital media can play through 'distillation and amplification' of service users' experiences, crucially giving a voice to those too often not heard.

In Chap. 14 'The Sheffield Carers' Voices Project: Was It Therapeutic?', Mark Shea used a range of theoretical psychological perspectives to analyse the process and impact of a Patient Voices workshop for carers in Sheffield for his MSc dissertation. He identified common themes, such as the impulse to help others, emotionally difficult revisiting of experience, group support and positive reframing. Though cautious about generalising, his findings suggest the potential for the experience to be cathartic and of long-lasting benefit through creating new, integrated narratives that give meaning to experiences of trauma or loss and create positive changes to participants' sense of identity.

In Chap. 15 'Building Healthy Teams: Digital Storytelling in NHS Organisations', Amy Stabler discusses the central importance of storytelling and listening to building healthy, resilient and effective teams, essential for patient safety. Honestly appraising her own desire for outcomes and reluctance to make her own story, she assesses the essential and positive experience of pre-workshop preparation and discussion of fears, especially of blame and exposure, and ethical issues of control and consent, for bringing healing and closure to team difficulties.

References

Baldwin, C. (2005). *Storycatcher: Making sense of our lives through the power and practice of story.* Novato, CA: New World Library.

Broyard, A. (1992). *Intoxicated by my illness: And other writings on life and death* (1st ed.). New York: C. Potter.

Payne, M. (2005). *Narrative therapy: An introduction for counsellors.* London: Sage Publications.

Pennebaker, J. W. (1997). Writing about emotional experiences as a therapeutic process. *Psychological Science, 8*(3), 162–166.

Pennebaker, J. W., & Seagal, J. D. (1999). Forming a story: The health benefits of narrative. *Journal of Clinical Psychology, 55*(10), 1243–1254. doi:CCC 0021-9762/99/101243-12.

White, M., & Epstein, D. (1990). *Narrative means to therapeutic ends.* New York and London: W. W. Norton and Company.

13

Healing Journeys: Digital Storytelling with Service User Educators

Julie Walters

Introduction

Two of the labels I identify with are mental health professional educator and mental health service user. I am an occupational therapy lecturer and have a diagnosis of cyclothymia, for which I choose to take mood-stabilising medication.

Sometimes I have disclosed my service user status within my professional role and sometimes I have not, such is the perceived risk of stigma and discrimination within the caring professions. However, whether I choose to admit it or not, a great deal of the knowledge I bring to my teaching work is expertise by experience: experience not gained from my professional role but because of having experienced mental health services myself, as both patient and carer. I have witnessed some great practice as a service user and carer, but some terrible things have also happened, which have left deep personal wounds.

J. Walters (✉)
Faculty of Health and Wellbeing, Sheffield Hallam University, Sheffield, UK

© The Author(s) 2018
P. Hardy, T. Sumner (eds.), *Cultivating Compassion*,
https://doi.org/10.1007/978-3-319-64146-1_13

199

The cornerstone of good mental health care is good relationships. Trust, rapport, respect—nothing can be achieved without these. But the process of professionalisation, necessary though it may be, can get in the way of one human being relating to and accepting another. Barriers form because of the biomedical paradigm so dominant in healthcare and in part because of the under-acknowledged emotional labour of caring (discussed elsewhere in this book). In my job, I try very hard to influence the attitudes and behaviours of the next generation of health professionals, so that they understand that their own humanity is their greatest asset, and also understand how they can use this in their work.

Peter Beresford is someone who also walks a similar road and writes extensively about service user involvement within health and social care practice, education and research (Glasby and Beresford 2006; Beresford 2001, 2002). I met him once, and he challenged me by saying that we must bring everything that we are to everything we do in this arena. It was the desire to find a way to achieve this—to bring everything I am to my professional role that sparked my interest in Patient Voices. I knew I had a story I needed to tell. What I did not anticipate was the depth of personal healing that would occur as a result of going through the process: digital storytelling as a healing activity, a concept I found extremely interesting as an occupational therapist. In my role, I recognise that engaging in activities that are meaningful promotes health and wellbeing and can be used for therapeutic purposes.

So, this chapter is about my interest in digital storytelling as an explicit therapeutic activity, and it is in three parts. It starts with an account of the making of my first Patient Voices story and then discusses the subsequent workshop at Sheffield Hallam University. Finally, it outlines some of my thoughts about what it is about digital stories that makes them therapeutic.

The First Story

It was a dark, rainy Friday night in November 2007. I was driving from Sheffield to Cambridge to my first encounter with the Patient Voices Programme. I was hoping for the opportunity to tell a story in a special way with a bunch of people I had never met. Would I feel safe enough? It felt scary.

I arrived in bedraggled fashion at a large comfortable house and was warmly welcomed at the door. I was led through to the sitting room. The introductions had already started, but I was in plenty of time for the story circle. Thus began my first digital storytelling workshop.

The story I thought I was going to tell sits in the middle of the finished story—it's the part about going psychotic. I had gone into hospital for help and sanctuary, but found that I had put myself in the most dangerous place I could possibly be. It seemed to me that I barely made it out alive. This was the story I told in the story circle—an illness experience so dark and horrible, so jumbled up, a sticky tangle of emotions of stigma, grief, misunderstanding, loss, anger and madness. During the workshop, my story was carefully listened to, and with help and encouragement, I made sense of, processed and presented it. It was therapy by presentation—years and years of therapy packed into one intense weekend. The process was transformative, cathartic—a release. The product was an emotionally powerful piece of communication. But much of my outpouring was left on the cutting room floor because, through the facilitated group, I came to understand that I needed to tell another story—the grieving story about my sister. That was the bigger story. You may wish to pause here and watch my story, *Surviving* (Walters 2007). I am still very pleased with it.

Healing Journeys

I returned to work absolutely evangelical about digital storytelling. As an occupational therapist educator, it was natural for me to want to promote the service user and carer voice within health and social care education. I also knew that the output of the workshops created many resources that would support my role as an educator. But the experience I had had making my story was so profound that I made it my mission to give others like me the opportunity to make digital stories with the Patient Voices Programme and that is what motivated me to organise a workshop at Sheffield Hallam University.

The money came from faculty funds set aside to support service user and carer involvement in health and social care education, research and curriculum development. The project involved collaboration between occupational therapy and social work subject groups at Sheffield Hallam University. The service users and carers approached were already involved in supporting teaching and learning activities within our faculty. In promoting the planned workshop to potential storytellers, I emphasised the healing that had occurred for me through the process and showed them the digital story I had made.

Patient Voices came up to Sheffield to facilitate the three-day workshop in March 2008, and we decided to call it 'Healing journeys.' It was my privilege to facilitate the workshop with Pip and Tony from Patient Voices and to see our workshop participants relax, enjoy and benefit from the experience.

Healing Journeys Feedback

Here is what some of the storytellers said about the experience at the time, as reported in the dissemination newsletter:

Writing and remembering about the events from my childhood was far from easy, however there was so much support from fellow storytellers and Pip and Tony from Patient Voices, and most of all from Sheffield Hallam staff, that the story has been told … Would I recommend it to others? Yes, I would. Thanks. (Ian)

This workshop was to be a big adventure for me. We took an unforgettable, emotional journey together … I discovered the film editor in me. I had not realised how creative this work would be and how much it would soothe my soul. After the three days it took a while to get over the excitement of it all. I found myself wanting to tell everyone about what I had done and felt immensely proud of myself. I have been touched by other people's response to my story. I had not anticipated how much my story would reach into people's hearts or how much insight and depth of understanding it would give. (Pep)

At first I didn't know what my story would be, I knew it was going to be about our situation, but how do you choose a piece out of a 21-year-old jigsaw? … The telling of the story and the making of the DVD … was a wonderful

experience and has enabled us finally to bring this hurt to the surface and deal with it in a most positive way, in that we feel some good will come out of our despair. Digital storytelling certainly has a place in the healing arena. (Muriel)
When it came time for me to relate my story my first few words trickled out, but then the gates opened wider and my thoughts spilled out like a torrent from my lips and rain fall from my eyes. I was shaking when I finished speaking. But I felt no embarrassment because there were reassuring smiles from all the other storytellers; they understood. I hope that people suffering from depression and lack of self-esteem might benefit from seeing my story. We can all feel very isolated at times, but by sharing stories we can begin to understand that we are not alone. (Paul) (Coleman 2008)

The Stories: Five Years On

It is clear that making the stories had a big impact at the time, for example:

> *I have been asked to show my DVD to two or three different audiences including over 70 social work students and a big meeting for stakeholders in the revalidation process. I feel the DVD has been a powerful tool already in presentations to a lot of people.* (Nev)

But want about since? Both Nev and Ian have continued to use their stories to support their service user educator activities at Sheffield Hallam University and other organisations. Ian and Pep went on to make second stories with Patient Voices at another workshop in Sheffield. We succeeded in creating a lot of interest in the Patient Voices stories generally, and my academic colleagues continue to ask me from time to time if I know of a story that fits a particular message or subject. I can often direct them to a suitable story from the many on the Patient Voices website. I have occasionally shown my first story to students, after some thought about the impact of it on students who might see me in a particular role.

I recently contacted the original storytellers and asked them for their reflections five years on.

Here is what some of them said:

I still look back on my videos from time to time, when I'm not very well. It does happen every so often, especially if it is something like the Jimmy Saville business. I get very annoyed and frustrated, that the same things are said by all those people who should have done something, but didn't. They all come up with 'we should have listened.' To me it's same old, same old. Other times it's more personal things that affect me, but then it's back to the good base coping strategies that I learnt from my occupational therapy, and some of the community psychiatry nurses and social workers I've had (not all helpful workers), and the digital stories, the students and the staff I've worked with, plus a little sleep and then everything is put back into the right context.

My GP used to say how much I had come along the road to better health, and I never realised it, not until after the digital stories and doing things at Hallam. I should probably do one final digital story—"Into the light". Like I said at the end of the second one, "What happened to me will always affect me, but it will not control me anymore." If doing the stories has helped to get me to that stage (which I believe they did), then the more they are used, as part of therapy for service users and carers, the better. (Ian 2013)

My son died at birth, and no one talked to me about it at the time. Instead I was sedated and I did not know what happened. When I was invited to make the digital story I thought I was going to do it just on myself but changed my mind. It was listening to everyone else's story during the workshop that gave me the courage. It clicked in my head that I would do it about my son. Making the DVD has been absolutely brilliant for me. It is really good that I have had a chance to heal and understand what happened even though it was a bad experience. I did not know you could express your feelings in this way. I have my DVD and I watch it all the time. I have shown it to my friends and my other son and daughter and because of the digital story I feel there are three children and not two and that my lost son is always with me … I am so grateful for this healing for my heart. Thank you to Pip and Tony and to all the other storytellers at the workshop. I get great comfort from how they have managed to deal with things and I am still in touch with many of them. (Christine 2013)

I still remember making my digital story with much affection. I thought that it would be tucked away and forgotten but instead it has become a useful tool—a way of explaining my life situation to people. I am an advocate for my sons, which means I attend many meetings, talk to many professionals and fill out many long and complicated forms. When I am asked what it has been like living

*with children (now adults) on the autistic spectrum, I have pointed them in the
direction of the Patients Voices website. My digital story seems to communicate
far more than my words and in a far more powerful, experiential way. What a
relief to have a way of communicating it all that doesn't necessarily involve me.*
(Pep 2013)

Some Thoughts

I have thought a lot about therapy and digital storytelling. Below is some
of my thinking so far.

StoryCenter make it clear that they would not pretend to have license
to function as a therapeutic encounter, but they do acknowledge the
emotional and spiritual consequence of making digital stories (Lambert
2006).

If we are to consider the value of digital storytelling as therapy, then we
need a definition of the word 'therapy.' The *Oxford English Dictionary*
(*OED*) offers two: 'Treatment intended to relieve or heal a disorder, e.g.
a course of antibiotic therapy' and 'the treatment of mental or psychological disorders by psychological means, e.g. "he is currently in therapy"'
(Jones 2010). Both of these have the suggestion that therapy is something
that is done to a person who has first been diagnosed with a condition of
some sort; the person is not active in this process—it is the therapist who
takes the action. There is no 'therapist' in the digital story process. The
storytelling facilitators take the place of therapist—implying a different
kind of relationship.

The definition offered for the word 'therapeutic' is more promising—
'having a good effect on the body or mind; contributing to a sense of
wellbeing' (OED 2013). A more equal power dynamic is implied here as
there is no 'being done to.' This is the kind of therapy we do for ourselves.
For example, I do a lot of bread making. I choose to take part in this
activity because I find it relaxing and I value the end product, so I might
describe this activity as therapeutic for me. It is this meaning of 'therapeutic' that occupational therapists are interested in.

So, digital storytelling can be conceptualised as therapy if occupational
therapy philosophy is considered. Occupational therapists believe in the

power of meaningful, creative occupation. We believe that engaging in such activities is inherently therapeutic (Wilcock 2006). Occupational therapists support people to engage in occupations through skilful collaborative goal setting, activity adaptation and grading. We may get involved if the person is experiencing some sort of occupational disruption or deprivation, through illness, disability or social disadvantage, but we act as facilitators. It is the people themselves who drive this process. As one of the important theorists of our profession states, 'Man, through the use of his hands, as they are energized by his mind and will, can influence the state of his own health' (Reilly 1962).

As an occupational therapist, I would recommend carefully facilitated digital storytelling (such as a Patient Voices digital storytelling workshop) to clients who need help to make sense of difficult experiences. What is more meaningful than crafting aspects of who we are into something tangible? As occupational therapist and medical anthropologist Cheryl Mattingly puts it: 'When occupational therapy is most effective, it connects treatment intervention to those areas of deep concern to clients' (2013).

Distillation and Amplification

But what is it about *digital* storytelling that makes it such a powerful and healing creative activity for storytellers? I should gratefully acknowledge my PhD supervisor, Professor Ian Gwilt, here for his input into the development of these ideas.

Here is another quote from Cheryl Mattingly:

> *Attention to human suffering means attention to stories, for the ill and their healers have many stories to tell. The need to narrate the strange experience of illness is part of the very human need to be understood by others.* (Mattingly 1998)

This quote draws attention to the fact that illness is a strange experience and that experiencing illness can isolate us from others who may not necessary relate to or understand it. It is listening and being listened to—giving attention and receiving it, and valuing that human experience. This is the key to a therapeutic relationship. Everyone has a story to tell, and it is through being listened to in the right way that a person finds it. This listening, and being listened to, may well stay as a dialogue, as is the case with friendships, forms of counselling and talking therapies. But illness experiences are often strange and painful. They are difficult stories to tell and difficult stories to hear. This is why therapy often stays confidential and private.

What makes digital storytelling so powerful is what I have come to conceptualise as a *distillation* and *amplification*: painful stories are crafted into the understandable and digestible. Similar processes of distillation occur with other forms of creative activity which utilise narratives such as poetry or creative writing. However, the output of the digital story process is a short film. It is this use of multimedia that amplifies the message.

Distillation

Distillation involves the extraction of the essential meaning or most important aspects of something. The story circle is key in the distillation process. It begins with careful, active listening within a closed group, made safe by skilled facilitators such as Pip and Tony. Occupational therapists understand that, while many activities have potentially therapeutic aspects, what is important is the way the client and therapist approach the activity, not the activity itself. This is a subtle and complex matter. The way the therapist creates an atmosphere of trust, openness and acceptance results in the disclosure which, in turn, results in healing. The process of distillation is shaped by the feedback that storytellers receive from facilitators and other storytellers.

Amplification

Amplification involves making something more marked or intense. This amplification is achieved through the production and subsequent presentation of a media object—which in the case of a Patient Voices digital story is a very short film.

There are several layers of amplification involved. The first is taking the time to do it in the first place. It takes at least two intense full days of work to craft a digital story, not including work on the story once the workshop is finished. The encouragement from the facilitators to take the time to make a story is a special, amplified form of listening.

The second is the inherent power of multimedia—the combination of images, video and sound (the storyteller's voice and evocative music). This amplification is the result of the crafting or design of the media elements of the story—it is a film we are making—a high-status, creative activity that has both technical and artistic attributes. A picture tells a thousand words. Joe Lambert talks about the inherently spectacular nature of projected and amplified media. Audiences love movies, so it is the short film that is the medium: punchy, easily absorbed by today's short-attention-span generation (Lambert 2006).

The other layers of amplification happen through presentation of the end product: showing the completed story to an audience and the impact of that on the storyteller. I will never forget the impact of seeing the story I had created on a large projector screen, being viewed by the other storytellers in an atmosphere of celebration—the pride and sense of accomplishment. It was the equivalent of the feeling of peace you get when you have had a massive spring clean and you are looking at your tidy house—with all the cobwebs and clutter gone and everything in its place.

Then there is the amplification that occurs as a result of who the storyteller chooses to show their story to. I showed my story to a friend who had heard me relate the account of my sister's suicide and my subsequent hospital admission. When she had finished watching it, she said that although she had heard me talk about it, she now understood the impact of those events on me. The digital story built a bridge of understanding between me and my friend and helped us feel more connected to each other.

Finally, there is the amplification of everyone else being able to see it. With the consent of the storyteller, digital stories go on the Patient Voices website and can be viewed anywhere in the world in any context. My story might be viewed by someone else who has gone through a traumatic bereavement or gone mad taking antidepressants. Like Paul, I really like the fact that they may be comforted to know that they are not alone. It is not well known that some antidepressants turn some people completely crazy, and if a health professional sees my story, they might be able to spot that this is happening with someone else. It is important to me that this message is out there.

Conclusion

This chapter has outlined some of my journey with digital storytelling and the Patient Voices team and my subsequent thinking about making media objects as therapy. I have found that the Patient Voices digital storytelling process is a powerful way in which multimedia can be used to validate a person through the amplification of their voice. It is important to note that digital storytelling is only therapeutic in the hands of skilled and trained facilitators, such as Pip and Tony, who both understand the media they are working with and the methods by which they can use themselves and the small group processes for therapeutic ends.

It is important to point out that there are ethical issues to consider around a therapy technique that involves presenting the output of therapy to a global audience. Professionals perceive therapy as a private, confidential activity. However, are therapists and professionals in danger of paternalism that negates a person's right to be heard? After all, one of the key things that makes digital stories powerful is that they are designed and crafted as pieces of communication. Patient Voices has a robust consent process, and the storyteller must always make a considered and informed choice, free from pressure, as to whether they decide to publish their story for this to be considered ethical practice.

If, like me, you have gone through the strange, often frightening and sometimes alienating experience of being ill and using mental health services; if you feel that you were ignored or not listened to, or misunderstood or not believed; if you struggle to make yourself heard—then it is your right to engage in the meaningful occupation of digital storytelling and to have your voice amplified across the globe. I would certainly recommend it if it feels right for you.

Key Points

- In the field of mental healthcare, it is important that professionals are able to confidently and appropriately acknowledge their own humanity and operate out of an attitude of respect and acceptance.
- The biomedical paradigm and the concept of professionalism itself can present barriers to this process of one human being relating to another.
- Making a digital story can bridge the personal and professional and allow us to bring everything that we are to our professional roles.
- Making a digital story can be a profound and life-changing experience if facilitated in the right way by skilled people. It is of interest to occupational therapists because the profession believes that engaging in activity that has meaning is inherently therapeutic.
- Making a digital story can be experienced as 'therapy by presentation.' It involves the processes of distillation and amplification. There are ethical issues to consider regarding confidentiality and vulnerability, but these need to be weighed against the storyteller's need and right to be heard.

References

Beresford, P. (2001). Service users, social policy and the future of welfare. *Critical Social Policy, 21*(4), 494–512.

Beresford, P. (2002). User involvement in research and evaluation: Liberation or regulation? *Social Policy and Society, 1*(2), 95–106.

Coleman, J. (2008). *Digital storytelling at health and wellbeing (dissemination newsletter)*. Sheffield: Sheffield Hallam University.

Glasby, J., & Beresford, P. (2006). Commentary and issues: Who knows best? Evidence-based practice and the service user contribution. *Critical Social Policy, 26*(1), 268–284.

Jones, A. (2010). Attachment, belonging and identity are important to effective health curricula. *Nurse Education Today, 30*(4), 277–278.

Lambert, J. (2006). *Digital storytelling: Capturing lives creating community* (2nd ed.). Berkeley, CA: Digital Diner Press.

Mattingly, C. (1998). *Healing dramas and clinical plots: The narrative structure of experience* (Vol. 7). Cambridge: Cambridge University Press.

Mattingly, C. (2013). Staff Profile University of Southern California. Retrieved May 2017, from http://chan.usc.edu/faculty/directory/Cheryl_Mattingly

OED. (2013). Oxford English Dictionary online. Oxford University Press. Retrieved May 2017, from http://oxforddictionaries.com/definition/english/therapeutic?q=therapeutic

Reilly, M. (1962). Occupational therapy can be one of the great ideas of the 20th century. *American Journal of Occupational Therapy, 16*, 1–9.

Walters, J. (2007). *Surviving*. Pilgrim Projects Limited. Retrieved March 2014, from http://www.patientvoices.org.uk/flv/0168pv384.htm

Wilcock, A. (2006). *An occupational perspective of health* (2nd ed.). Thorofare, NJ: SLACK Incorporated.

Julie H. Walters is an occupational therapist with experience in Forensic Psychiatry and Housing, and a senior lecturer at Sheffield Hallam University. She has research interests in mental health and creative media and has been involved in research on community interventions for people with psychotic conditions. She was a founder member of Hackney Patients Council, one of the first patients' councils in the UK, and identifies with the mental health system survivor movement.

14

The Sheffield Carers' Voices Project: Was It Therapeutic?

Mark Shea

Introduction

This chapter explores the experience of digital storytelling with a group of people who took part in the Sheffield Carers' Voices Project in June 2009. Elsewhere in this book, there is lots of information about how digital stories are being used to improve and transform health and social care services, but I have taken a different perspective.

This chapter describes my MSc dissertation, rather than a piece of published peer-reviewed research. It looks at how the *process* of making a digital story impacted onstorytellers and how it affected them subsequently. This subject had not been covered explicitly in the psychological literature, and consequently my research project was exploratory. The chapter provides a very brief overview of my study and only covers the main points. 'An exploration of personal experiences of taking part in a digital storytelling project,' the dissertation I prepared for

M. Shea (✉)
Sheffield Health and Social Care NHS Trust,
Sheffield, UK

© The Author(s) 2018
P. Hardy, T. Sumner (eds.), *Cultivating Compassion*,
https://doi.org/10.1007/978-3-319-64146-1_14

the psychology MSc thesis, Sheffield Hallam University, can be seen on the Patient Voices website (Shea 2010).

The Sheffield Carers' Voices Digital Storytelling Workshop

This story begins with Ian enthusing about a Patient Voices project called 'Healing Journeys' (described in the previous chapter) and a little scrap of paper on which he'd written the details. Ian was a long-term mental health service user who'd used his own experiences to help others by setting up a user support group, which in turn was helping to shape the development of mental health services in Sheffield. Our paths crossed when I was working for adult social care services as a commissioner of mental health services. As I recall, the scrap of paper sat on my desk for several weeks because I didn't really understand what Ian was trying to describe to me. It was only when I visited the Patient Voices website that things started to fall into place, and I remember being impressed and moved by the stories I watched. As a result of this, I contacted Patient Voices and set about commissioning a project in Sheffield for carers of people with mental health problems.

The workshop was held over three days at Whirlow Grange, a retreat centre near Sheffield, UK, in June 2009. People who use mental health services and those who care for them were invited to attend, and the event was sponsored by Sheffield City Council. For a relatively small project, there seemed to be an awful lot to sort out, including recruiting participants, finding the money and organising the venue.

However, the project was a great success: it highlighted carers' experiences in a novel and powerful way, and the participants really seemed to benefit from the workshop.

Several months later, I decided to look into the impact on participants of digital storytelling for my psychology MSc dissertation. At first, the subject seemed a bit off the wall, difficult to ground in a theoretical basis and thus an unlikely subject for a master's dissertation. Fortunately, I found an enthusiastic and supportive supervisor and got stuck in.

Aims of the MSc Research

I wanted to explore the experiences of people who took part in the Sheffield Carers' Voices workshop during which they produced digital stories about emotional and traumatic experiences. The study was concerned with the participants' experiences before and during the workshop and its subsequent impact.

The Patient Voices workshop is a complex process and has consequently been investigated from several disparate but complementary psychological perspectives. Synthesising these approaches, the study investigated how the participants made sense of their traumatic experiences through producing coherent stories and the underlying processes that helped them to construct meaning from these experiences. The study focused on how the digital storytelling workshop affected the participants' views of their loss or trauma, their core or deeply held beliefs about the world, and consequently their sense of themselves. Although the study was concerned with individual subjective experiences, it aimed to reflect the group context and identify common themes across the group.

The project is described in detail in my thesis (Shea 2010), and so I want to focus here on what I learned about the therapeutic potential of digital storytelling.

My research project was exploratory, in that I set out to see what the data suggested rather than to prove a particular hypothesis. So what did the data suggest? Basically, that people benefited from telling their story as part of the Patient Voices Programme.

The next question was why, and this led me to explore a wide range of theoretical perspectives, considering how stories form part of our identity and how they help us make sense of our world.

Theoretical Perspectives

Storytelling features heavily in narrative psychology, and so this is where I started my literature review. Narrative psychology highlights the relationship between storytelling and a person's experience of themselves and their world (Murray 1997). The literature suggests that reflecting on the past, present and future to produce narratives requires people to develop coherent accounts of their experiences. From this perspective, people can also be conceptualised as actively constructing their world through narratives, and the study of these narratives can provide insight into how people understand their worlds.

I also looked at the life story model of identity, which suggests that narrative is a means of identity development (McAdams 2008). The model emphasises the link between the stories that people tell and their sense of identity. Significant memories, such as traumatic events, are key components of narrative identity. According to the model, if a person changes their view of such events, their sense of identity will also change, but through the use of narrative, they can maintain a coherent sense of themselves over time.

The digital storytelling process starts with writing about emotional experiences; theories about emotional writing suggest that this activity is psychologically and physically beneficial (Pennebaker and Seagal 1999). The findings show that the benefits are contingent upon participants using emotional words and positive words, and producing a coherent story. The studies suggest that three main processes are involved:

1. positively reframing past events,
2. being able to express emotions more openly, and consequently
3. enabling people to access social support more easily.

The social element of the group is also important, both in terms of the group environment and the stories' potential audience. These factors can help to give meaning to difficult experiences, which can impact positively on the storyteller's wellbeing (Davison et al. 2000). I also looked at how people make sense of loss. The constructivist literature suggests that finding meaning in negative events is important for subsequent wellbeing (Neimeyer et al. 2010). It has also been shown that talking about loss experiences in ways that integrate the loss into a person's own ongoing life stories can help the grieving process (Walter 1996).

In conclusion, my review showed that a range of disparate psychological approaches are relevant to the study of digital storytelling. It also showed that a number of psychological processes can help people successfully adjust to loss and trauma. These include reflecting on the past, present and future; writing about emotional experiences; forming a coherent story that integrates views of loss, world and self; making meaning out of the loss by finding some positive outcome; and sharing the story with others.

The Participants and Their Stories

Ian is a long-term mental health service user and has made two digital stories: one in 2008 about his struggle to overcome his antisocial personality disorder; his second story, *A clearer road ahead* (Porritt 2009), describes the therapeutic impact of creating his first story.

Pep cares for her two autistic children and also made two digital stories: one in 2008 that focused on her role as a carer; her second story, *Tell me your story* (Livingstone 2009), describes how her first story has helped her to respond to life's challenges more creatively.

Maureen cares for a son with psychosis, and her story, *Coming out the other side* (Skayman 2009), describes his first major psychotic episode. During the storytelling process, she became liberated from unconscious feelings of guilt which she had experienced for many years.

Jan cares for a son with psychosis, and her story, *A lost life* (Carder 2009), describes how she feels her son is dying over and over again. In the interview, she describes her feelings of guilt and grief.

Lyn's son suffered from depression and took his own life in December 2006. Her story, *When services fail* (Mansfield 2009), describes the circumstances leading up to his death. She made her story so that services could learn from the mistakes that she feels were made with her son's care.

Tim had a near-fatal industrial accident, and his story, *My struggle* (Kirk 2009), describes his accident and subsequent struggles. The workshop helped him to make sense of these events, and he found the storytelling process very therapeutic.

Mia's story, *I love you more* (Bajin 2009), describes her mother's life and eventual death. Producing her story helped her to realise how she had blamed herself for not being with her mother when she died, and she found the storytelling process cathartic.

The Research Findings

The themes identified through the analysis of interview data fit together to form a coherent narrative. The data suggest that difficult life experiences motivated the participants to help others with similar challenges; revisiting these experiences was emotionally difficult and was possible because of the supportive context. The whole process enabled the participants to positively reframe these difficult experiences, and this has subsequently had a positive impact on their life. Within these themes, I identified subthemes which were common to a subset of the group, but for brevity, these have not been included here. The main themes are described below.

Wanting to Help Other People

The first theme summarises how the participants described their reasons for taking part in the storytelling workshop. All the participants talked about wanting to make stories that would help other people; for example, Tim told me, 'I wanted to do it to help me and help other people and Maureen said, I thought if this can help anybody in anyway, I'm just going to go for it.'

This theme reflects the aim of the workshop, and so is not surprising. From a narrative perspective, good self-narrative needs a guiding reason or 'story goal,' and all the participants described their goal as wanting to help others.

An Emotional Experience

All participants described the workshop as emotionally very difficult, using terms such as *very painful, exhausting, upsetting, unsettling* and *very traumatic*. In the workshop, most of them found talking about their experiences difficult. For example, Lyn recalled that:

> we were told that some people would feel it was like a cathartic experience …
> at the time it didn't seem like that, it just seemed as though I'd been through hell
> and back again.

Mia explained that it was

emotionally a really challenging journey … this felt really painful because you're taking the plaster off … getting to the very root cause of what's going on.

Jan described how she found it very difficult to talk about my experience.

This theme reflects emotions such as sadness, despair, anger, frustration and helplessness, in response to stories about loss and trauma, which are consistent with grief theories and thus to be expected. However, it is interesting that the participants felt able to experience and express these emotions despite being with strangers and not in a formal therapeutic group. Narrative perspectives conceptualise the participants as revisiting dysfunctional life stories, that is, looking back to a world that doesn't make sense and experiencing the resultant feelings of loss and confusion. Finally, from a constructivist perspective, the workshop is not simply a difficult experience that participants endure, but part of an ongoing process of constructing meaning.

A Supportive Context

All the participants described the workshop context as very supportive. They described support from the facilitators and the rest of the group, feeling safe and being listened to attentively and empathically. These factors help to explain why people were able to experience and express the difficult emotions described above. The data suggest that they were able to have their experiences understood and validated by the facilitators and other group members. Jan enthused that the facilitators and group members were marvellous and they were so sensitive. Mia described how she felt very, very safe in the group. Tim also enthused about the group:

I think it's because people were that interested in me and what had happened to me … I think the group we were in really cared about each other … I thought they was absolutely fantastic … you couldn't wish for a better group of people to do anything like that with so they just made you feel at home.

Jan was also very positive about the group:

*To have people listening and being supportive was a wonderful experience …
and I think that was the only time I've ever had that … so it was good, yes, it
was very positive.*

Although the workshop is not offered as a form of therapy, it meets
many of the conditions found in therapeutic self-help groups:

* shared objectives
* a supportive context for emotional disclosure
* clear boundaries
* empathic listening
* opportunities for members to compare their experiences with others
  and see that they weren't alone in struggling with challenges.

Several of the participants contrasted the experience with other forms
of therapy. For example, Pep explained:

*I'd had … loads and loads of therapy … I've had Gestalt therapy where you …
do lots of creative things but not in as a concentrated powerful way.*

Tim also had therapy prior to the workshop:

*I did cognitive behaviour therapy and I did a lot of writing about … from
when I were born and it didn't work … so I think the workshop had more of
an impact.*

In summary, all the participants described how much they valued the
support from other group members and the facilitators, and how this
helped them to tell their story. Although the workshop was ostensibly
focused on producing digital stories, the above analysis demonstrates that
a supportive context is not only fundamental to the process but an important
outcome in itself. Moving away from the group context, the next
theme looks in more detail at the storytelling process.

Positively Reframing Difficult Experiences

There is clear evidence in all the participants' interviews of varying degrees of positive reframing. This theme allows established theory to be applied to digital storytelling in an original way and provides useful insights into the participants' experiences. The data provided good examples of the storytelling process, helping people to make sense of their worlds. Reframing took different forms for each participant and is illustrated by the following examples.

Mia talked about blaming herself for not being with her mother when she died. The workshop gave her a rare opportunity to reflect on the events surrounding her mother's death, during which she developed a more positive view of herself and no longer feels burdened by guilt. Mia described how making her story:

> just helped me reflect on the positive which I think … is just … tremendous cos I just always viewed me as such as baddy who wasn't there for mum.

Applying a narrative approach highlights how Tim positively reframes a traumatic event through three stages: first, putting his experience into words helped Tim develop hope about the future. Second, he describes emplotment or a process of bringing order to the crisis through which, in this case, he is able to gain a more objective perspective on his accident: Doing a process like that helps you get it all into sequence. Finally, the data show that Tim's narrative has a progressive structure and is used to redefine a crisis as an opportunity for rebirth and development:

> My main objective now is to keep helping people … it's made me more want to help people as well.

This analysis also reflects that putting events into a coherent life story helps people to make sense of them and affirms life's meaning and purpose.

The next example considers narrative identity. Pep related how she realised that she had lost her previous identity as a result of continually telling her children's story, rather than her own. She had become consumed by an identity of being their carer and comments that this story had the power to control her for the rest of her life:

> *You realise that you can let your story control you for the rest of your life … but I suppose that as carers we rarely ever get the chance to tell our story.*

This illustrates how telling stories can contribute to a sense of narrative identity and that stories can be an essential part of being human. Prior to the first storytelling workshop, Pep's identity revolved around being a carer. Producing her first digital story helped her rediscover her previous identity. From a life story perspective, Pep's narrative identity was 'swamped' by her children's narratives; the storytelling workshop enabled Pep to rebuild a coherent narrative identity, which in turn enabled her to grow personally.

The final example illustrates how the process helped Maureen to make sense of loss. She realised that she had been carrying hidden feelings of guilt about her ability to bring up her children. The workshop helped her to see that in response to her son becoming ill, she had had to be strong. This realisation improved her self-confidence. She now feels liberated from feelings of guilt and is consequently happier:

> *It wasn't 'til weeks later that I realised that I had been carrying guilt feelings around with me … and it's released me of that … I think I'd buried those feelings and hadn't dealt with them … but doing that made me realise that, and I felt freer than I have in a long, long time.*

Using a constructivist perspective, it is speculated that prior to the workshop, Maureen made sense of her son's illness by developing a self-narrative as an inadequate mother, which enabled her to maintain core beliefs that the world is fair. The workshop helped her to see more of her positive qualities, enabling her to develop a more positive self-narrative.

In summary, a range of analytic approaches have been used to reflect the range of experiences, and this approach revealed common themes across the dataset. Overall, there is evidence that the workshop helped the participants to positively reframe negative experiences, which had a positive effect on their subsequent wellbeing.

A Positive Impact

All the participants described how the process had had a positive effect on their lives in the nine months since the workshop. There is consensus within the above theories that being able to positively reframe difficult experiences, however that process is conceptualised, is beneficial. For several participants, the experience was life changing and helped them break out of a long period of negativity. The participants generally described how negative events in their past had less power over them now than before the workshop. For example, Ian told me about: 'the confidence I've got from it … I've actually broken the chains … they were sort of holding me back from doing what I wanted to do.'

Pep reflected that she found the process affected her:

> I used to worry about the future all the time … now I don't … I'm a lot more at ease.

In conclusion, the variety and prevalence of data supporting this theme demonstrates its importance. Although the participants are very positive about the experience, the analysis was not able to address the sustainability or depth of the workshop's effect.

A Narrative Perspective Across the Whole Dataset

For most participants, their 'storytelling' story started many years before the workshop. Traumatic events shattered their lives and deeply affected them. A constructivist perspective suggests that to reconcile these events and assimilate the loss into their core beliefs, the participants changed their self-narrative to one that incorporated a greater sense of vulnerability than before. This allowed them to maintain core beliefs that the world is fair. These experiences motivated them to try to improve health and social care services, which helped to give meaning to their experiences and may have been part of their recovery. The workshop allowed them to re-examine their self-narrative and see how they had developed personally to overcome life's challenges. This process led to a more positive self-narrative incorporating a greater sense of strength and resilience.

The analysis suggests that having a coherent story both in their mind and on DVD enabled them to share their story with other people. Whereas previously they may have kept their feelings secret, through fear of burdening others or facing discrimination, they now find it easier to gain emotional support from others and experience release from the emotional strain of inhibition. Consequently, the participants are more able to tell their story to others and gain emotional support.

Researcher Influence

Reflecting on the study, I inevitably influenced the analysis, for example by asking certain interview questions, and the data was clearly jointly constructed by me and the participants. There is also a risk that the participants talked about the workshop more favourably as they knew that I had commissioned the project. To mitigate this effect, I encouraged the participants to be open and honest in their responses. Overall, these findings are particular to this Patient Voices workshop and this study, and caution should be exercised when attempting to generalise to other situations.

Conclusion

Overall, the study produced rich data, and I identified five themes which form a coherent narrative:

1. Difficult life experiences motivated the participants to make a digital story so that others could learn from their experiences.
2. The process was emotionally difficult.
3. The process was possible because of the supportive context of the group and facilitators.
4. The storytelling process enabled storytellers to positively reframe their difficult experiences.
5. The process has subsequently had a positive impact on their lives in general.

Although these themes could have been predicted, the strength of the themes is surprising, and this is particularly clear from the positive descriptions of the workshops and its subsequent effect. Rigorous cross checking with the data suggests that these themes are robust for this study.

In conclusion, all the participants talked positively about their experiences of digital storytelling and how they had subsequently benefitted. Many of the participants were consequently more optimistic about their future. By contrast, they also found it a difficult experience. The current study has not investigated whether these benefits can be sustained over the longer term, and for several participants, the benefits were relatively short lived. Synthesising the above theoretical perspectives, the analysis suggests that during the workshop the participants were able to reflect on their past, present and future. They were then able to form a coherent story, experience changes to their narrative identity and thus make meaning out of their traumatic experiences.

I found the project really interesting and exciting, and felt lucky to be able to gain an insight into people's personal experiences of making their stories. I am very grateful to the participants for giving up their time for the interviews and for being so open about not only the experience of making their stories but also the difficult experiences behind their stories.

I am also grateful to Pip Hardy and my supervisor, Rachel Abbott, who made the project possible.

Key Points

- The digital storytelling process can help participants to reframe their experiences and change their self-narrative to create a new, more positive narrative and identity.
- Digital stories can help people to resolve their distress and see that there is a better tomorrow—it might not be ideal, but it's better than what they've had.
- People can develop a greater sense of self-belief as a result of sharing their story.

- Digital stories provide a safe place to share difficult and personal issues.
- The process of making a digital story can lead a person to relive very traumatic feelings and is emotionally very demanding, but most storytellers describe the process as cathartic.
- Many storytellers describe the process as life-changing and one that enables them to break their cycle of negativity.

References

Bajin, M. (2009). *I love you more*. Pilgrim Projects. Retrieved May 2017, from http://www.patientvoices.org.uk/flv/0400pv384.htm

Carder, J. (2009). *A lost life*. Pilgrim Projects. Retrieved May 2017, from http://www.patientvoices.org.uk/flv/0396pv384.htm

Davison, K. P., Pennebaker, J. W., & Dickerson, S. S. (2000). Who talks? The social psychology of illness support groups. *American Psychologist, 55*, 205–217.

Kirk, T. (2009). *My struggle*. Pilgrim Projects. Retrieved May 2017, from http://www.patientvoices.org.uk/flv/0403pv384.htm

Livingstone, P. (2009). *Tell me your story*. Pilgrim Projects. Retrieved May 2017, from http://www.patientvoices.org.uk/flv/0402pv384.htm

Mansfield, L. (2009). *When services fail*. Pilgrim Projects. Retrieved May 2017, from http://www.patientvoices.org.uk/flv/0397pv384.htm

McAdams, D. P. (2008). Personal narratives and the life story. In O. P. John, R. W. Robins, & L. A. Pervin (Eds.), *Handbook of personality psychology: Theory and research* (3rd ed., pp. 242–262). New York: Guilford Press.

Murray, M. (1997). A narrative approach to health psychology: Background and potential. *Journal of Health Psychology, 2*, 9–20.

Neimeyer, R. A., Burke, L. A., Mackay, M. M., & van Dyke Stringer, J. G. (2010). Grief therapy and the reconstruction of meaning: From principles to practice. *Journal of Contemporary Psychotherapy, 40*, 73–83.

Pennebaker, J. W., & Seagal, J. D. (1999). Forming a story: The health benefits of narrative. *Journal of Clinical Psychology, 55*(10), 1243–1254.

Porritt, I. (2009). *A clearer road ahead*. Pilgrim Projects. Retrieved May 2017, from http://www.patientvoices.org.uk/flv/0388pv384.htm

Shea, M. (2010). *An exploration of personal experiences of taking part in a digital storytelling project*. MSc dissertation, Sheffield Hallam, Sheffield. Retrieved May 2017, from http://www.patientvoices.org.uk/pdf/papers/MarkSheaMScThesis.pdf

Skayman, M. (2009). *Coming out the other side*. Pilgrim Projects. Retrieved May 2017, from http://www.patientvoices.org.uk/flv/0398pv384.htm

Walter, T. (1996). A new model of grief: Bereavement and biography. *Mortality, 1*, 7–25.

Mark Shea currently works as a cognitive behavioural therapist within the Sheffield Adult Mental Health Services. Prior to this, he worked in a range of roles within commissioning, business management and finance within the NHS and Social Care Services. Mark started his career in the private sector.

15

Building Healthy Teams: Digital Storytelling in NHS Organisations

Amy Stabler

Introduction

At the time of writing this chapter, I was a member of an Organisation Development Team in a large NHS Foundation Trust. Our work involved facilitating service improvement, leadership development and team effectiveness. Provision of support to front-line teams for their emotional resilience was core to our team's effectiveness. Sometimes those teams found themselves in a dark place, a place of torn relationships, mistrust and broken spirits. We sought to support them to repair their relationships and to regain equilibrium and confidence both individually and as a team. This process could take a number of years and was always an emergent and multi-faceted process. Our Trust was committed to this uncertain and emotionally demanding path because we knew that poor teamwork undermined patient safety. When teams fall apart, we saw it as a duty to intervene to protect our patients and our staff and do so openly and transparently. Shame and heartache always accompanied us on this journey.

A. Stabler (✉)
Northumbria University, Newcastle upon Tyne, UK

© The Author(s) 2018
P. Hardy, T. Sumner (eds.), *Cultivating Compassion*,
https://doi.org/10.1007/978-3-319-64146-1_15

My colleague, Dr Maxine Craig, had been leading and developing our work with teams in difficulty since 2003. Maxine made a connection with Pip Hardy from Patient Voices through Twitter during 2013. She was interested in how digital storytelling might support the emotional resilience of individuals and teams in our Trust. Having observed some digital storytelling work, she commissioned Patient Voices to run a workshop to support individual and team resilience following difficult times. She asked me to lead and evaluate the project. I had been collaborating on some action research, involving individual and shared team stories, and believed that the stories teams tell each other are their lifeblood. So I was really interested in how digital storytelling might provide emotional closure for teams that had emerged from difficulty.

The commitment of our colleagues from all disciplines to improving team relationships was always inspiring. We recognised that poor communication endangered our patients directly and that it also blighted life at work for our colleagues, leading to increased stress and absence due to sickness. This created a vicious circle in which the resulting heavier workload led to further stress and resentment for those remaining and further fragmentation of team relationships. Michael West and his colleagues' in-depth research (West et al. 2006) into team effectiveness in healthcare convinced us of these links. Poor relationships and communication had been highlighted in all public inquiries into failures in the NHS since the Bristol Inquiry in 2001 (Kennedy 2001). Most recently, the report of the Mid Staffordshire NHS Foundation Trust Inquiry highlighted:

> *a culture of fear in which staff did not feel able to report concerns; a culture of secrecy in which the trust board shut itself off from what was happening in its hospital and ignored its patients; and a culture of bullying, which prevented people from doing their jobs properly. Yet how these conditions developed has not been satisfactorily addressed.* (Francis 2013)

We knew that fear, secrecy and bullying existed in some teams in our organisation and that individually and collectively it took courage for these teams to face and speak about it. For my team, it involved working below the surface with what is sometimes termed the 'shadow organisation,' with the collective memory of teams that is spoken, never written, felt rather than thought and passed around through everyday conversation and gossip.

Since 2003, we had been researching and practising methods to support team resilience as a means of prevention as well as cure for team difficulties. We learned that resilience—the ability to bounce back from difficulty or challenge—is crucial if a team is to function healthily and effectively. We had explored the use of stories in a number of projects and took the philosophical position that individual stories and meanings needed to be heard and respected for team dynamics to change. As Paul Bate discovered in an intervention in a UK hospital:

> *stories and storytelling are therefore not only crucial to establishing group identity; they are equally crucial to implementing change, especially cultural change.*
> (Bate 2004)

Storytelling is critical to engaging and mobilising people to change (Ganz 2011). At an individual and team level, the stories people tell themselves and each other create and recreate the beliefs, values and relationships of team culture: *the development of narratives is a constructive and re-constructive process* (Aranda and Street 2001). Given the evidence that clinical microsystems at a ward or department level are the most potent unit for healthcare delivery (Ham and Dickinson 2008; Toussaint and Berry 2013), then the ward or department's narratives are a vital resource for building and maintaining resilience. If the stories are ones of deficit and hopelessness, individuals become disillusioned, disempowered and teams fragment. In our work with teams in difficulty, we seek out appreciative stories of hope and care that help team members to reconnect to their core values and motivation for working in healthcare and to reconnect with each other.

Aims of the Workshop

This chapter was initially written one week before the workshop was due to take place, so what follows is an account of my experience of engaging with Pip and with potential storytellers for the six months leading up to the workshop during the process of preparation for a digital storytelling workshop. I hope that the reader will find something that may be useful about introducing digital storytelling to staff in healthcare organisations. This is my story.

My first thought about the workshop was that it would be an opportunity to gather and share stories that might be liberating to other teams who found themselves in dark places. I also believed that it would provide us with some rich qualitative evidence with which to evaluate the ways in which teams emerged from and felt about their experiences having been through intensely tough development processes. So I hoped to obtain an educational resource and evaluative material. I was enchanted by this new method that Maxine had found and Pip eloquently described, and I assumed that potential participants would be captivated too. Assumption is always a tripping hazard for me. My focus was on the potential stories—the outputs of the workshop and their value to me and to others in the organisation. My focus was neither fully on the potential storytellers nor on the process of making their stories. In my experience of working with teams, when I have overlooked the people involved and how they might experience the process, in favour of outcomes, I haven't helped matters. Disempowering others comes to mind. Not a long way from bullying.

What Happened

Getting a handle on digital storytelling wasn't obvious. At first I thought it was the same as telling a story speaking directly to camera. Having spoken with Pip and watched some digital stories, I was struck by their emotional force and the subtle layers of communication to the viewer. Whilst I had worked with oral narratives in the organisation, the combination of the spoken word with visual metaphor was new to me in this context. I spoke with and wrote to potential storytellers to invite them to a briefing session with Pip. I invited people who had participated in completed organisation development interventions for teams in difficulty.

Only 4 people turned up from a potential 30. My assumption bubble burst as I listened to these four people and Pip's careful handling of their fear and uncertainty about the project. What was it for? How would the stories make a difference? Who would see them? They were frightened about how the stories would be used and unsure about going back to a bad place again. Pip assured them that the stories would belong to them and they could choose never to release them. We also agreed that the workshop needed to happen off-site from the Trust and to create a place of retreat and contemplation. They began to engage with the idea.

Pip offered to hold a second briefing session as the four attendees felt it would be helpful for their colleagues to meet her and understand the nature of the workshop and the digital storytelling process. I began a series of conversations with members of those teams that were stimulated by the digital storytelling discussion. They expressed deep feelings of grief that remained unresolved about their experiences of being in a team in difficulty. They also demonstrated deep care for each other. The second briefing session deepened these discussions, and Pip offered the workshop as a way of coming to terms with difficult experiences and recognising personal resilience. Each time Pip came, I felt that hope and understanding were created. Certainly I was learning from her and from potential participants that the introduction of digital storytelling to this group was a complex and challenging emotional experience.

Through my discussions with potential participants, I learned that whilst each individual had their own story in relation to past events, they also felt that others held part of the story that they hadn't heard. In this way, storytelling was linked to the collective memory and meaning making of the team. I was reminded of the importance of making meaning in response to traumatic events. In my experience of working with healthcare teams, the bonds of attachment between team members are generally deep and enduring, even if unhappy. The breaking of these bonds is traumatic and can be accompanied by intense feelings of distress and disillusionment. Healing requires contact, connection and an integration of experiences into a new sense of self and of team (Schore 1994). It seemed to me that digital storytelling was an experience that could offer this possibility, and I hoped that the team members might take the emotional risk to participate.

Through a process of several group discussions and individual reflection, all the potential participants from one team eventually chose not to continue with the digital storytelling project. The team was no longer working together and they agreed that the moment had passed when the work would have been most constructive. In reaching this decision, I felt they had reached a resolution. I had learned an enormous amount from them and was grateful to have been part of their deliberations. I felt that some closure had been gained from the consideration of the workshop and the meetings it engendered. The possibility of participation tapped into a collective experience that has touched me deeply. I felt the fear and disempowerment that might attend publicly giving voice to one's own experience: the fear of not being understood or being manipulated by me or others within the organisation. In contrast to this, I saw the pull of reconnecting with oneself and others. The team that has chosen to participate still works together and therefore has the opportunity to build on their learning from the digital storytelling workshop as they continue their collective development. Members of this team wavered about their participation until their leader committed to participating herself. To my mind, this gave formal legitimacy to the process and has allowed their stories to come out of the shadows and into the light.

Reflection/Critical Analysis

One of the key points I have taken from reading the Mid Staffordshire Inquiry is that:

> *blame will perpetuate the cycle of defensiveness, concealment, lessons not being identified and further harm.* (Francis 2013)

Making a digital story as a member of the NHS can feel like a high-risk activity if blame is experienced as a possibility. It links to risks of isolation or job loss that might be associated with whistle-blowing or other forms of speaking truth to power. Control over the making and release of a digital story is therefore critical, and the three-stage participant consent and release process used by Patient Voices addresses this ethical issue. It creates psychological safety as far as possible. And yet it cannot address internal memories and feelings of blame from others, or oneself. In my view, shame is an intensely private emotion, and evoking it in a group situation, such as a storytelling workshop, may have been too daunting for some potential participants. Thinking about making such feelings public through releasing a digital story added an increased degree of challenge.

It was important to me to be clear with all potential participants that I would respect their choice to participate or not, and to value that they had considered taking part, which in some cases had been intensely painful in itself. I felt that to allow choice was reparative, as it permitted freedom and self-agency, which are central tenets of a healthy workplace culture (NPSF 2013). However, I am left wondering, if I had paid more attention to the possible jeopardy that the process represented in my initial invitation to potential participants, whether they might have felt safe enough to take part.

I was so keen to see the outcomes that I overlooked the potential effect of the fear of blame and shame on participants. If I were to approach this project again, with the benefit of hindsight, I would pay attention to my initial invitation to participants by stressing the importance of the process, its essentially appreciative and constructive nature and the power of the storyteller to determine what happened to their story. It is clear to me that the process of digital storytelling has the capacity to strengthen and build individual and team resilience and that the stories themselves are a gift that only the teller can give freely and without fear.

Pip asked me on a number of occasions if I planned to make a digital story at this workshop. I felt that the available places should be offered to colleagues from teams in difficulty and that my participation may have compromised the openness of participants. So I declined—even when there was a single place left available. However, in doing so, I was also defending against the challenge of making my own digital story and the fear of shame and exposure that I also feel in thinking about it. In order to accompany people through the process, perhaps it would have been better if I'd said 'I'll be there with you and I also have a story to tell.' I'm not sure which was the best path, but I do think there is value in going through development processes that I invite others to experience, understanding them from the inside out. If I had been ready to make my own digital story, perhaps I could have helped the organisation of which I was part to become more ready too. I am glad that one team leader and four members of her team have been bold enough to lead the way. Readiness is a gradual change of state, and together we have been gradually getting ready for telling the story of our difficulties, their transformation and our resilience.

Conclusion

As someone introducing digital storytelling to NHS teams, I have learned (again!) that I am as much a part of the process as anyone else. I began as a project manager interested mainly in the outcomes of the project. This may have been my own defence against involvement in a challenging process with teams I didn't know well. Whatever semi-conscious feelings drove my position, meeting Pip and experiencing her care in setting up the process, as well as her listening to, hearing and responding to the emotional cues of potential participants, led me to consider the situation more deeply and to explore what was going on beneath the surface with these teams. As I moved through the process, taking the time to meet and consider many thoughts and feelings, the potential participants took control and guided me to their own conclusions that were appropriate for them. I am grateful that they did, as I now look forward to next week's workshop from which it is possible I may never see a story but from the setting up of which I have gained deep learning. That would be a fitting end to this story.

Postscript

I found myself, three days after the workshop, sitting in the late September sun, appreciating the memory of five digital stories I was privileged to see. Following consultation, the storytellers had invited me to join them to view their stories for the first time together. 'I didn't know how hurt they all felt,' the team leader said to me as I arrived at the end of the workshop. Stories of grief, loss, courage, care and the beauty of relationships with family members, patients and colleagues that transformed their lives, gave them insight and the ability to heal, each one individual and connected, like different themes in a piece of music. I was reminded of something Pip said about each story being connected to one story. And I felt my own story echo in their words, pictures and music.

Each affects the other and the other affects the next and the world is full of stories and the stories are all one. (Albom 2003)

I kept in touch with the team over two years following the workshop. Participants reported profound and enduring effects from their digital storytelling experiences. A number spoke to me about feeling a renewed engagement and pride in their work. One spoke of finally experiencing closure on the worst period of her long professional career. The team leader arranged a second workshop for other team members so that they could experience a similar catharsis. The ward has continued to go from strength to strength receiving a Quality Mark amongst other awards and innovating ways to improve the experience of patients and their families. It is a lovely place to visit—calm, welcoming and reassuring. Sadly, over-use of the term in healthcare policy has devalued compassion, and yet I believe it is central to healing for staff as well as patients. I experienced deep compassion between colleagues on the digital storytelling work-shops and, via their stories, for and with their patients. The stories gave voice to their individual and collective compassion, which enhanced the team's healing and their motivation and pride in their service to others. Their story acts as a beacon to those involved in healthcare: clinical teams need time to reflect on difficult experiences together as well as celebrating what they do well, and, above all, their voices need to be heard.

Key Points

- Engaging participants in getting ready for a digital storytelling work-shop is part of the overall process.
- There is significant emotional and professional risk for healthcare workers engaging in digital storytelling, so choice to participate or not is key.
- It was important to allow time and several opportunities to discuss the implications for potential participants to reflect on whether they were willing to participate.

- As project leader, I was on a journey with the digital storytellers and making my own might may have helped others feel psychologically safe.
- Digital storytelling can provide healing and support resilience for teams following a period of difficulty.

References

Albom, M. (2003). *The five people you meet in heaven* (1st ed.). New York: Hyperion.

Aranda, S., & Street, A. (2001). From individual to group: Use of narratives in a participatory research process. *Journal of Advanced Nursing, 33*(6), 791–797.

Bate, P. (2004). The role of stories and storytelling in organizational change efforts: The anthropology of an intervention within a UK hospital. *Intervention Research, 1*(1), 27–42.

Francis, R. (2013). The final report of the Mid Staffordshire NHS Foundation Trust Public Inquiry.

Ganz, M. (2011). Public narrative, collective action, and power. In S. Odugbemi & T. Lee (Eds.), *Accountability through public opinion: From inertia to public action* (p. 273). Washington, DC: The World Bank.

Ham, C., & Dickinson, H. (2008). Engaging doctors in leadership: What we can learn from international experience and research evidence? NHS Institute for Innovation and Improvement.

Kennedy, I. (2001). The report of the public inquiry into children's heart surgery at the Bristol Royal Infirmary 1984–1995. Stationery Office.

NPSF. (2013). *Through the eyes of the workforce: Creating joy, meaning and safer healthcare – Report of the Roundtable on Joy and Meaning in Work and Workforce Safety*. National Patient Safety Foundation Lucien Leape Institute, Boston, MA.

Schore, A. N. (1994). *Affect regulation and the origin of the self: The neurobiology of emotional development*. Hillsdale, NJ: Lawrence Erlbaum Associates.

Toussaint, J. S., & Berry, L. L. (2013). The promise of lean in health care. *Mayo Clinic Proceedings, 1*, 74–82.

West, M. A., Guthrie, J. P., Dawson, J. F., Borrill, C. S., & Carter, M. (2006). Reducing patient mortality in hospitals: The role of human resource management. *Journal of Organizational Behavior, 27*(7), 983–1002.

Dr Amy Stabler is a senior lecturer in corporate and executive development at Newcastle Business School, Northumbria University, with research interests in work cultures, team development and coaching. She has worked in National Health Service organisation development and consulted nationally and internationally in leadership development and coaching for 20 years.

Part V

Contributing to Evidence: The Evidence of Experience

Pip Hardy and Tony Sumner

Stories are always true – it's the facts that mislead. (Winterson 2007)

Until recently, stories did not have a place in the generally accepted hierarchy of evidence. However, as patient experience data is becoming increasingly more frequently gathered in the search for evidence to underpin initiatives within care, and a widening range of approaches and technologies are being applied to the task, this is gradually changing, and digital storytelling is included within the methodologies discussed in the literature (Coulter et al. 2009).

Most methodologies that involve the use of patient stories capture or harvest accounts of patient experience and then the processing of that data to extract meaning is done by professional researchers or academics. The reflective digital storytelling process used within a Patient Voices workshop allows patients to do more than simply provide their experiences as data. The processes of reflection, sense-making and distillation used within the workshop empower them to become analysts of their own experiences. Their stories become auto-analysed data, 'facilitated digital micro auto-ethnographies' (Sumner 2014) that turn patient experience data into patient experience information that carries the meaning important to them.

Part V moves to consider Patient Voices stories as a valid form of evidence, the evidence of experience. By its very nature, the impact of qualitative evidence on change is difficult to quantify, but evidence of patient experience, in particular through patient stories, is gradually being acknowledged as a way of promoting patient-centred change. Digital stories provide a rich and multi-layered resource for research into patients' true concerns and needs and into the effects of personal development training that places empathy and compassion at the centre of the therapeutic relationship.

In Chap. 16 'Measuring What Counts: The Stories Behind the Statistics', Karen Taylor describes the power of digital stories to place patients—and not just statistics—at the centre of high-level debates and at conferences where a large number of people, including policymakers, can be reached. She believes that stories commissioned by the National Audit Office about stroke, neonatal nursing and end-of-life care have contributed greatly to changes and improvements, and will continue to do so as the stories are increasingly used in teaching and board rooms. She argues for the greater use of technology to drive change and improvements and shift the balance of power.

'What *Really* Matters to Patients? Digital Storytelling as Qualitative Research' is the subject of Chap. 17. Carol Haigh and Eula Miller find this question is best answered through the emancipating medium of Patient Voices digital stories, enabling patients' concerns, rather than the researcher's agenda, to emerge. Using two case studies, the authors describe first a workshop with six 'survivors' of mental health services, with clear messages of forgiveness and the need for reassurance from their experiences of failures in the health services. Faced with an impenetrable wall of 'protectiveness' barring vulnerable patients from being heard, the authors then found stories on the Patient Voices website provided those voices and valuable post-hoc data for research, often in unforeseen directions.

In Chap. 18 'Increasing Empathy: Digital Storytelling in Professional Development', Nick Harland's personal awareness of the transformational benefits for staff to take time out to reflect, together with his belief that the empathic relationship between therapist and patient is key in defining the clinical outcome in physiotherapy, led to his setting up a research project centred around a Patient Voices workshop for physiotherapists. The conflicting strands of a research and personal development training project produced some anxiety pre-workshop, but Nick believes, despite the difficulties of measuring such experiences, that they have the potential to affect real change from the personal to the organisational, and perhaps even cultural level.

References

Coulter, A., Fitzpatrick, R., & Cornwell, J. (2009). *The point of care: Measures of patients' experience in hospital: Purpose, methods and uses.* London: Kings Fund.

Sumner, T. (2014). *From data to insight: Obtaining the patient/service user voice.* Paper presented at the Independent Information Governance Oversight Panel, London.

Winterson, J. (2007). *The stone gods.* London: Hamish Hamilton.

16

Measuring What Counts: The Stories Behind the Statistics

Karen Taylor

Introduction and Background

The most important things cannot be measured.
Measure what counts. Don't count what is easy to measure. W. Edwards
Deming

From 2002 to 2011, I was the Director of the Health Value for Money (VFM) Audit at the National Audit Office (NAO), responsible for investigating whether England's Department of Health (referred to as 'The Department') and National Health Service (NHS) organisations were spending government funding in an economic, efficient and effective manner. While the NAO Act 1983 gave the NAO relatively unfettered access to data and information, for most of the 1990s and early 2000s the paucity of centrally held data meant that we used surveys to collect and

---

This chapter is based on a conversation between Karen Taylor and Pip Hardy.

K. Taylor (✉)
Stonecutter Court, London, UK

© The Author(s) 2018
P. Hardy, T. Sumner (eds.), *Cultivating Compassion*,
https://doi.org/10.1007/978-3-319-64146-1_16

245

benchmark NHS performance data. Survey data was supplemented with structured interviews, literature reviews, financial analysis and economic modelling. In this way, my team and I were able to obtain a pretty unique understanding of how healthcare organisations were deploying their resources and the priorities and concerns influencing their decision-making. Where relevant, we would also triangulate this information with qualitative information from surveys or focus groups of staff and service users.

As a result, our reports were strongly evidence based. However, the human side could often be overshadowed by the facts and figures on the size of the problem and the amount of money that was being spent. The challenge, therefore, was how to give sufficient weight to the patient voice and make the patient experience more tangible to the reader.

Patient Stories and Their Use in Understanding the Efficiency and Effectiveness of NHS Services

Reconnecting with Life: Stories of Life After Stroke

In 2005, we published our hard-hitting report on the paucity of NHS stroke services (National Audit Office 2005). Although very critical of the services then on offer, the Department accepted the report findings and, in response, developed the national stroke strategy. Our report generated a huge amount of interest and we decided to hold a conference to platform the report findings. We also used the conference to promulgate more widely the many examples of good practice we had identified, including innovative approaches from Australia and Sweden.

While it was easy to get people to talk about the various aspects of stroke services and to present examples of good practice, it was more difficult deciding how to make the patient story central to the conference. Given the different types of stroke and the impact stroke can have it was not easy to get a single patient perspective that could convey all the issues we wished to raise. There was also the fact that some strokes do, literally, rob people of their voice or, at least, the voice that could tell their story as they might want to tell it.

In response to this challenge, I commissioned Pilgrim Projects to develop a DVD of digital stories on the key issues raised in the report, as seen through the eyes and voices of patients and their carers. Our key aim was to show policymakers and politicians that it really was worth investing in stroke services because of the potential to improve and, indeed, save lives, and that many people can recover and go on to lead meaningful lives.

The result was 'Reconnecting with Life: stories of life after stroke' comprising a number of digital stories about stroke survivors, including overcoming aphasia, which is common to many strokes and where the inability to express thoughts or words or understand thoughts as expressed in the spoken or written word causes a great deal of distress and depression in stroke survivors. These stories were very powerful in demonstrating how people can overcome the debilitating after-effects of a stroke. There were also two stories that illustrated quite starkly the difference in outcomes between 1995, when stroke was treated as an inevitable part of ageing with nothing much that could be done to alleviate the condition: *Imagine* (Whitehead 2006), and the impressive outcomes that can be achieved by treating stroke as a medical emergency *A vision of the future* (Newell 2006).

We played the DVD throughout the conference, including on the main screen during the intervals. Copies of the DVD were also provided to everyone who attended the conference. A number of people subsequently told me that they took those DVDs back to their organisations and used them in their training and teaching of staff. This, my first experience of Patient Voices, convinced me that the use of digital stories was a worthwhile investment.

The Power of Digital Stories in Illustrating the Impact of Effective Neonatal Services

While the stories on stroke were aimed at ensuring that the patient experience was central to the conference, a few years later, when designing my study of neonatal services (National Audit Office 2007), I commissioned another DVD of digital stories to accompany the report publication. The aim was to reinforce the point that, while neonatal services are needed, thankfully, by only a small percentage of people, they are an incredibly important service whose effectiveness (or otherwise) has lasting repercussions. Again, we particularly wanted to demonstrate to politicians and policymakers—the people who could do something about the findings in the report—that it was about more than just wasted or poorly spent resources and that the deficits in the system could have a significant impact on people at a vulnerable time. As a reader, it is often easy to gloss over a statistic or a figure about a shortage of neonatal nurses or availability of beds in the Neonatal Intensive Care Unit but it is much harder to do that if you see a story that reveals the impact of that shortage, such as Vanessa's story, *Thank you very much* (Lett 2007).

Every year, for as long as I've been working with the health sector, I've read reports about the lack of midwives. Indeed, I examined this issue in 2001 as part of the report on *Educating and Training the Future Health Professional Workforce* which identified that the NHS wasn't training enough midwives (National Audit Office 2001). While the numbers of midwives did increase, the Department has acknowledged recently that the NHS still hasn't trained enough. So it was no surprise to find in the neonatal services report that a lack of neonatal nurses was a particular problem. The impact of this was brought to life emphatically by the digital stories, in particular that the impact is not just on the individual but on the whole family, and not just in the short term but, often, for life. In publishing the report we drew attention to the digital stories and subsequently held a conference where, once again, the stories were an integral part of the proceedings.

Simple Things Make a Difference: The Challenge of End-of-Life Care

The third project to use Patient Voices was on end-of-life care services (National Audit Office 2008). Once again, the stories were used to illustrate some of the challenges that are encountered in caring for people in their last weeks, days and hours of life. In preparing this report, we drew on the knowledge and experiences of a wide range of health and social care staff involved in the delivery of end-of-life care; and also of people approaching the end of their life and those caring for them. In addition to commissioning surveys of commissioners, hospices and care homes, Patient Voices digital stories were used to illustrate the impact that both good and bad care can have, and how sometimes it's the simple things that make all the difference. This DVD was, for me, really important and I defy anyone to watch the stories and not want to do something about improving end-of-life care services. For me, the most poignant story is *Can I have a hand please?* (Pang 2008) where, as the only male professional on the ward, Wee Haan is at first frustrated, but then patiently responds to the final requests of a dying man. As before, the stories were part of the publication of the report and also formed part of our conference on end-of-life care.

An Evolution in Evidence Collection

For me, the Patient Voices stories were part of an 'evidence evolution' aimed at improving the information base underpinning our reports. However, my first encounter with Pilgrim Projects was not in relation to Patient Voices, but was actually in commissioning them to undertake a survey of service users as part of our review of Clinical Governance in Primary Care. Pilgrim Projects helped us in this endeavour by bringing together focus groups of patients and carers to identify what more needed to be done to involve them in designing and evaluating primary care services (Pilgrim Projects 2006)

Indeed user surveys and focus groups were common in many areas of NAO research, but the use of Patient Voices digital stories was and remains a very unusual thing for the NAO to have done. Meanwhile, in the health service more generally there is an increasing recognition of the need to listen to patients and carers. Of course, the outcome of failing to do so has been evidenced, starkly, by the Francis report (Francis 2013) and subsequently the report on the government-commissioned review of NHS complaints handling (Clwyd and Hart 2013). In these and other high-profile examples of service failure, patients' and staff's views of the service were evident, if only people had been listened to. In a way, that's what the Patient Voices stories provide: they illustrate in an accessible way the public and staff's experience of health care. Moreover, the current

NHS climate is such that the opportunity to harness patients' views and get patients' stories mainstreamed has never been more important.

One of the interesting things about the Patient Voices stories is that they are relatively timeless. It is not just about the here and now as they don't lose impact over time. It is, however, somewhat challenging to make a direct link between the stories and changes in policy and practice, and therefore difficult to demonstrate, unconditionally, their worth. I am personally convinced that the stories do make a difference. For example, I know that the stroke stories were used in teaching and training of people delivering stroke services and, given the impressive changes that have been made to stroke services in recent years, I believe that something changed as a result of the evidence we provided, which included the stories.

Likewise, when we presented the neonatal study to the Committee of Public Accounts, I was called in to speak to two of the MPs on that committee who had looked at the stories on the DVD. They had clearly obtained more insight into the report because they'd seen the stories, so I know it brought the report to life and gave them a focus for their questioning.

Further Opportunities and Challenges

In 2013, I did a piece of work on end-of-life care with the Institute for Global Health Innovation at Imperial College London. The research comprised a review of end-of-life care policies and practices across the world, which was presented to government representatives from across the globe at the World Innovation Summit for Health in Qatar in December 2013 (http://www.wish-qatar.org/app/media/386). It was a challenging study as the situation with regard to end-of-life care is so very different in so many countries and there is a need to ensure the research report is relevant to each of them. However, regardless of the different cultures and approaches there is a need to support everyone to live well until they die and, in dying, to die with dignity and compassion.

While achieving this aim is challenging in our own health and social care system, achieving a good death is an even bigger challenge in many low- and middle-income countries where the causes of death are changing dramatically: latest estimates suggest that 60–80 per cent of deaths are now due to life-limiting chronic diseases (Alwan et al. 2010). Yet dying in many of these countries is poorly supported, particularly in relation to pain relief and, depending on the country, has very different cultural and social taboos. I can't help thinking that something akin to Patient Voices, because of their ability to shine a light on the patient experience, could be valuable in demonstrating the huge challenges involved. For example, stories can convey the impact of a lack of pain relief in a way that the written word can never hope to achieve.

In October 2014, I published a further report on *Transforming Care at the End of Life* (Taylor 2014) in my new role as the Research Director at the Deloitte UK Centre for Health Solutions. While I did not commission any more stories for this report, I was able to draw on my previous experience and the stories we had already developed as well as others that have since been published on the Patient Voices website.

The Genie's Out of the Bottle

For many years, hospital boards have reviewed copious amounts of data and information, questioned staff about key issues whilst reflecting on the impact of their services on the patient, but often without direct access to the patient voice. As the power of patient stories has gathered momentum, many NHS Boards now do start their Board meetings with a patient, carer or staff story. The Board on which I am a Non-Executive has, for the past five or so years, started every meeting with a patient or staff story. Everyone agrees that this is an important part of the evidence needed to provide assurance on performance. This information is also supplemented by executives and non-executives being twinned with parts of the hospital and being encouraged to visit and develop an understanding of what the patient experience is like on the 'shop floor,' gathering patient stories directly.

Today, an increasingly popular medium for gauging the quality of care is through social media. Indeed, the use of social media in healthcare is increasing exponentially and has the potential to transform our understanding of disease and how we deliver care. Social processes tend to underpin our lifestyle choices, including health-related decisions. Our social networks help define who we are, but social networks have, as a result of the internet, changed beyond recognition, expanding horizons and changing the way we interact with each other. Now that patients and the public have seen the value of exchanging information, especially through patient stories, the historical imbalance in access to information is being turned on its head and the genie is well and truly out of the bottle! There has never been a better opportunity to get patients' stories mainstreamed.

Harnessing Technology

The NHS has historically been extremely slow to learn lessons or to stop re-inventing the wheel. It has also been the last service industry to embrace the use of technology in its daily interaction with service users. Indeed, most service industries use technology to improve the efficiency and effectiveness with which they deal with customers, capturing the customers' experience, expectations and needs, enabling them to be more responsive to the customers' needs. The NHS is only now catching on, for example with technology-assisted care initiatives, like Telehealth and Health Apps and, of course, patient stories, such as Patient Voices.

It is debatable, however, to what extent patients can be considered customers or consumers—terms that are increasingly being applied and debated—but, by and large, patients (in the UK at any rate) do not really have much in the way of choice. However, as recipients of a service, they need to be treated as though they do have a choice and are not just passive recipients of care. Technology could really improve this experience. This doesn't mean replacing people with technology, but using technology to make things easier, more efficient and effective. Technology can also make care more convenient and personalised, supporting self-monitoring and self-management and giving people back control over their own health and wellbeing. Patient stories have a role to play in providing other service users with examples of what works and what doesn't.

In my first report as Director of the Centre for Health Solutions, *Primary Care Today and Tomorrow*, (Deloitte 2012b), we acknowledged general practice as the foundation upon which different models of primary care should be built. However, we also identified why and how primary care needs to work differently if is to respond effectively to the rising demand-and-supply challenges it is currently facing. Furthermore, we highlighted technology as a key lever to support primary care to work differently. We have since followed this up with a further report, *Primary Care Today and Tomorrow: Adapting to survive*, which again highlighted the importance of technology to help manage the increasing demand, but also to improve convenience and consistency of advice to patients (Taylor and Hinsch 2016).

Both reports propose that GPs should use technology to deal with issues that don't require a face-to-face discussion and reserve longer face-to-face time for those people who really need it. At the same time patient stories could be used either in consultations or on GP websites to illustrate to patients how others are dealing with similar issues. In our 2012 report on Telehealth and Telecare, we explored the power of technology to support service re-design and, importantly, to restore the information deficit between patients and clinicians by providing patients with the information to self-manage their conditions more effectively (Deloitte 2012a). Again some of the most powerful illustrations of how technology has helped change lives is in the sharing of individual stories.

While the healthcare powerbase is shifting, assisted by technology, it remains an uphill struggle to mainstream the use of technology and to get staff to work differently. This is relevant to the issue of patient stories as it's the same sort of resistance that undermines the wider-scale development and use of patient stories.

Some of this resistance comes from the fact that clinicians believe each patient and patient experience is different and every story is therefore going to be different, so what can possibly be learned from just one story? There is also a suspicion that the people prepared to share their stories will be of a particular type and won't be representative of the patient population. So, even those who want to change, remain reluctant to acknowledge the power of the patient story.

For example, many non-executive directors, who are perfectly comfortable attending audit committees and finance committees, feel ill-equipped to challenge clinical issues. In the absence of effective education and training for non-executives, one or two really well-chosen patient stories could give non-executives the chance to discuss how to raise concerns in order to obtain the necessary assurance that the actions proposed will reduce the risk of similar problems happening in the future. Stories can, of course, also provide reassurance that things are going well.

Shifting the Balance of Power

In terms of changing cultures and shifting ideas, I think that the Patient Voices approach does provide an opportunity for a shift in power, allowing the storyteller to tell the story that he or she wants to tell rather than the story a structured interview would generate. I'm a strong advocate for appreciative inquiry, which is a much more open approach to questioning, letting the interviewee say what's important to them and why, rather than being led. I think this approach empowers the storyteller, which shows in the Patient Voices stories. Indeed, I think the particular power of Patient Voices and why they are so impactful lies in their directness and simplicity and because the approach adopted enables the patient's story to stand alone, without any sense of being directed or led by the interviewer.

Conclusion

This chapter started with my use of Patient Voices stories in my reports for the National Audit Office. This wasn't straightforward, as it required a business case to demonstrate that this was an effective use of the resources available in the study budget. At the time, and now with the benefit of hindsight, I believe that investing in Patient Voices was worthwhile and, indeed, good value for money.

As I have sought to illustrate in the final sections of this chapter, the potential use of digital stories is even greater if developed as part of the health technological and social media revolution where they can be shared more widely and have more impact as a force for change.

Key Points

- Patient Voices stories are timeless, multifaceted and have many uses.
- They are particularly useful in capturing the attention of people with time-limited attention spans.
- A single story can convey important and universal messages.
- They allow a patient or carer to actually resolve their concerns, be it anger, distress or gratitude, by telling their story.
- The stories have the power to elicit compassion and transform culture.

References

Alwan, A., Maclean, D. R., Riley, L. M., d'Espaignet, E. T., Mathers, C. D., Stevens, G. A., & Bettcher, D. (2010). Monitoring and surveillance of chronic non-communicable diseases: Progress and capacity in high-burden countries. *Lancet, 376*(9755), 1861–1868. doi:10.1016/S0140-6736(10)61853-3.

Clwyd, A., & Hart, T. (2013). A review of the NHS hospitals complaints system putting patients back in the picture.

Deloitte. (2012a). *Primary care working differently: Telecare and telehealth – A game changer for health and social care*. London: Deloitte Centre for Health Solutions.

Deloitte. (2012b). *Primary care: Today and tomorrow – Improving general practice by working differently*. London: Deloitte Centre for Health Solutions.

Francis, R. (2013). The final report of the Mid Staffordshire NHS Foundation Trust Public Inquiry.

Lett, V. (2007). *Thank you very much*. Pilgrim Projects Limited. Retrieved March 2014, from http://www.patientvoices.org.uk/flv/0142pv384.htm

National Audit Office. (2001). *Educating and training the future health professional workforce for England*. London: The Stationery Office.

National Audit Office. (2005). *Reducing brain damage: Faster access to better stroke care*. London: The Stationery Office.

National Audit Office. (2007). *Caring for vulnerable babies: The reorganisation of neonatal services in England*. London: National Audit Office.

National Audit Office. (2008). *End of life care*. London: The Stationery Office.

Newell, O. (2006). *A vision of the future*. Pilgrim Projects Limited. Retrieved March 2014, from http://www.patientvoices.org.uk/flv/0071pv384.htm

Pang, W. (2008). *Can I have a hand, please?* Pilgrim Projects Limited. Retrieved May 2017, from http://www.patientvoices.org.uk/flv/0262pv384.htm

Pilgrim Projects. (2006). *Improving quality and safety: Progress in implementing clinical governance in primary care patients, carers and voluntary organisations* (Report prepared by Pilgrim Projects Limited). London: National Audit Office.

Taylor, K. (2014). *Transforming care at the end-of-life: Dying well matters.* London: Deloitte Centre for Health Solutions.

Taylor, K., & Hinsch, M. (2016). *Primary care today and tomorrow: Adapting to survive.* London: Deloitte Centre for Health Solutions.

Whitehead, D. (2006). *Imagine.* Pilgrim Projects Limited. Retrieved March 2014, from http://www.patientvoices.org.uk/flv/0070pv384.htm

Karen Taylor OBE is Research Director of Deloitte UK's Centre for Health Solutions. Until 2011, Karen was the Director of Health Value for Money Audit at the National Audit Office, reporting to Parliament's Committee of Public Accounts. Since 2011 she has also been a non-executive director at Dartford and Gravesham NHS Trust where she chaired the Board's Quality and Safety Committee.

17

What *Really* Matters to Patients? Digital Storytelling as Qualitative Research

Carol Haigh and Eula Miller

Introduction

It can be argued that the entire focus of qualitative research is about teasing information about a specific experience from individuals. Information is coaxed from participants in a number of ways, many of which involve the telling of stories, sometimes via the use of interviews and sometimes in less sophisticated ways, such as twitter feeds. However, it is also possible to contend that, even in the most unstructured of unstructured interviews, the agenda and the direction of the stories shared by participants are in the hands of the researcher. This chapter will explore the concept of using digital stories to permit research participants to share what really matters to them through the emancipatory medium of digital stories. It looks at digital stories as both a form of data collection and as an information source of post-hoc analysis, using two specific research studies as reflective case-study examples. The aim of the chapter is to explore how

C. Haigh (✉) • E. Miller
Faculty of Health, Psychology and Social Care, Manchester Metropolitan University, Manchester, UK

© The Author(s) 2018
P. Hardy, T. Sumner (eds.), *Cultivating Compassion*,
https://doi.org/10.1007/978-3-319-64146-1_17

the information provided by storytellers can illuminate and illustrate research questions. This is of particular personal importance to one of us (C.H.) because what was obvious when viewing their first digital story, *For the Love of Lee* (McGlinchy 2006), was that this was a medium that allowed the storyteller to communicate the message that was the most important thing they wanted people to know. It could immediately be seen that this had enormous potential to drive healthcare research in a new and exciting direction. The power of the stories is such that the first one you see is one that stays with you forever.

Case Study 1: Mental Health

As this specific study is the focus of another chapter, only a brief synopsis will be offered here. The study focused upon the experiences of six survivors of mental health services. The key words that were fundamental to the stories were 'dignity' and 'respect.' We assisted in the three-day workshop, and as we did so a number of extraneous research issues were highlighted in our minds. Although all of the stories were very different, there were a number of messages that, as researchers, we would have loved to explore in more depth.

Forgiveness and Reassurance

First, the overwhelming message from the stories was that of wanting reassurance; although the experiences described by the storytellers varied in terms of environment and illness trajectory, there was one point in every story where it was apparent that what the storyteller had needed at some point was for someone to put an arm around them and tell them that everything was going to be OK, that they would do their best to keep them safe and help them towards recovery.

We were also surprised at the amount of forgiveness that ran through the telling of the stories. Some of the workshop participants were describing situations and experiences that, as healthcare professionals, we found disturbing and that reflected poorly on the care they had received.

However, none of the storytellers seemed particularly bitter about the incidents that they related and even the angriest of the group was keen that his story be heard so that others would benefit. Phrases such as 'life is too short to hold a grudge' and 'it's all water under the bridge' were used.

These notions of forgiveness and reassurance have been investigated in the past but often to inform the agenda of the researcher rather than the service survivor. Often, research around forgiveness centres upon the relationship between forgiveness and recovery (e.g., Maltby et al. 2004) or forgiveness of oneself (Ingersoll-Dayton and Krause 2005). There is a dearth of research exploring the concept of forgiveness towards professional care providers, yet this was an element of the stories that was extremely important to the storytellers. This is an example of how research that is nominally done to explore and enhance the patient experience often misses the important issues that patients would like to have explained in more detail and highlights the dangers of doing research *on* people rather than *with* people.

Reassurance is often seen by healthcare professionals as a key element of their role; however, as long ago as 1989, Teasdale was suggesting that nurses used the term 'reassurance' in 15 different ways but that the most common way was hopefully (Teasdale 1989). This was highlighted again by the stories of these service survivors. The reassurance that the healthcare professionals thought they were providing in no way met the needs of the individuals themselves at that particular time. The reassurance that the storytellers seemed to imply that they needed was less that of a qualified professional and more that of a kind human being.

We found being a part of the space in which these brave people shared their stories on that three-day workshop an illuminating and humbling experience—illuminating because it highlighted to us that these were the people who actually inhabited the theory/practice gap that nurse educationalists, in particular, are so keen to theorise about and expound upon. Their experiences were grounded in the gloomy hinterland between research that was done to either a national or an academic agenda and the practice environment that took such research and moulded and reinterpreted it to meet the clinical agenda. The issues of reassurance and forgiveness that were common across the varied and assorted stories shared by the service user would not be formally acknowledged because the research agenda of service survivors is not constructed, consulted or promulgated.

We found the entire encounter humbling because our own reaction to the incidents related was that of anger, frustration and the urge to apologise for the whole of our profession for the perceived shortcomings, and this reaction was in complete contrast to that of the group participants. Their calm acceptance that not all care experience will be positive and their willingness and ability to seek the good in such encounters, even if it takes years or decades to find it, were overwhelming and inspirational.

Case Study 2: Dementia and Cancer Care

This study used digital stories in a slightly different manner to the previous one. A study that was designed to ask vulnerable people who were undergoing chemotherapy for cancer how they thought healthcare professionals could better communicate with them. 'Vulnerable people' meant individuals perceived as vulnerable before they received their cancer diagnosis: people with mental health issues, with long-term debilitating conditions such as Parkinson's disease or those with a learning difficulty. One problem that was not anticipated was the over-protective stance that appeared to be the default setting of the healthcare professionals who were crucial to the recruitment of such people (Witham et al. 2013). For a myriad of reasons, service providers were unable or unwilling to identify potential participants, using excuses such as the fear that the identified patients would not be able to cope with the extra burden of taking part in such a study or being identified as requiring extra help. The position taken was that, for example, if an individual were diagnosed with dementia, the invitation to participate in a small research study would be too much for them to bear, in relation to the onset of other illnesses. There was also a significant reluctance to communicate explicitly the notion of vulnerability to patients, with healthcare professionals expressing concerns that the patient would challenge them for labelling them as vulnerable. There was a clear sense that this group of patients was burdened with cancer as well as their other issues and as such would be overwhelmed at being involved in a focus group. This protection appeared to exclude independent discussion with patients.

Fricker explored notions of how we communicate knowledge (epistemology) to others and also how we use it to make sense of our social experiences (Fricker 2009). She argues that when a group of people are disenfranchised or removed from this communication, it can be described as epistemic injustice. Fricker suggests that 'testimonial injustice' exists when the capacity of individuals as 'knowers' is diminished or undermined by, in this case, healthcare professionals. The inevitable outcome of this is that the beliefs and experiences of such participants are trivialised and marginalised.

This left a real problem. The voice of these patients was crucial to the success of the research project but this voice was being stifled by healthcare professionals who would argue that they had the patients' best interests at heart (although what the patients would think will never be known). The concept of the over-protected participant was one that had not been encountered before outside of an ethics committee. However, the success of the study needed insights into communication with and within cancer services from individuals with concomitant illnesses, and it seemed to the team that the best place to find this information was on the Patient Voices website.

A search was done on the site using the search terms 'people with learning difficulties', 'carers of people with dementia, stroke' and 'translator'. These provided sufficient stories to obtain insights into the experiences of users of cancer services in terms of how they were spoken to and the information they received.

The use of digital stories as a rich source of post-hoc data was one that had not crossed the collective mind of the research team before this episode. However, the most important element of using stories in this way is that the crucial message that the storyteller wishes to convey is clearly accessible. Most qualitative researchers are familiar with the 'through-the-door' phenomenon, where one has just spent the best part of an hour or more interviewing a research participant then, when all the recording equipment is packed away and literally as you are walking through the door, the participant adds 'and another thing …' and proceeds to give the best/most insightful/most interesting quotation of the entire study. You then have to desperately try to remember it as you sprint to the car to write it down. One of the things that struck us most about the stories we viewed was the immediacy of the message conveyed. Admittedly, it was a message we were searching for in the story so we would expect to see it but the strength and clarity of the stories made the data easy for us to find. Thus, for example, one of the stories sampled—*My Michael* (Spurden 2007)—was ostensibly about patient/carer and healthcare professional communication. However, the sub-theme of understanding a patient's backstory was one that came through loud and clear. Table 17.1 shows some of the stories accessed; the focus that the storyteller put upon the inherent message (as evidenced by the title and synopsis); and the research theme that they contributed to.

The use of digital stories in this way showed us two things. First, that the emphasis that Patient Voices put upon the open access sharing of the stories meant that service users and carers were given a research voice that is often denied them by the over-protective nature of the service providers and gatekeepers. This is an important issue since, when running a

Table 17.1 Digital stories and synopses

Theme	Synopsis	Story	Link
Protection	Sometimes professionals try to protect patients or carers, but patients don't always want that	She's fine, don't worry	www.patientvoices.org.uk/flv/0276pv384.htm
Backstory	Patients come with other healthcare experiences—they need to tell their backstory	My Michael	www.patientvoices.org.uk/flv/0088pv384.htm
Big picture	Patients have different needs when it comes to assimilating information	The worst day of my life	www.patientvoices.org.uk/flv/0582pv384.htm
Partnership	Patients need to feel they have a voice in the partnership	My Michael	www.patientvoices.org.uk/flv/0088pv384.htm
Safe space	Make the patient feel safe/try to make the encounter a happy one	Room 22	www.patientvoices.org.uk/flv/0567pv384.htm
Tension	Professional differences can affect the patient	She's fine, don't worry	www.patientvoices.org.uk/flv/0276pv384.htm

'vulnerable people' focus group (participants of which were recruited from sources external to the NHS), one of the participants said, 'I have never been invited to take part in research before, why is that?' before answering his own question by stating sadly, 'It's because I have learning difficulties, isn't it?' This highlights the second of Fricker's epistemic injustices, that of 'hermeneutic injustice' (Fricker 2009). In this case, the individual was prevented from making sense of an experience because of wider prejudice that having a learning difficulty implied that any opinion expressed was worthless. The lack of a voice for people with learning difficulties or mental health issues or long-term debilitating diseases such as dementia outside of topic-specific research should be a cause for concern for the serious researcher.

The second lesson that we learnt from this experience was how versatile the stories can be. Although they contain a clear message from their creator, they can be so nuanced that a researcher can find data in them that possibly others may not find. It can be argued that this is a highly subjective method of obtaining data, to which our reply would be 'well, what of it?' The very defining nature of qualitative research is that of subjective interpretation (Graneheim and Lundman 2004). Seeking unrelated subjective experience in previously collected data is a relatively new and unexplored approach to health-related research. Nursing research, particularly, is not a significant user of post-hoc data, but using patient stories in this way provided a broad data foundation upon which to build future data collection.

Conclusion

Even in today's research environment with its emphasis upon public involvement in the development, running and dissemination of research, and health-related research in particular, academics are still accused of being removed from the concerns of service users by virtue of their 'ivory tower'. The stories that are available on the Patient Voices website put the voice of the patient, and especially the voice of the over-protected patient, back into the centre of qualitative research by allowing what *really* matters to research participants and service users to be clearly articulated.

This leaves the recipient of the story in no doubt about what needs to be heard. This can also be balanced by the subtle nuances of the stories that can be teased out by a researcher working to a data-collection agenda—and that is one of their great strengths. Beneath the message of the story-teller are a myriad of themes, sub-stories and motivations that can be identified by interested parties. It can be argued, therefore, that the stories present a dichotomy, in that other, equally powerful material also supports the original and intended message.

This is exemplified by the observations that we report in the mental health service case study, where areas of enquiry, not necessarily reflective of the formal research agenda of the various research funding bodies, were signposted by the experiences of the service survivors. These are fruitful areas for further research that non-service users may never iden-tify, and lead to the question, 'Are the problems we research for patient benefit really the problems that service users care about or would see as making a difference to their encounters with organised health care?' This is not a trivial question: epistemic injustice helps to ensure that the research agenda is developed and supported by the dominant paradigm, which is generally white, male and middle class. One needs only to look at the healthy living advice to see evidence of this.

Being involved in the creation of a story at a Patient Voices workshop, either as a storyteller or a facilitator, encourages a bond and a trust between individuals that qualitative researchers would value in terms of disclosure of information; it allows for the discovery of new avenues of research and for data from the over-protected service user to be accessed. Much has been written about the theory/practice gap (Monaghan 2015), a gap which can also be argued to include research activity since it is this that informs the theoretical foundations of our practice. However, the rhetoric of this debate generally focuses upon how the bridging of this gap by researchers and practitioners can be brought about. It became clear that storytellers often inhabit this gap and are, therefore, best posi-tioned to understand the effects and consequences of this disconnect—things of great interest to researchers. The muting of these voices is a serious disservice to patients, practitioners and quality of care. The Patient Voices Programme gives a voice to those whose voices are often stifled and frees researchers from the confines of traditional thinking.

Key Points

- Digital stories provide a voice for the overprotected.
- They allow the storyteller's message to take centre stage.
- Digital stories can be used for research data.
- They signpost directions of research that are pertinent to service users.
- Digital stories have a versatility that is useful to researchers.

References

Fricker, M. (2009). *Epistemic injustice: Power and the ethics of knowing.* Oxford: Oxford University Press.

Graneheim, U. H., & Lundman, B. (2004). Qualitative content analysis in nursing research: concepts, procedures and measures to achieve trustworthiness. *Nurse Education Today, 24*(2), 105–112.

Ingersoll-Dayton, B., & Krause, N. (2005). Self-forgiveness a component of mental health in later life. *Research on Aging, 27*(3), 267–289.

Maltby, J., Day, L., & Barber, L. (2004). Forgiveness and mental health variables: Interpreting the relationship using an adaptational-continuum model of personality and coping. *Personality and Individual Differences, 37*(8), 1629–1641.

McGlinchy, Y. (2006). *For the love of Lee.* Pilgrim Projects Limited. Retrieved March 2014, from http://www.patientvoices.org.uk/flv/0054pv384.htm

Monaghan, T. (2015). A critical analysis of the literature and theoretical perspectives on theory – Practice gap amongst newly qualified nurses within the United Kingdom. *Nurse Education Today, 35*(8), 1–7.

Spurden, J. (2007). *My Michael.* Pilgrim Projects. Retrieved March 2014, from http://www.patientvoices.org.uk/flv/0088pv384.htm

Teasdale, K. (1989). The concept of reassurance in nursing. *Journal of Advanced Nursing, 14*(6), 444–450.

Witham, G., Beddow, A., & Haigh, C. (2013). Reflections on access: Too vulnerable to research? *Journal of Research in Nursing.* doi:10.1177/1744987113499338.

Dr Carol Haigh is Professor of Nursing at Manchester Metropolitan University and has over 30 years' experience of working in healthcare settings and. She maintains strong links with the wider clinical disciplines, facilitating improvements in patient engagement and experience using social media. Her research interests centre on ethics, social media and technology in relation to health.

Dr Eula Miller is a registered adult and mental health nurse, with over 30 years' experience. She is a senior lecturer at Manchester Metropolitan University and a Senior Fellow of the Higher Education Academy (SFHEA). Her research has focused on developing the emotional resilience of professionals working in public facing services.

18

Increasing Empathy: Digital Storytelling in Professional Development

Nick Harland

Introduction

There is merit in encouraging practitioners to study the therapeutic relationship and to seek reflexivity to improve their own contribution to it. (Dixon et al. 2010)

I am a physiotherapist specialising in back pain, particularly its psychological and social aspects. I first heard about Patient Voices in a monthly physiotherapy news journal; it described how digital stories were being used in a university to help teach students about the importance of communication and the therapeutic relationship. At that time I was working as a research fellow and as a spinal assessment clinic lead. Over the years spent working clinically, teaching students on placement and starting to research back pain, it had become increasingly obvious to me that in the treatment of chronic pain, the relationship between patient

N. Harland (✉)
Teesside University, Middlesbrough, UK

Physiotherapy Department, Friarage Hospital, Northallerton, UK

© The Author(s) 2018
P. Hardy, T. Sumner (eds.), *Cultivating Compassion*,
https://doi.org/10.1007/978-3-319-64146-1_18

and clinician defined the outcome as much as any other factor. As a result of the article, I spent some time looking at stories on the Patient Voices website and, like many, was surprised by the depth and honesty of the storytelling and the resulting power the stories held.

At the time, I was also taking part in an intense leadership training programme aimed at researchers leading teams. This programme was non-didactic and was based on a personal transformational change model. After years of non-stop clinical practice and fitting in a PhD and follow-on research into the mix, taking time out of my usual high-pressure work to do the programme was invaluable, and was indeed transformational. My mother used to call it a 'fur lined rut,' that is, you are doing well, progressing, working hard, but you are actually stuck in a rut and not moving forwards, missing the big picture. Others, more dramatically, describe working for institutions like the NHS as being 'in the trenches.' My leadership training gave me time and allowed me to climb out of my rut; taking time to reflect on myself and share these reflections with others in a protected environment allowed me to transform.

My investigations into the Patient Voices model led me to believe that attending a Patient Voices workshop could be another way for others to do what I had been able to do: take time out to reflect and share in a protected environment. It seemed to me that if all clinicians could be given that opportunity, they would probably be better clinicians for it. The researcher in me took over and I wanted to test my theory: I wanted to see if attending a Patient Voices workshop would change clinicians and maybe even change how successful they then were when treating chronic back pain patients.

I looked at the research literature and was unsurprised to find what my heart already knew—that such things as empathy and communication skills could not only define a therapeutic relationship but also affect the health outcome of that relationship. I found empathy was often a lacking component of therapeutic relationships and that clinicians 'scientifically' and theoretically appreciate the importance of empathy as a concept, but are unable, unwilling or simply unused to using it (Mercer and Reynolds 2002; Reynolds and Scott 1999; Taylor 1997). I spoke to a post-doctoral physiotherapist whose PhD was in communication training with physiotherapists. She confirmed that clinicians know what empathy is, and even recognise it when shown a video of a good and bad consultation, but they still tend not to use it themselves.

I felt that in this case, 'knowing it' and 'feeling it' were different things and that is why the leadership training I had undergone had worked and why I thought Patient Voices worked, because the stories evoke feeling and reflection rather than just knowledge. To take the analogy one step further, those in the trenches could be given a report on activity in no-man's land and the opposing trench, but unless they stuck their head over the top, they could never feel what it was like or truly understand it. Seeing the courage of the storytellers whose stories I had watched on the Patient Voices website made me sure they had stuck their heads above the trench. I set about finding funding for what I wanted to do and eventually received a grant from the National Institute for Health Research.

The Project

I designed a personal development training programme with attendance at a Patient Voices workshop as the catalyst for the programme. A total of 18 physiotherapists from 3 hospital Trusts would be randomised so that 9 would receive the training and 9 would not. Their clinical outcomes with chronic pain patients would be measured before and after the training. Those receiving the training would also be interviewed on the subject of communication, empathy and the therapeutic relationship several weeks before and after the training and colleagues would complete a 360° questionnaire about them after the programme. Finally, on completion of their treatment, patients would complete a Personal Impact Factors Questionnaire (PIFQ) about their therapist, although patients would not know if the therapist they saw had received any training and therapists would not know if the patients they were seeing were providing information to the trial. The project was designed and funded as a relatively small feasibility project to enable assessment of whether a much larger piece of work along similar lines could be undertaken in the future. The project was not powered to be able to define the effectiveness of the training programme as such, but to support larger bids for research money in the future.

The Training Programme

In line with the concept of therapists needing to 'feel it' rather than 'know it,' the Patient Voices workshop was the first part of the training programme. The purpose was to give the physiotherapists time out to reflect and share their story—related to the subject of the therapeutic relationship—in a protected environment, and to record that story. The intention was that this time out would enable them to reflect and learn about themselves, perhaps for the first time in years, and to discover what was important to them and therefore perhaps to others. The other difference was that there was no final assessment of information they thought they needed to remember to complete the required task, a rarity in the NHS.

The second part of the training programme was to facilitate a transition from pure self-reflection to more directed reflective learning using OATEC (Online Awareness Training for Empathy and Communication). This online package of short modules contains information about the importance of concepts like empathy and communication but is not written in the usual dry scientific language. The OATEC modules contain edited video footage of patients being interviewed about their positive and negative experiences of receiving healthcare to ensure clinicians stay in touch with how it feels to care and be cared for and what impact this might have.

Having been re-acquainted with the process of self-reflection through the Patient Voices workshop, the OATEC modules were also intended to carry on the 'feel it' theme and participants were asked to complete some short self-reflective learning outcomes attached to each OATEC module.

The final part of the training programme was a more traditional advanced communications workshop to provide those additional skills the therapists would now hopefully be open enough to use, having been given the opportunity to both feel and understand their importance.

Organising the Training Programme

Recruiting physiotherapists to the trial was relatively easy and no one had issues regarding whether they ended up in the training or control group, as should be the case if adequate information has been given. Although the Patient Voices concept and process had been explained to the participants and they had been directed to the Patient Voices website, we felt it was necessary for Pip from Patient Voices to visit all the staff members to talk to them, show them some stories, answer their questions and gain their initial consent for the workshop that was to follow. Pip and I visited the three intervention group therapists from each of the three Trusts and spent about half an hour with each group.

Organising time out from clinical duties to hold these meetings was difficult and the time we had was more limited than we would have liked. We would have preferred to meet all nine therapists as a single group for a longer meeting, so they could meet each other and all ask questions and learn from the answers. Unfortunately, the logistics of organising this with therapists with different schedules who worked in locations long distances apart proved to be too difficult.

Although each therapist had been given information about the workshop and been directed to look at the website (which some had not done), having the reality of the situation presented to them was a different matter. I had also agreed to be a full member of the group undertaking the workshop and found this quite a worrying time because it became apparent that there was a significant level of trepidation as staff were presented with the reality of what they were being asked to do. The groups of three were talked through the process and shown a couple of stories and slides from a workshop that had taken place. It appeared that only now this had been presented to them face to face did they better understand the nature of the workshop and they all seemed very nervous and asked very few questions. Nonetheless, all the staff signed the initial consent form for the workshop and promised to work on their draft scripts. Given the opportunity to organise another workshop, I would spend more time ensuring more comprehensive briefing. However, organising such things within the NHS, particularly between several different Trusts, remains very challenging.

Another factor that caused additional pressure was that the workshop had to take place over two days, rather than the usual three days, due to the restraints of getting Trusts to agree to give staff time off from work, even though this time was being paid for as a research cost. Although the therapists were plainly nervous about the undertaking, no one pulled out and all seemed to find the courage to engage actively in the process. At this stage, I felt at one with the group as I was also nervous about taking part in a workshop. I felt this would be a more intense process than I had undertaken so far in my development training and was really unsure about what story to tell. Here are some comments made by therapists about the anxiety they felt before the workshop:

> *When I first looked at it I thought this is taking me right out of my comfort zone. I was incredibly nervous about it.*

The Workshop

The workshop was held in February 2013 as part of the overarching programme of research. The success of the study and the workshop depended on everyone turning up and thankfully everyone did. Although the groups of three from each Trust knew each other they did not know any of the other therapists and were, hopefully, about to share a personal story with them. Organising the venue and catering had been a problem but all went well and the main room and two smaller break-off rooms served their purposes well. The only hiccup was that although I had asked for a couple of the rooms to have couches in them, to facilitate the informal nature of the workshop, apparently when you order a room with a couch within a hospital you get a medical examination plinth!

Before the workshop, Pip had said that many people attending a workshop plan to bring their 'safe' story—one they feel comfortable with that doesn't give too much away, one that they don't need to bare their soul to tell, and I think that this is perhaps especially true of NHS staff more than patients. She also said that, on the day, most people end up telling a deeper story, the one they know they *need* to tell.

The Story Circle

After introductions and a discussion about what makes a good story, the workshop moved into the story circle where each participant read aloud to the group the script of the story they had prepared so far. From this point of the workshop, I was a participant rather than a researcher and had gained the verbal consent of all the therapists to be part of the group rather than part of the research team. I had agonised for weeks about what story to tell, not so much struggling with what I was prepared to share but simply with having anything interesting to say. I felt under pressure to match the high-impact emotional stories held on the website; to match the honesty and courage of the storytellers: patients and clinicians alike.

My story was called *People person?* (Harland 2013) and was about my introversion and difficulty in school. Feeling the pressure to get the ball rolling and wanting to get it over with, I was the first in the story circle to read my script. I found it difficult to get through it and everyone could tell I was obviously a little emotional.

The other nine then shared their stories and it was clear that no one had settled on a 'safe story.' All the stories were personal and thoughtful and there was silence during each reading. We were each invited to say a few words after reading our story and what most people said touched at least to some degree on the common themes of it being difficult to decide what to say, difficult to say it, and being a new experience to share such things in a group of comparative strangers.

Developing Our Stories

We were introduced to the computer program we would be using to put our digital stories together and this went well. People then worked on developing their rough scripts, with many being much longer than they needed to be, thus detracting rather than adding to their impact. I observed here something I have observed in many other settings, from PhD students and the authors of peer review articles to undergraduate students and non-clinical staff: most people find writing difficult. Even if they have had to write essays at degree level, few people are confident with their writing. By the end of the day the group had bonded and everyone seemed fully engaged with the process and was working hard. Most people had managed to audio record their scripts. People left obviously exhausted and several commented it had been the hardest day they had had for a long time.

On the second day, we continued to work hard on building our digital stories, with people working in the different rooms and wandering occasionally to chat or get help with aspects of the computer editing. Having regular short breaks and refreshments available almost all the time was helpful and everyone appreciated that we had not scrimped on the lunch! Despite being a two- rather than three-day workshop we all completed a working digital story in time for everyone to see them at the end of the second day. The stories were all emotional and courageous, just like the other stories on the Patient Voices website, and I was happy to have made the workshop happen.

How the Stories Have Been Used

The stories were used to change the storytellers. They may also be used as a qualitative research output but very little guidance exists regarding how to analyse such stories and this will be a challenge.

I understand from Pip and Tony that the vast majority of people are proud to put their name to their story and to release it to the website, so it is perhaps a function of the means by which the storytellers came to the workshop that has meant almost none of them have agreed to the final release of their story. I feel this is because staff were recruited to a research study after being given information and were then randomised to receive the training, and therefore take part in a workshop, or not. Workshop participants were therefore, to some degree, there as a matter of chance, by default. Although they seemed to engage fully with the process, they perhaps saw participation as learning for themselves, as indicated in the research paperwork, rather than an opportunity for others to learn from them. This was unexpected but also interesting.

If I were to do it again, I would spend more time ensuring participants had a better idea of what they might be asked to undertake and would make sure they had seen and discussed a few stories before consenting to the study, rather than just providing written information and asking them to visit the website. I wonder if this has affected their experience of the workshop and perhaps what they learnt from it, though from the interviews several weeks later almost everyone felt they benefited, as the following quotes show:

> *I think it's quite a personal thing, it's quite engaging at a personal level, if you are of a sensitive disposition. I think there are some people it won't work for, because they will think "what absolute nonsense, a waste of my time", but I think if you give it a try it is very useful. Before I did it I thought "what on earth is this, what is it going to do for me?" The Patient Voices is more of an insight thing, a personal insight, and if you are willing to give it a try it will give you an insight into yourself and insight into other people.*
>
> *It gave me a better appreciation of maybe the impact certain things have on other members of staff, in particular the more junior members of staff, who haven't had as much experience.*
>
> *I thoroughly enjoyed it, and I didn't expect to.*
>
> *It certainly made me realise the importance of reflection.*

Conclusion

Discovering, learning about, designing a project around, and taking part in a Patient Voices workshop has been rewarding both personally and professionally. With 'quality' and 'patient experience' slowly rising to their deserved place in the hierarchy of NHS outcome indicators, phenomena like digital storytelling become invaluable and have the potential to affect real change from the personal to the organisational, and perhaps even cultural level. Using digital storytelling within a mixed research methodology remains a challenge, and the process of using stories as qualitative data remains in its very early infancy, but I would recommend anyone in any setting to get involved.

The research was successful in meeting its goals of developing and testing the training programme and proving the feasibility of undertaking larger scale research to fully explore the benefits of such a programme. One publication (Harland 2014) and two applications for further funds were undertaken after the research, but unfortunately neither of the funding bids was successful.

Key Points

- When using digital storytelling as a research intervention, patients and staff should be specifically briefed about digital storytelling in person, prior to the process of giving their consent to the overall study involvement.
- Giving staff 'time out' to undertake learning without didactic content or an assessed outcome has great value, but remains rare within institutions like the NHS.
- When it comes to concepts such as the therapeutic relationship, 'knowing it' is entirely different from 'feeling it,' and teaching it therefore also needs to be entirely different.
- Including digital storytelling within a research methodology is challenging and the development of evidence-based knowledge on the matter remains in its infancy.
- Given the opportunity, patients and clinicians alike can be courageous in telling their story and that courage can help and inspire both themselves and others. There should be more opportunities within organisations for junior staff and patients to show this courage.

References

Dixon, A., Appleby, J., Ruth, R., Burge, P., Devlin, N., & Magee, H. (2010). *Patient choice: How patients choose and how providers respond.* London: Kings Fund.

Harland, N. (2013). *People person.* Pilgrim Projects. Retrieved March 2014, from http://www.patientvoices.org.uk/flv/0682pv384.htm

Harland, N. (2014). Does specific training of Physiotherapists improve clinical outcomes: Feasibility study consideration and results, a brief report. *Journal of Physiotherapy Pain Association, 36*, 10–14.

Mercer, S. W., & Reynolds, W. J. (2002). Empathy and quality care. *British Journal of General Practice, 52*, S9–S13.

Reynolds, W., & Scott, B. (1999). Empathy: A crucial component of the helping relationship. *Journal of Psychiatry Mental Health Nurse, 6*(5), 363–370.

Taylor, M. B. (1997). Compassion: Its neglect and importance. *British Journal of General Practice, 47*, 521–523.

Nick Harland is a clinical research consultant physiotherapist specialising in back pain. He has been a post-doctoral NIHR Research Fellow and was the first Allied Health Professional to become a fellow of the National Institute for Health and Care Excellence. Dr Harland is also a speciality group lead for the clinical research network in the North East.

Part VI

Doing It Together: A Model for Co-production

Pip Hardy and Tony Sumner

One major change to care services design and improvement during the life of the Patient Voices Programme has been the rise of co-design and co-production methodologies, which seek to involve service users in the design and improvement of services. Almost coincident with the start of the Patient Voices Programme, the Design Council published their Red Paper *Health: Co-creating Services* (Cottam and Leadbeater 2004), which would presage the development of Experience Based Design, later Experience Based Co-design, approaches in healthcare. The National Nursing Research Unit review of the process (Donetto et al. 2014) reports the success of this approach and notes that approximately 50% of the projects surveyed used patient videos in their initiatives, which are said to offer 'an emotionally and cognitively powerful starting point for the co-design process'. The process for gathering these videos as described in the *Experience-Based Co-design Toolkit* (Dale et al. 2013) involves filming 1–2-hour interviews with around ten patients. These videos are then edited down independently of the patients to form one 30-minute composite video. Decisions regarding sense-making, chronology and prioritisation of elements of the interview are taken by the researcher, and then the edited interview replayed to the patient for approval. The patient's role in the development of their contribution to the evidence that will be used in co-design is largely passive and reactive.

This approach echoes a remark by one of our first storytellers, Monica Clarke, who expressed her concern about the way researchers and interviewers tended to 'dismember' her story, picking out the bits that were important to them, regardless of what really mattered to her. We agreed with the authors of a paper that was to influence the early development of Patient Voices that 'to treat stories in this way is to fail to respect the tellers of these stories. It is to make the assumption that our interpretation of the patient's experience is more valid than their telling of it' (Hawkins and Lindsay 2006).

Hence one of our major drivers in the development of the Patient Voices approach was to bring the ethos of co-production and co-design into the patient storytelling process, ensuring that what really mattered to the storyteller was the most important thing. This part highlights the collaborative nature of making and using digital stories and some of the issues and challenges that can emerge in relation to purpose, authorship, power and control. Keeping these issues alive for the facilitators and educators ensures that the stories and the people who make them remain authentically at the heart of the process and gives them their power to move and become effective in teaching the compassion and awareness of patients' issues that is fundamental to a caring health service.

In Chap. 19 'Finding Our Voices in the Dangling Conversations: Co-producing Digital Stories about Dementia', Jo Tait and Rosie Stenhouse explore how writing about giving other people a voice also meant discovering their own voices and uncovering the relationship between voice and power in possibly conflicting roles. Did adaptations to the Patient Voices workshops to provide support for storytellers with early stage dementia affect the control usually held by the storytellers and the eventual films? They discuss how the flexible, reflective, emergent form of facilitation, aiming to balance the creation of 'effective' stories for student nurses and academics, whilst retaining the authentic voices of the participants, eventually revealed the person behind the illness.

Chapter 20 'Learning Together with Digital Stories' concentrates on how digital stories created by service users are used to educate healthcare students to become effective and compassionate health professionals.

Elspeth McLean details the various ways the storytellers and the stories they created as part of the 'Fit 4 the Future' project enrich the training environment and stimulate active learning in small-group sessions, lectures and a virtual learning environment. In turn, the stories help learning to become student-led. Elspeth sees the value of the stories in their quality, the knowledge that they were made under the storyteller's control, and that they are stories. They bring 'people' back into learning.

Chapter 21 'Cultivating Compassion in End of Life Care: Developing an Interprofessional Learning Resource Based on Digital Stories' reports on a collaborative project designed to offer clinicians and carers an opportunity to develop some of the so-called softer skills to enhance their care of those facing the end of their lives. Elizabeth Howkins, recent Chair of the Centre for the Advancement of Interprofessional Education, and Pip Hardy consider the need for staff working in this challenging and sensitive area to develop self-awareness and resilience as well as empathy and compassion. The focus on interprofessional collaboration is underpinned by a collection of digital stories created by staff as well as service users.

Chapter 22 'The DNA of Care: Digital Storytelling with NHS Staff' focuses on the value of digital storytelling for NHS staff, acknowledging the inextricable links between staff wellbeing and patient care. Head of Staff Experience for NHS England, Karen Deeny, and Pip Hardy describe the challenges facing healthcare staff and their need to be cared for with compassion so that they can, in turn, offer compassionate care. Digital storytelling offers staff a much-needed opportunity to reflect on their personal and professional lives, providing valuable insights into what really matters.

In their conclusion to this book, Chap. 23 '*The Stories Are All One*: Care, Compassion and Transformation', Pip Hardy and Tony Sumner pull together their key learning and salient outcomes from developing and running the Patient Voices Programme, the contributions and experiences of project sponsors and participants, and their hopes for a future that will be characterised by greater humanity and compassion for everyone.

References

Cottam, H., & Leadbeater, C. (2004). *Health: Co-creating services*. RED Papers. London: Design Council.

Dale, C., Stanley, E., Spencer, F., & Goodrich, J. (2013). Experience-based co-design toolkit. *King's Fund*. Retrieved June 2017, from https://www.kingsfund.org.uk/projects/ebcd

Donetto, S., Tsianakas, V., & Robert, G. (2014). *Using experience-based co-design to improve the quality of healthcare: Mapping where we are now and establishing future directions*. London: King's College London.

Hawkins, J., & Lindsay, E. (2006). We listen but do we hear? The importance of patient stories. *Wound Care, 11*(9), S6–14.

19

Finding Our Voices in the Dangling Conversations: Co-producing Digital Stories About Dementia

Rosie Stenhouse and Jo Tait

Introduction

Student nurses are required to engage with the art as well as the science of caring. A desire to offer an opportunity for student nurses to develop aesthetic knowledge that would, in turn, support the development of empathy and a sense of compassion for people with dementia led to the decision to create a set of Patient Voices stories for use as an e-learning resource. The stories were created with seven people experiencing 'early stage' dementia and one paid carer during a four-day workshop in the community resource centre that the participants regularly attended. This chapter explores the themes of co-production, power and voice

R. Stenhouse (✉)
Department of Nursing Studies, School of Health in Social Science, University of Edinburgh, Edinburgh, UK

J. Tait
Wayside, Whiteway, Stroud, UK

© The Author(s) 2018
P. Hardy, T. Sumner (eds.), *Cultivating Compassion*,
https://doi.org/10.1007/978-3-319-64146-1_19

arising in this project. In writing the chapter, we ourselves learned first-hand about the challenges of co-production, power and voice.

We were all thrilled with the outcomes of the project. At the launch of the stories, the audience—storytellers, their families, academics and nurse educators—were visibly moved. Feedback from student nurses gave us confidence that the stories provided a valuable resource that helped them see the people behind the diagnosis of dementia.

But writing this chapter about the process of making those stories has challenged our comfortable sense of a shared and an individual voice. Neither of us was happy with that first draft. At different points in the writing process each of us had felt that our voice had been silenced. Jo experienced a profound sense of being silenced by an academic writing style that she had managed to avoid, even in writing a PhD thesis. It was not until Pip Hardy commented (in her editorial capacity) that they had not been able to find my voice in the text that I (Rosie) realised that academic writing conventions had silenced us both.

When Jo and I first met to discuss the content of the chapter, we were collegiate and energetic. We identified some of the obvious issues and found ourselves bouncing ideas off each other, drawing on our different experiences and theoretical understandings. We started writing whilst still together: Jo pulled together some quotes and useful ideas from the literature and I started drafting a possible introduction. We were pragmatic and division of labour seemed to be the most useful way forward. Before we parted we divided up the writing task, agreeing that we would use email to comment on drafts until we were happy. We had assumed that, because we seemed to think along the same lines, our two separate voices could easily be blended into one, coherent voice.

Our experiences in trying to write this chapter illuminate the subtle ways in which writing practices, as forms of representation, give privilege to one version of reality over another. Feminist critiques suggest that traditional academic writing styles claim their authority through the representation of an objective, authorless reality (Haraway 1991; Lather 1991). We both needed to be present within this text, but our voices differ, as we come from different positions. I sit within discourses of academia and nursing, with the inherent need to be recognisable as a competent member of both. Jo, as a retired academic, sees her writing position as a 'grandmother'—nurturing and guiding, asking questions to clarify and cut to the chase. To this end, we have written sections of the text in conversational form, honouring the value of each of our voices.

Power, as embodied by the concept of voice, is key to the digital storytelling process. This chapter offers an insight into our reflections on how power operated within the digital storytelling workshop with people with early-stage dementia. This workshop differed from others in many ways (see Table 19.1) as we worked together to support the storytelling process. Our process of negotiating our writing voices has mirrored the issues of power and representation in digital storytelling workshops. Our discussions at the end of each day of the workshop constantly returned to the question, 'How can we be sure that the voices of the storytellers are heard?' This was the underlying question for our reflections during the workshop and is the question that motivated us to write this chapter.

Table 19.1 Daily tasks during the workshop

Day 1
- Introductions and showing exemplar Patient Voices digital stories
- Discussion of process of workshop
- Work individually to find and develop stories
- Write script
- TS scan all images into computers

Day 2
- Read scripts to the group in story circle
- Practice reading scripts in preparation for recording
- Record voiceovers
- Choose images to go with script
- Collect additional images—photographs or video—that participants identified as necessary for their stories

Day 3
- Listen to voiceovers and drop images in to make digital story using video editing software
- Choose music and decide whether it plays in background under voiceover
- Facilitators tidy up transitions between images in digital stories

Day 4
- Participants, staff and facilitators gather mid-morning for premiere showing of all stories
- Cake and celebratory lunch

Storytelling, Co-production and Power

Storytelling is the most common form of representing experience, both to ourselves and to others (Gee 1985; Riessman 1993; Polkinghorne 1988). Storytelling is, however, representative: stories do not offer a mirror image of what happened, but are subject to the interpretive processes of both storyteller and audience. Stories are told within the context of a social relationship between the storyteller and the audience (present or imagined) and in a particular context. This relational aspect of stories leads them to be influenced by the reactions (real or imagined) of the audience to the story, as well as the context in which the story is told—in this case for teaching student nurses.

If stories are constructed within a social relationship, then within that relationship power will operate. This power may operate in subtle ways during the storytelling process, influencing the version of events that is presented. The storyteller's version of events is, in a sense, their *voice*—the story as he or she wishes to tell it. In this context, *voice* is not simply to do with the auditory experience of hearing someone speak, but constitutes issues of *whose* story is heard.

The Patient Voices digital storytelling process aims to support the voice of the storyteller through the facilitation of group processes that empower each storyteller to take control over story production. The aim is co-production, where stories are produced within a facilitator–participant relationship: the participants, as a group, share the power, and each person leads the creative process. However, in our workshop with people with dementia we adapted the usual process of digital storytelling in order to provide the support that we felt would enable the participants to create their stories (Stenhouse et al. 2013). Without our adaptations to the process, I don't think the creation of digital stories with these people would have been possible. We also wanted them to be created so they were effective, but of course that is a subjective judgement, and most of what supports the creation of effective digital stories is in the structure that the Patient Voices process provides. It is arguable that one of the issues for us (and creating some of my anxiety) was precisely because we moved away from that normal structure.

People with dementia experience negative social interactions shaped by societal understandings of dementia marked by expectations of loss of capacity and capability (Kitwood 1997), leading to disenfranchisement and social exclusion. As facilitators, we were aware of these understandings and the potential for us to act in a way that embodied such beliefs, particularly in a context where we were unsure of the true capabilities of the participants. We realised that there was an increased risk of our assumptions influencing the process of making stories.

Rationale for the Project

The project aimed to develop a learning package for student nurses to enable them to engage with the experience of people with dementia. A couple of chance conversations with colleagues took me to digital stories, and in particular the Patient Voices website. From the stories that I watched, and my subsequent experience of making a digital story with Patient Voices, I identified a number of attributes of digital stories and digital storytelling that made this method suitable for the development of the learning package. First, the storytelling and story creation was participant controlled, fitting with my desire to open up spaces for the voices of the participants (rather than researchers) to be heard. The relationship between storyteller and workshop facilitator appeared to be one of co-production where power was shared or the process was participant led. Second, the product (digital story) was multi-layered and appeared to engage audiences on both cognitive and emotional levels. I therefore commissioned Patient Voices to work with people with early-stage dementia to make a set of digital stories.

The workshop was run over four days and the eight participants (including one paid carer who made a story) each attended only the morning or the afternoon for its duration. The workshop was facilitated by Tony, Pip and Jo from Patient Voices, and me. Although there was some brief reminiscing about first jobs or holidays at the beginning of the first workshop, we did not begin with a story circle. Instead the workshop began with individuals working one-to-one with facilitators, and it was only at the beginning of day two that we had a story circle in which the participants had an opportunity to read their scripts to the whole group. Participants' stories were inspired by the photographs that they had brought with them, with facilitators drawing the threads of the story together and developing the script in collaboration with the participant. During the phase where images were inserted onto the timeline to accompany the voiceover, the facilitators worked with the participants, who directed their use of the technology. The support provided by facilitators varied for each participant and was responsive to their level of engagement and ability (see Table 19.2). All of these deviations from the normal digital storytelling process gave facilitators more opportunity than usual to shape the developing digital story.

The discussion that follows illuminates our understandings of how the adaptation of the normal Patient Voices digital storytelling format supported, but might also have put at risk, the co-productive, participant-centred storytelling process.

Discussion

Commissioner/Facilitator Role

Involving the project commissioner as a facilitator is unusual. I had not considered that my presence would be problematic due to my previous experience of carrying out narrative interviews. However, Jo was curious about its impact on how I/we worked:

Jo: But what about the production of the stories, the making of the *artefacts* if you can call them that, which is different from the listening and the first bit of writing? There is a primary audience, the student nurses for whom the stories were being made. And then, as it turned out, there were psychiatrists and academics at the public premier, which brought home to me the layers of authority that can be affected by these stories. Did knowing that this was the direction of travel affect you as the 'owner' of the project?

Rosie: As I was working with Rob and Wallace, I guess in the back of my head I was aware of issues of engagement: how was the audience going to engage with the story we were making? I was probably thinking about the most powerful transitions [between images]. I think that is a bit where we all exerted more power

Table 19.2 Vignettes of different strategies used when working with each story teller

---

Still fit (Kerr 2011)

Rosie negotiated what she called a 'freestyle' approach, drawing on conversations and pictures about Wallace's life. This was perhaps the closest to an open-ended interview: the free-flowing voiceover was Wallace's recorded response to four themes that then made up the story. This was partly a solution to the fact that his failing eyesight limited his ability to read a script. As Rosie said, once she asked the question, she had no control over what Wallace spoke into the recorder. The pictures were then added at appropriate points with Wallace's full involvement.

It's a different world (A. Smith 2011; R. Smith 2011)

Rob had a great time making his story with Rosie. Again, there was a freedom about the way they worked. The idea of going out and making an actual video of using his bus pass was Rosie's idea, based on what Rob had been telling her. He read a script written by Rosie based on a story that was formed from pictures of his early working life and what he told her from there. It took a lot of rehearsal for him to gather confidence to read the script, because of a lack of confidence in speaking. Voice was important to him and yet it was the one thing he had lost.

It's the art (Third 2011)

Gerry was perhaps the most aware of the purpose of the project, so did reflect on his diagnosis. Gerry's voiceover was read and recorded. His script was made up of words about his pictures and his life that Jo noted down as they were speaking, but she reconfigured them into a more structured 'story'. She tried to alleviate her anxiety about this by checking out interpretations and offering simple alternatives. Gerry chose the pictures himself (and actually decided to take another, more up-to-date picture for inclusion in the story) but was not interested in sitting at the computer ordering the images or lining them up with the script. Although this made Jo anxious, she had to respect that choice.

Some things don't change (Hynd 2011)

Etta loved telling her story and generated a lot of words in a sort of free-association process. She also kept bringing more pictures to illustrate the multiple threads of her story, which became unmanageable. With some difficulty, Tony worked with her to shape these into a story and she read the script without too much trouble.

Making the most of life (A. Smith 2011)

Aileen worked with Pip, using a limited number of pictures. There were problems with reading more than one line at a time so they printed the story out in large font, then cut up the lines and handed them to her one at a time, recording the story sentence by sentence.

It's home (Duff 2011)

(continued)

Table 19.2 (continued)

Bill came with a pre-prepared story and a set of pictures, created by his wife as a sort of potted biography. Working to edit was impossible from this 'finished' place and Bill was largely disengaged throughout the process.
The lad fae Norrie's pend (Whynne 2011)
Alex was a natural spinner of yarns and, in the early forming of the group, starting to tell stories, came up with some amusing anecdotes. But he didn't see the point of a script, so, after a couple of run-throughs, simply improvised his voiceover in response to the pictures as they came up on the screen. For the purposes of a lively story, it might have been better to record his first telling and edit that. Rehearsal was not helpful as he didn't see the point.

(or influence), but definitely I was thinking, 'how does that [transition] increase the impact of the material that comes before/after/during the transitions between the images'?

You can see the effect of a transition in Fig. 19.1.

Rosie: Despite my presence as commissioner of the workshop, and therefore the potential for my motivations to shape the workshop products, the stories made by the participants do not all directly address the experience of having dementia.

Generally, people make digital stories for a purpose—because they want their stories in the public domain and they want their voice to be heard. In this instance, that was less the case. I think, that perhaps shows in the stories we got—stories about people's lives rather than stories about living with a particular illness:

Jo: As the commissioner you were the person primarily responsible for the outcomes of the project. Did that affect how you worked?

Rosie: I do remember experiencing some conflict about whether these stories were going to be any use for teaching student nurses about dementia. And it was only by showing them to people who said they were great that I thought then, 'They do the job'. And I think they do the job because the audience hears the story knowing that the storyteller has dementia. That's what makes them powerful, because it is not the dementia that's presented, it's the person. And that's the bit that the students fed back in the

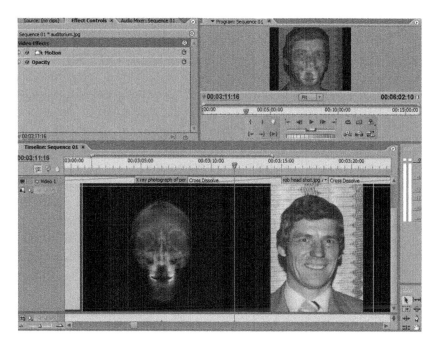

Fig. 19.1   Screen grab showing a cross dissolve transition in Rob's story

evaluation—the benefits of watching stories about their lives and 'seeing the person behind the illness'. And nobody's ever said to me, 'why did you bother making those stories?'

Jo: For me, listening for a story in what Gerry and Alex said to me in our one-to-one sessions was so engrossing and such a complex task that the story itself became the motivation for the work. The overarching purpose—creating a learning resource—was far from my thoughts. I agree that the stories, once created, do the job.

Process

The digital storytelling process in the workshop was person centred, focusing on the relationship between storyteller and facilitator and how it might best support the creation of the digital story. Whilst the process was somewhat emergent and responsive to participant needs, we were conscious of the support offered by the usual digital storytelling structure (see Chap. 4). It may be helpful for readers to have a clearer idea of what actually happened during the workshop, as shown in Table 19.1.

Jo: Sitting beside people, with their pictures, giving them atten-
           tion, seemed to motivate them. It is unusual to spend that
           number of hours, one-to-one, listening to someone's story,
           without the ebb and flow of the group process that you get in
           most digital storytelling workshop settings.
Rosie: It's difficult to say that at the beginning the participants had
           bought into making digital stories because they did not really
           engage with any of the exemplar stories. But the evidence from
           watching them grow over the four days makes me believe that
           there was something in that whole process, and in the dynamic
           between the one-to-one and group interactions that was hugely
           validating.
Jo: In our earlier discussions we saw the form of the story as a con-
           straint, that it could have a negative impact on the storytelling pro-
           cess because it was a way that we, as keepers of that format, could
           exert power. But, on reflection, perhaps it was also liberating.
Rosie: Yes, the boundaries provide a secure space to play. If you know
           where the boundaries are you can work to them, push against
           them if you want, but it needs someone to set the boundaries
           and hold onto them. If we think about Etta's story, and how she
           went off on tangents and Tony had to hold onto the threads of
           that story to try and develop some coherence, it felt as though
           we were exerting control, and yet for people to engage with a
           story, it needs to have some sort of a recognisable form.

Reflection

These adaptations to the normal process of digital storytelling did not occur randomly, but were part of a reflexive process in which we, as facili-tators, were continually engaged. We experienced tension between the need to work within the digital storytelling process and the need to allow participants to have control over their story. Not to forget, keeping within the time constraints of a four-day workshop!

Rosie: The reflective meetings at the end of each day helped give us space to discuss what we each saw happening in the workshop, the impact of our presence and interventions on the participants and the overall digital storytelling process. It was in the reflective group that we decided to do the story circle on day two because it felt like, by that time, we were ready to move from working as individuals to sharing across the group.

Jo: So the shape or process of the workshop was emergent. That takes confidence—to risk flexibility.

Rosie: It also required us [as facilitators] to be engaged with the dynamics of what was happening in the workshop. We were all engaged with the participants and able to analyse and think about our interactions in a way that informed how we worked. And although it was pressured, we needed Tony's structures to keep some sense of the journey and a timetable for us to work within.

Jo: Those reflective sessions at the end of the day felt a bit like peer supervision: checking in with how the stories were going; trying to find a story that would hang together while respecting the voice of the storyteller, but also supporting each other in our uncertainties.

Table 19.2 summarises the different strategies we adopted with each storyteller and includes links to their completed stories.

Conclusion

In this chapter, we set out to interrogate the influence of our actions on the co-production of the digital stories in our workshop. We were particularly keen to consider how the alterations to the usual digital storytelling process might have influenced the stories told. Unusually, the project commissioner was present in the workshop occupying what might be considered conflicting roles of commissioner and facilitator.

We concluded that, without a purpose, digital storytelling (or this project) would not happen. In that sense, the commissioner and the potential audience for the stories are 'in the room' during every digital storytelling workshop. However, in this workshop we had to be aware that the storytellers might not share our motivation, and be vigilant about the impact that this might have on the power dynamics in our relationship with them.

The extent to which the digital stories might be considered as co-produced is determined by the power dynamics of the relationship between workshop participants and facilitators. Working from where the storytellers were was important in keeping us focused on their voices, facilitating co-production.

As facilitators, we missed that first story circle, where the group starts to see a collection of stories that hang together. As the workshop progressed in its modified form, the usual dynamics of mutual support and feedback that establish themselves from the story circle onwards were not present in the group: we created them for ourselves in the reflective space at the end of each day. But by the end of the workshop, we all had a strong sense that a motivated group had produced these stories.

Working reflexively with the digital storytelling process helped us to support each storyteller in a way that enabled them to create their story. We were able to play with the process, within the boundaries of the Patient Voices digital storytelling genre, and create stories that work. When I introduce the stories in the 'Dangling Conversations' e-learning package that was developed from them, I talk briefly about how they were made, as I feel that is important for anyone using the package to understand.

Writing this chapter has allowed us to really interrogate the process in relation to its social context and allows the reader to make a judgement about the validity of the stories as representations of a reality. Acknowledgement of the stories as representations of reality created within a particular historical and social context and the transparency created by the account of the digital storytelling workshop allow digital stories to be considered a valid method of enquiry.

Despite anxieties about the stories not directly addressing issues of living with dementia, and therefore their value for teaching nursing students, adherence to the principles of co-production and allowing people to tell the stories that were important to them enabled development of a set of stories that convey far more than simply the experience of living with dementia. The feedback from practitioners, academics and nursing students who have seen them is that they reveal the person behind the illness: an aspiration of person-centred care.

This chapter has attended to issues of co-production of meaning within the digital storytelling process. The co-production of meaning does not stop at the development of the digital stories. Audiences engage with stories and enter into a relationship with them where personal knowledge is co-produced. You, as our audience, will engage with our discussions within a co-productive relationship, and for each reader particular points will be given priority. It is in this spirit that we invite you to take a moment to consider your own personal learning through engagement with this chapter before reading the key learning points that we have identified from writing this chapter.

Key Points

- When working with people who don't have a voice, or whose voices are marginalised, we need to attend to the power dynamics of our interactions throughout the process of digital storytelling, adjusting the usual process in order to maximise partnership and co-production.
- Using an appropriately adapted version of the Patient Voices method of digital storytelling required us to sit with the story that people wanted to tell rather than the one that we wanted to hear. This approach generates rich stories that offer the audience multiple layers with which to engage.
- Finally, it became clear to us in writing this chapter that it is not possible to think about giving others a voice without working out how we negotiate our own voices within the text.

References

Duff, B. (2011). *It's home*. Pilgrim Projects. Retrieved May 2017, from http://www.patientvoices.org.uk/flv/0548pv384.htm

Gee, J. P. (1985). The narrativization of experience in the oral style. *Journal of Education, 167*(1), 9–35.

Haraway, D. J. (1991). *Simians, cyborgs and women: The reinvention of nature*. New York: Routledge.

Hynd, E. (2011). *Some things don't change*. Pilgrim Projects. Retrieved May 2017, from http://www.patientvoices.org.uk/flv/0549pv384.htm

Kerr, W. (2011). *Still fit*. Pilgrim Projects. Retrieved May 2017, from http://www.patientvoices.org.uk/flv/0552pv384.htm

Kitwood, T. (1997). *Dementia reconsidered: The person comes first*. Maidenhead: Open University Press.

Lather, P. (1991). *Getting smart: Feminist research and pedagogy within/in the postmodern (critical social thought)*. New York: Routledge.

Polkinghorne, D. E. (1988). *Narrative knowing and the human sciences*. Albany, NY: State University of New York Press.

Riessman, C. K. (1993). *Narrative analysis*. Thousand Oaks, CA: Sage.

Smith, A. (2011). *Making the most of life*. Pilgrim Projects. Retrieved May 2017, from http://www.patientvoices.org.uk/flv/0546pv384.htm

Smith, R. (2011). *It's a different world*. Pilgrim Projects. Retrieved May 2017, from http://www.patientvoices.org.uk/flv/0551pv384.htm

Stenhouse, R., Tait, J., Hardy, P., & Sumner, T. (2013). Dangling conversations: Reflections on the process of creating digital stories during a workshop with people with early stage dementia. *Journal of Psychiatric and Mental Health Nursing, 20*(2), 134–141. doi:10.1111/j.1365-2850.2012.01900.x.

Third, G. (2011). *It's the art*. Pilgrim Projects. Retrieved May 2017, from http://www.patientvoices.org.uk/flv/0550pv384.htm

Whynne, A. (2011). *The lad fae Norrie's Pend*. Pilgrim Projects. Retrieved May 2017, from http://www.patientvoices.org.uk/flv/0547pv384.htm

Rosie Stenhouse is a Lecturer in Nursing Studies at the University of Edinburgh. With a background in mental health nursing, her research interests relate to peoples' experience of health services and illnesses/disease with a particular focus on issues of voice and re/presentation and the use of digital stories to explore experiences of people with dementia.

Jo Tait graduated in independent studies at Lancaster, which gave her a solid grounding in experiential learning and a creative approach to academic structures. A doctorate with the Open University led to work in educational developments in universities and NHS trusts. She is now retired, apart from occasional digital storytelling projects.

20

Learning Together with Digital Stories

Elspeth McLean

Introduction and Background

My job as Staff Development Officer in the School of Health Sciences at the University of Liverpool had two strands. One was around supporting teaching staff to find and develop the best ways to help students to learn to be effective and compassionate nurses, radiotherapists, physiotherapists, occupational therapists, orthoptists and diagnostic radiographers. We know that learning is more likely to be successful where the student is an active partner (Biggs 2003), where there are opportunities to try out new ideas and to get some feedback (Race 2010) and where there are resources and approaches that catch students' attention and suit their various learning styles (Rogers 2001). My job was to draw on what we

---

This chapter was written with the help of storytellers Judy Bowker, Kath Corrie, Stephen Cronin and Pat Lavery and lecturers Bev Ball, Joy Burrill, Cath Gordon, Maria Tiffin and Louise Waywell.

E. McLean (✉)
School of Health Sciences, University of Liverpool, Liverpool, UK

© The Author(s) 2018
P. Hardy, T. Sumner (eds.), *Cultivating Compassion*,
https://doi.org/10.1007/978-3-319-64146-1_20

know about making learning happen to encourage and help staff to develop effective and engaging learning within the university context.

The second strand was around creating opportunities for students to learn from and with people with experience of using health and social services. Students have always met patients, service users and their families and carers while on practice placements. Inviting people to join the team at the university, however, is a relatively recent, very successful and now standard development (HCPC 2013) that has located people's knowledge alongside the rest of the evidence base for good practice.

The two strands met at the Patient Voices workshop at University of Central Lancashire's 2007 Authenticity to Action conference. I could see how digital storytelling allowed people to tell their stories in a way that kept them in control. I could see how making a digital story could also be an excellent means of communication about difficult issues that might be hard to explain in person to a group of students. And I could see a resource that could be used flexibly to promote active learning. So I was ready with a bid when, in 2009, a funding opportunity came by from NHS North West.

In preparation for the workshops, I asked Health Sciences colleagues to suggest areas where they had had difficulties finding appropriate ways for people to share their experiences or where there were no suitable audio or video resources. We identified experiences of mental health, living with cancer and/or a long-term condition, and the experience of being a young carer, as areas where digital stories would be a helpful resource for staff and students. People with relevant experiences were invited to an introductory day and five people signed up for the workshop. They were joined by a university colleague who wanted to find out more.

Making Digital Stories: The Workshop

Additional funding from the University of Liverpool Centre for Excellence in Teaching and Learning enabled us to hold the workshop in a comfortable and accessible venue outside the university. This really helped because although the workshop was very enjoyable, it was a steep learning curve for all of us, especially on the technical side, and we all struggled at times. When asked for written comments afterwards, people said:

> *It was a huge challenge—in a positive way.* (Workshop participant)
>   *Facing things I hadn't thought of for a while was cathartic—but I felt better afterwards.* (Workshop participant)

Most of us who attended the workshop are still in touch and still working together. Sadly, Pat Lavery passed away during the writing of this book. She was a key member of our team, and is much missed.

Learning Together with Digital Stories

Enriching Face-to-Face Sessions with People Who Have Experiences to Share

At the heart of the development of people's involvement in student learning is the creation of opportunities for students and people with experiences to share to meet each other in a context where learning can take place. People tend to think of the lecture as the standard context for student learning, but there are other options that are more appropriate when interaction is a priority. To maximise opportunities for engagement and active learning, Radiotherapy lecturers Bev Ball, Louise Waywell and Cath Gordon developed Q&A sessions where small groups of students met people who have experienced radiotherapy. One of our aims in making our own digital stories was to create a resource that people could use when meeting and engaging with students in these sessions.

The storytellers of *My friend autopilot* (Corrie 2009) and *One woman's life* (Lavery 2009) met undergraduate and postgraduate Radiotherapy students, usually before they went on their first practice placement. The year group was divided into smaller groups and each group had an informal Q&A session with a person about their life and experiences. The aim of the session was for students to gain an insight into the experience of living with cancer and having radiotherapy, and an understanding that their patients are real people with lives and experiences outside of hospital and cancer treatment.

Pat used to show her story (*One woman's life*) as an introduction to the session and then invited students to ask questions. Showing the story saved her having to explain all the details, and communicated a great deal in a short time. Pat found that the story itself was '*a bit of a conversation stopper*', which she then complemented by talking about her very positive approach to life and her experiences as a patient and as a carer. To avoid awkward silences, students were asked to prepare questions beforehand, but could also pick up on themes that interested them from the digital story. Student comments on evaluations of the session have included:

> *Health professionals tend to forget to see patients as people with lives outside hospital—to be able to understand this will help me provide better support and more empathy.* (Year 1 Radiotherapy student)
>   *It taught me to see the patient, not the cancer, and I will put this to good use on my placement.* (Year 1 Radiotherapy student)

Kath (*My friend autopilot*) also met Radiotherapy students but preferred to introduce herself and talk with the students first. Sometimes she showed the story at the end of the session and sometimes she suggested students watch it afterwards.

Either way, using digital stories in these sessions enriched the learning environment by offering students a variety of ways to learn, creating opportunities for active learning and widening the scope of the session by introducing themes that may not otherwise emerge from the discussion.

Getting Students Thinking in Lectures

It is important that students are motivated to be really good at working in teams when they graduate as health professionals. This was an aim of a session on teamwork I delivered for a variety of modules across the school. After an introductory exercise where students thought about their own experience as team members and leaders, I showed *Bicycle clips* (Sumner-Rooney 2006) and asked them to make a note as they watched of who is involved in the support and treatment of the young storyteller. The list is long, and discussion of it brings out how many people are involved even in a simple encounter with the health service. The session can then lead on to how the team can ensure they communicate and work effectively.

Bligh (1998) and others have identified a dip in students' attention after 15–20 minutes of a lecture. Showing a digital story creates a useful change of pace at around this point. A digital story is short and personal and helps students to think about and engage with what they have been listening to. I had wondered if *Bicycle clips* was too simple or too childish for this exercise, but students at all levels have found it a helpful way into the issues. The exercise also succeeds because there are quite a few answers to jot down, so the students are finding answers all the way through. This has worked better for me than simply asking them to watch a story and then discuss it afterwards.

Technical resources are improving these days, but showing a digital story successfully in a lecture theatre does depend on students being able to see and hear it. Checking in advance that there is internet access and sound that works has been essential!

A Starting Point for Problem Solving

In a long-standing and innovative programme devised by Occupational Therapy lecturer Joy Burrill (Burrill 2012; Hughes and McLean 2006), small groups of Year 1 Occupational Therapy students meet three times with a person living with a physical or mental health issue, and work with them on possible ways to tackle some of their current or past barriers to daily living. Explaining the impact of mental health issues is not easy, and when Judy has taken part, she has shown her story, *Darkness* (Bowker 2009), to her group of students as a starting point for their work together. This has broken the ice and given students a variety of ideas for their work. Judy has used the story in a range of contexts and comments:

> *One thing that sticks out for me in the digital story making is the need for sounds to go with the narrative as opposed to music. This was really important to me and for me it works beautifully. Mine is the shortest story but I have shown it to many students in my presence so they can ask me questions later. It comes as quite a surprise to them and I think they really do feel a 'deeper meaning'.*

Using Digital Stories in a Virtual Learning Environment

All new Health Sciences students take part in an introductory programme on professional communication skills. Much of their work takes place in small interdisciplinary groups, but the programme used to be launched with a lecture for all students from a health professional and a person with experience of communicating with health professionals. The aim of the lecture was to demonstrate and explain the crucial importance of communication in health and social care.

The introductory lecture used to involve cramming hundreds of students into a huge lecture theatre. It was hard for lecturers to ensure they could be heard at the back, and it was hard for students to find the lecture room and a seat, and then to settle down and think.

Pedagogical as well as practical problems led module leader Maria Tiffin to move the introductory session onto the university virtual learning environment (VLE), and to include some introductory exercises for students to complete and then discuss online and in their small groups. The exercises were created around some brief profession-specific podcasts and Stephen's story, *Blink once for yes* (Cronin 2009). Students were simply asked to note down examples of where communication was taking place, and this was the starting point for a discussion in the small group of why communication is important. Group facilitators reported that this was an effective starting point for achieving the aims of the module, and that a wide range of issues emerged in the discussion of the story.

Stephen has used the story with a variety of student groups and comments that:

> *I often use the "Blink" story with university students and it seems to go down great. I tell it in the context of motivation in those times when students may feel they are on a treadmill. It reinforces the importance of both communication and also thinking/acting independently and the positive impact it can have.*

There were, however, some technical problems. The VLE could not cope with large numbers of students all trying to access the story at the same time (an hour or so before the small groups met). Had we anticipated this we could have taken steps to make sure the story remained accessible.

Later in the programme each small group met and worked with a person who had experiences, both good and bad, about communicating with healthcare professionals. The aim was that the students would develop their understanding of what is good and bad practice in specific situations. To complement this session, a second exercise was created around Lynne's story, *She's fine don't worry* (Currie 2008). By then we had ironed out the technical problems and found that this too was an effective way to stimulate thought, discussion and the application of theory to practice.

Looking Forward, Looking Back

Creating ways to use our own digital stories to enhance student learning has led us to look for and use digital stories that others have made too, for example, Cathy Jaynes' *Go around* (Jaynes 2007), Lynne Currie's *She's fine don't worry* (Currie 2008) and Imogen Sumner-Rooney's *Bicycle clips* (Sumner-Rooney 2006).

It has also given us the confidence to create our own audio recordings of people telling their stories of encounters with health professionals. These have been made into short podcasts and are part of the Communication Skills resource.

Some of our storytellers are keen to make another story—there is more to tell.

Four questions were raised by various people at the beginning of our digital storytelling journey:

1. Do digital stories enhance student learning and help students to become better health professionals?

 Our experience of using digital stories in a variety of contexts has been that students find them interesting, so they pay attention and engage with them. It is not easy to separate out a digital story from its context in order to evaluate its impact, but it does seem to us that using digital stories has been helpful in enabling students to learn from and reflect on other people's experiences, and that digital stories have enriched the learning environment. Using a digital story does 'push the pedagogy' by making us think about what exactly we are helping the students to learn, and how we are going to do it. Students have a range of responses to the digital stories we have used, some of them unexpected. These unexpected responses can lead discussion and reflection in new and student-led directions.

2. Can we cope with the technology?

Technical issues have at times been a problem. Lecture theatres and group rooms are not always equipped with the appropriate equipment and internet access that makes using a digital story easy. VLEs cannot always cope with large numbers of students accessing the same story at the same time. It is not always possible to get into a lecture room beforehand to check all is well, or to find somebody to help, and minor issues such as a lack of curtains on a sunny day can create a problem. A Plan B may occasionally be required!

3. Do digital stories offer something we cannot already find on the internet?

It is very easy to find video clips on the internet on every subject under the sun, and to use them in our teaching. It would seem that these days there is no need to add our own digital stories to the existing resource. However, making and using digital stories has made us aware of a couple of issues about using video clips we have found on the internet.

A properly made digital story is made by the storyteller, so you know they have chosen what to include (and leave out) and they have been in control of the process. In contrast, there is usually no way of knowing whether the people in video clips on the internet have given their consent or if they knew what they were consenting to. And digital stories are engaging because they are just that—stories. Many video clips do not have a story-based structure and do not engage the way that a story does. We have used our digital stories consistently in the five years since they were made and that is because of their quality, which in turn reflects the quality of their creation. It took a great deal of time, effort and funding, but it has paid off.

4. Will digital stories replace people?

Developing digital stories together has helped us to develop the ways we work with people who have experience of health and social services. Working together in the workshop to co-produce digital stories broke down barriers and has built strong relationships. Exploring ways to use the stories has enabled us to find better ways to work with students. There were some concerns expressed at our introductory workshop that once we had made some stories, the University would no longer need to arrange for real people to meet and work with students. The reverse has turned out to be the case—using digital stories has been a way for some of the people who work with us to enhance their teaching, and using digital stories has created more and more interesting ways for us to work together.

Key Points

- Using digital stories enhances the student learning environment and makes lectures and seminars more interesting and effective.
- Using a digital story can be the catalyst for improving and updating the ways we create learning opportunities for and with students.
- Showing and discussing a digital story can enrich encounters between students and service users.
- Digital stories are different to most video clips that can be found on the internet, and are often more appropriate for educational use.
- Digital stories will not replace people; rather, they help us to create new ways for us to work together.

References

Biggs, J. (2003). *Teaching for quality learning at university* (2nd ed.). Maidenhead: Open University Press.

Bligh, D. (1998). *What's the use of lectures?* Exeter: Intellect.

Bowker, J. (2009). *Darkness.* Pilgrim Projects. Retrieved March 2014, from http://www.patientvoices.org.uk/flv/0370pv384.htm

Burrill, J. (2012). *The influence of service user involvement in an academic module on the learning and professional development of first year occupational therapy students.* Liverpool: University of Liverpool.

Corrie, K. (2009). *My friend autopilot.* Pilgrim Projects. Retrieved March 2014, from http://www.patientvoices.org.uk/flv/0371pv384.htm

Cronin, S. (2009). *Blink once for yes.* Pilgrim Projects. Retrieved March 2014, from http://www.patientvoices.org.uk/flv/0374pv384.htm

Currie, L. (2008). *She's fine, don't worry.* Pilgrim Projects. Retrieved March 2014, from http://www.patientvoices.org.uk/flv/0276pv384.htm

HCPC. (2013). *Consultation on service user involvement in education and training programmes approved by the Health and Care Professions Council.* Health and Care Professions Council.

Hughes, R., & McLean, E. (2006). *An evaluation of the get involved 2 project.* School of Health Sciences, University of Liverpool, UK.

Jaynes, C. (2007). *Go around.* Patient Voices.

Lavery, P. (2009). *One woman's life.* Pilgrim Projects. Retrieved March 2014, from www.patientvoices.org.uk/flv/0373pv384.htm

Race, P. (2010). *Making learning happen.* London: Sage.

Rogers, J. (2001). *Adults learning* (4th ed.). Buckingham: Open University Press.

Sumner-Rooney, I. (2006). *Bicycle clips.* Pilgrim Projects. Retrieved March 2014, from http://www.patientvoices.org.uk/flv/0045pv384.htm

Elspeth McLean was, until recently, Staff Development Officer in the School of Health Sciences at the University of Liverpool. Her role included the development of collaborative and interdisciplinary work between staff, students and people with experience of using health and social services. Her background is in education and social work.

21

Cultivating Compassion in End-of-Life Care: Developing an Interprofessional Learning Resource Based on Digital Stories

Elizabeth Howkins and Pip Hardy

Introduction

The way care is given can reach the most hidden places and give space for unexpected development. We frequently see how both patient and family may find peace and strength for themselves when we know we have given so little. There are possibilities in people facing death that are a constant astonishment. We will see them more often if we can gain the confidence to approach our fellows without hiding behind a professional mask, instead meeting as one person to another, both aware of the depths of a pain that somehow has its healing within itself. In this discovery we may find out as much about living as about dying. People at the end of their lives will then be our teachers. Dame Cicely Saunders (Saunders 2007)

E. Howkins (✉)
Centre for the Advancement of Interprofessional Education (CAIPE), Portchester, UK

P. Hardy
Patient Voices Programme, Pilgrim Projects Ltd, Landbeach, Cambridge, UK

© The Author(s) 2018
P. Hardy, T. Sumner (eds.), *Cultivating Compassion*,
https://doi.org/10.1007/978-3-319-64146-1_21

Care at the End of Life

The provision of care at the end of life that is dignified, respectful, appropriate, and compassionate presents a considerable number of challenges, but as Dame Cicely Saunders reminds us, we should not be daunted by the challenge.

The complexity of care at the end of life requires a variety of professionals, spanning a range of care providers. This brings both benefit, in terms of the breadth of expertise, and frustration (intrusion and confusion about who does what) for patients and families. From the provider's perspective, the same is true: there is great benefit from an interprofessional approach but there is also the challenge of providing coordinated care and supporting seamless care across provider boundaries. Palliative and end-of-life care is the one area where an 'interprofessional team approach to care is necessary to meet the physical, spiritual, and psychological needs of the patient and their families' (Hall et al. 2006). Interprofessional education (IPE) offers a framework that supports different professionals learning together, sharing experiences, valuing each other's contribution, and thus improving collaboration and the quality of care. The Centre for the Advancement of Interprofessional Education (CAIPE 2002) definition of IPE, widely used around the world, is: *when two or more professions learn with, from and about each other to improve collaboration and the quality of care.*

A New Approach to Educating Staff

Traditionally, medical and healthcare education has focused on knowledge and skills-based learning, with less attention given to exploring the broader aspects of care delivery (GMC 2009), that is, the human factors, such as empathy and compassion, emotional intelligence (EI), willingness to face personal challenges, and resilience. However, the importance of these qualities is highlighted in the NHS England document: *Actions for End of Life Care: 2014–16*, which specifies the need to educate staff in ways that enable them to meet the emotional demands of end-of-life care, as well as the practical and intellectual demands. The impact of professionals' own experience, values, assumptions, and prejudices on the decisions made within consultations is probably significantly underestimated, while the experience of both patients and professionals in the consultation is insufficiently understood. Reflection is underutilised, certainly within the medical profession, despite being required by the General Medical Council (GMC 2009), as is recognition of the need to develop emotional resilience.

There is a breadth and depth of experience within the various professions involved in end-of-life care, including the ambulance service, nursing homes, social services, mental health services, allied health professionals, acute and secondary care, commissioners, hospice workers, specialist palliative care services, faith groups, the voluntary sector, and primary care teams. However, training is usually delivered piecemeal to individual professional groups, or to small interprofessional groups. It is unusual to see training offered for or by both health *and* social care, or by interprofessional teams of health professionals working together, and even more unusual for service users to be integral to training opportunities. It is also useful to note that the 'training' is the term most commonly used, reflecting an emphasis on the acquisition of specific skills and knowledge rather than the development of empathy, EI, critical awareness, resilience, and the capacity for reflection. The authors feel it is useful to distinguish between 'training' and 'education' and, in doing so, are reminded of Socrates' words: *Education is not the filling of a vessel, but the kindling of a flame*—in this case, we hope to spark the desire to become more reflective, more empathic, more self-aware, more resilient, and so on.

The Evidence of Experience

Central to the design of patient-centred care is the 'evidence of experience' that can only be provided by service users and their carers, and it is through their stories that it is possible to gain some insight into their values and beliefs. We recognise that these individuals play a crucial role in determining what constitutes good care and they are an integral part of the interprofessional team.

Since the turn of the century, there has been a growing consensus about the importance of partnership working across teams and care providers, together with the need to engage more fully with service users. This aspiration is clearly indicated in strategic documents, including *The Health and Social Care 2012*, which advocates 'a greater voice for patients' (DH 2010, 2012) and is also reflected in the requirements of statutory regulators of professional courses, such as the GMC and the Health and Care Professions Council. NHS England (2014) has further developed this theme, with an intention to promote development of communities of practice, across health and social care boundaries, learning from each other in order to build resilience and capability.

Accordingly, a proposal was submitted to Health Education England in the North East (HEENE) for the development of an educational resource intended to acknowledge and utilise the wide range of expertise that resides in the providers of end-of-life care, as well as the experiences of patients, service users, and carers and that would also support the development of compassion, EI, and resilience in the care of the dying. The resource would be innovative and was, at the request of HEENE, to be co-produced with patients. It was to be capable of delivery in face-to-face teaching sessions as well as online.

Aligning Education with Policy

A key requirement of the project was to align the resource with themes identified by Health Education England in *delivering high-quality, effective, compassionate care: Developing the right people with the right skills and the right values* (DH 2015), including:

- greater integration of services across boundaries, including health and social care and between primary and secondary care
- developing transferrable, generalist skills
- developing training which reflects the pathway of care, rather than relating to exclusive professional groups
- a focus on behaviours and skills to enable safe, dignified, and compassionate care

- offering an effective voice for patients, service users, and the public
- utilising technology to support and deliver education and training
- an approach which is inclusive of key staff groups, for example, health-care assistants

Designing the Resource

The resource was intended to consist of a number of short, flexible learning modules based around a suite of digital stories created by service users/patients, carers, and professionals that would illuminate key issues and themes.

Designing an educational programme for such an emotionally charged and complex area of learning presents a challenge, but through the use of narrative and digital storytelling participants would be enabled to explore the human side of caring at the end of life.

IPE provided the ideal educational framework to underpin the resource which 'employs interactive learning methods to enhance mutual understanding of each other's roles and responsibilities' (CAIPE 2011).

The core design team consisted of Pip Hardy and Tony Sumner from Pilgrim Projects/Patient Voices; Colette Hawkins, a palliative care consultant working in the North East of England; and Elizabeth Howkins of the CAIPE. A steering group consisting of representatives from HEENE and a range of professional groups was established to guide and support the project.

Aims of the Resource

The programme set out to improve the quality of care delivered at the end of life. It would:

- promote an interprofessional approach to end-of-life care that supports compassion, insight, EI, reflection, and resilience and holds patients and their stories at the heart of care
- recognise, acknowledge, and share the wide range of experience and expertise that can contribute to high-quality end-of-life care

- ensure that user engagement is central to the design, development, delivery, and evaluation of the resource
- foster an approach to learning that has real impact on practice
- build and strengthen a community of practice committed to learning and practising the skills and qualities that will contribute to improved experience of care for those delivering as well those as receiving it

To ensure that the learning resource accurately reflected the interprofessional nature of end-of-life care, we would gather and share the stories of a selection of people who had been involved in care of the dying from both a professional and personal perspective. These stories would form the core of a learning resource that would, in turn, build on Chochinov's (2007) work on dignity-conserving care which highlights aspects of attitude and behaviour while acknowledging the importance of listening to stories as a stepping stone to providing compassionate and dignified care. Values of co-production would lie at the heart of the process of creating the resource and would also strengthen the interprofessional nature of the resource, reinforcing the need for teams to work together to achieve the best outcomes for patients.

The Digital Storytelling Workshops: Some Physical, Emotional, and Intellectual Challenges

Recruiting storytellers to the workshops proved more challenging than anticipated. The willingness to talk about dying and death for someone who is terminally ill needs courage and careful preparation by the facilitator to enable that person to feel comfortable in sharing end of life thoughts, fears, and hopes when time is very precious.

Despite the best efforts of the team, and patients who expressed interest in participating, it was not possible to find anyone nearing the end of life who was able to take part. One patient became quite poorly just before the workshop and one patient did attend the first morning of a workshop but was so exhausted by coffee time that she was unable to continue.

In addition, staff across the professional range found it difficult to take three days away from work. The solution was to hold three smaller, two-day workshops; these took place during July 2015. The standard Patient Voices briefing was accompanied by an invitation to contribute to the development of the educational resource, as follows:

The resource will be firmly based on what really matters to people receiving and delivering care. We believe that the best way to discover what matters most to people is by listening to their stories. We know that real change rarely comes about as a result of reading reports and scouring statistics alone and so we want your stories to form the foundation of our new resource. To that end, we would like to invite you to share your stories of end of life care with us so that important lessons may be learned from your experiences. (From the Invitation to participate in a Patient Voices workshop)

Storytellers included four family carers and representatives from the interprofessional workforce, including: a district nurse, a domiciliary carer, a social care educator, a general practitioner, a funeral director, a paramedic, a chaplain, a solicitor, a community respiratory nurse, a community specialist palliative care nurse, a consultant in palliative medicine, and a palliative care physiotherapist. The workshops followed the well-established Patient Voices Reflective Digital Storytelling process described in Chap. 4; 18 stories were created in the workshops and one audio story was developed outside the workshops. While it was no surprise that the family carers created stories about their experiences with loved ones who had died, what was not entirely expected was the number of stories made by professionals that focused on personal, rather than professional experiences of death.

One explanation may be found in the process of composing a digital story. Flannery O'Connor, a twentieth-century American writer, comments that every good story needs a dragon: *No matter what form the dragon may take, it is of this mysterious passage past him, or into his jaws, that stories of any depth will always be concerned to tell* (O'Connor 1969).

Patient Voices storytellers are always encouraged to find 'the dragon' in their stories. We explain that our understanding of the dragon in this context is 'the challenge that is faced by the 'hero' or 'heroine' of the story—the illness, the accident, the despair, the grief, the loss—that must be overcome in order for the hero or heroine to demonstrate his or her courage, strength, wit, wisdom, kindness, resourcefulness, or whatever quality it is that contributes to that person's humanity' (Hardy 2016). Without a dragon, O'Connor suggests, the story will lack depth and the audience will fail to be engaged.

The process of examining one's own professional practice, together with the ability to reflect on a professional experience that has an emotional and/or a personal impact can present an even more difficult challenge than reflecting on a personal experience. The creation of a digital story about a professional experience requires careful consideration of issues such as confidentiality, anonymity, professionalism, and ethical issues, all in the context of the current NHS culture which is often characterised by blame, competition, high pressure, increasing demands on time and resources, and a lack of compassion (Ballatt and Campling 2011; Francis 2013).

So, although the professional storytellers found the experience emotional, they welcomed the opportunity to reflect on their experiences and many related their personal experiences of death to their professional roles, as in the following two examples:

- In one particularly affecting story, *Don't wait* a palliative care physiotherapist recalls what really matters in life through reminiscing about his uncle John, and reminding himself and his viewers of the importance of attending to priorities before it's too late (Bayer 2015).
- In *All hope is gone*, a palliative care nurse reflects sadly on the poor care her own mother received following a diagnosis of cancer (Kingston 2015).

In the end, having faced some dragons, many of the storytellers reported that the creation of their digital stories had been cathartic and, perhaps more importantly, their stories had focused on what really mattered to them as people and as professionals. It is difficult, we have come to understand, to separate the personal from the professional. In order to deliver compassionate, high-quality care to patients, it is essential to care for oneself; this in turn relies on the ability to integrate personal and professional selves, as you will see in the next chapter.

Analysing Stories and Identifying Themes

Two months after the digital storytelling workshops, a one-day event was held to analyse the stories and identify themes that would shape the learning resource. In total, 16 people—a mix of storytellers and Steering Group members—attended. The Effective, Affective, Reflective model of reflection (Sumner 2009) was used to prompt responses to the stories: as each story was shown, individuals were invited to note down their thoughts in relation to the questions, 'What was the story's effect on you (or, what did you think)?' 'How did the story affect you (what did you feel)?' and 'What are your reflections in relation to your own practice (what will you do differently)?' The group then divided into three smaller groups that attempted to pull out key ideas and themes and relate these to individual stories; these were captured on flipcharts and then presented back to the larger group. One group's flipcharts is shown in Fig. 21.1.

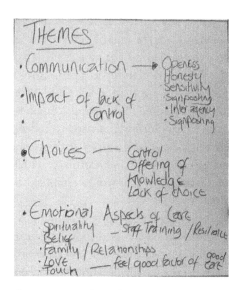

Fig. 21.1 Flipchart from story analysis day

All the data were then gathered and analysed with a view to coming up with the main themes that would form the structure of the resource. In total, 12 themes were identified:

1. Communication
2. Compassionate care
3. Holistic care
4. Prognosis
5. The Mental Capacity Act
6. Shared decision-making
7. Clinical decision-making at end of life
8. The effective interprofessional
9. The professional as a person
10. Advance care planning
11. End-of-life care at home
12. The experience of informal carers

Developing the Educational Resource

Since this resource was intended to reflect what really matters to people receiving and delivering care at the end of life, the content of the resource must necessarily be determined by the stories. This approach had been used by Patient Voices in the past, firstly in a project for the Royal College of Nursing intended to develop an e-learning resource designed to improve continence care. Rather than trying to make the stories fit the curriculum, the entire curriculum was revised to reflect what really mattered to patients as revealed in the stories they created (Hardy 2007). Similarly, the Manchester Mental Health project, which is the subject of Chap. 8, set out to collect stories that would establish the 'curriculum' for an e-learning resource.

The first task in developing the learning resource was to create a matrix to guide the use of stories in particular modules. The aim was to ensure that each story was used at least once and not to overuse any one story, although some stories seemed to have almost universal applicability. It was sometimes a challenge to select the most appropriate story or stories for a particular module but a matrix was eventually drawn up to ensure that the most relevant stories were used in the most appropriate context. The matrix is shown in Table 21.1. Dignity, respect, compassion, and interprofessional working were to be woven throughout the resource.

An Interprofessional Approach

The model used to develop the educational resource is one that has been used over many years by Pilgrim Projects and relies on pairing up a subject expert (in this case, Colette Hawkins) with an open learning editor (in this case, Pip Hardy) and a specialist subject advisor, (in this case Elizabeth Howkins). Content was drafted by Colette and edited by Pip to ensure that the materials were active, motivating, engaging, reflective, stimulating, reassuring, and learner centred; the modules were then reviewed by Elizabeth to ensure that they complied with the principles of IPE, which enshrine and extend those of adult learning by stating that any IPE activity must reflect values, process, and outcomes (CAIPE 2011).

IPE offers a framework to underpin educational programmes where different professions learn together, share experiences, value each other's contribution and thus improve collaboration and quality of care. Crucially, practitioners must be competent to work collaboratively. In a seminal paper from the Lancet Commission Report (Frenk et al. 2010), which examined health professional education, the authors concluded that the *'attainment of specific competencies must be the defining feature of the education and evaluation of future health professionals.'*

A competency statement is a strong, overarching statement that guides behaviour and lasts over long periods of time. The model used to analyse the digital stories for IPE and interprofessional collaboration was based on the competency statements that have been generated in countries around the world, including Canada (CIHC 2010) the United States (Schmitt et al. 2011) and in the UK, the Sheffield Capability Framework (Gordon and Walsh 2005).

Although the specific competencies vary from country to country, they all have similar core competencies, including: role clarification, team

Table 21.1 Cultivating compassion in end-of-life care story/module matrix

Module/story	Not coming home	All hope is gone	The crack down on pull-up pants	Just a care worker	Fancy dress, of course	Everyone's family	No someone's time to talk	My dad	Last mountain	Who cares?	Legal care at end of life	A Chasm	A family or a team	Choices (After the end)	Don't wait	Time to go home	Between a rock and a hard place	A chaplain's tale	Forever young
01 The personal professional					X														
02 The effective interprofessional			X							X		X	X	X	X	X			
03 Communication	X		X	X			X	X		X		X			X	X	X		
04 Compassionate care	X	X	X			X	X	X	X	X	X	X	X	X	X	X	X		X
05 Holistic care						X	X				X			X			X		
06 Prognosis	X												X		X		X		
07 The Mental capacity Act	X								X	X							X		
08 Shared decision-making	X														X				
09 Clinical decision-making			X			X	X	X	X		X	X	X	X	X	X	X		X
10 The professional as a person			X	X		X	X				X	X	X	X	X	X	X	X	X
11 Advanced care planning/DNR	X	X									?			X	X		X		
12 End-of-life care at home	X	X	X	X		X	?	X	X				X	X			X		

working, developing supportive relationships, reflection and self-awareness, working across boundaries, interprofessional conflict resolution, interprofessional communication, and interpersonal skills.

A specific competency framework was developed to analyse the digital stories developed for this project, as shown in Table 21.2.

While this resource was not intended to provide competency-based training, we did want to ensure that an interprofessional approach was embedded in the modules. Each digital story was therefore analysed for aspects of interprofessional work and collaboration. An example of the analysis is shown in Table 21.3 but applied to only three of the digital stories.

Table 21.2 Competency framework for interprofessional collaboration and interprofessional education: analysing digital stories for the end-of-life care project

Communication	Interprofessional communication, learning from others, showing respect for other professional roles and experience. That is, is there a level of trust, evidence of collaborative work?
Patient centred	Is the patient/carer at the centre of care? Is the patient/carer part of the team? Are the professionals working to meet the needs of patient/client and their interests above all else? Is there empathy to patient/carer situation?
Role clarification	Professionals understand their own role and those of other professionals and are able to use this knowledge appropriately to establish and meet patient/carer/family goals and needs
Team functioning	Professionals understand the principles of team dynamics and group processes to enable effective interprofessional team collaboration
IP conflict resolution	Professionals actively engage self and others, including the patient/client/family, in dealing effectively with interprofessional conflict
Collaborative leadership	Professionals work together with all participants, including patients/clients/families to formulate, implement, and evaluate care/services to enhance health outcomes
GOAL: interprofessional collaboration	A partnership between a team of health providers and a client in a participatory, collaborative, and coordinated approach to shared decision-making around health and social issues

Table 21.3 Analysis of stories for IP competencies

	All hope is gone	Choices	A family or a team?
Communication	Medical team did not communicate in a manner that was reassuring, it was one of fear	A level of trust and empathy shown throughout	Communication could certainly have been more open and honest
Patient centredness	Diagnosis was lung cancer: a medical approach and **not** person centred	Lovely examples of how the family's needs and worries were met	N/A
Role clarification	N/A	N/A	N/A
Team functioning	N/A	N/A	N/A
IP conflict resolution	N/A	N/A	Conflict was not addressed and time was not prioritised for family to talk together and share these very difficult end of life issues
Collaborative leadership	N/A	N/A	N/A

As the modules were developed, feedback from the IP competency framework analysis was incorporated to ensure that learners were encouraged to explore IP issues as they undertook the reflective tasks. Questions and activities guided learners to work, share, and discuss with other professionals, to learn more about each other's roles, address conflict, and be always patient/client centred. In addition, the 12 themes encouraged learners to realise that end-of-life care involves a large number of organisations and professionals and that a collaborative, coordinated approach to shared decision-making should be the goal.

Piloting the Resource

At this point the materials were piloted. A piloting questionnaire was devised and modules were delivered to 179 people in seven groups, including medical students, physician associates, social care practitioners, nurses, and one interprofessional group. Stories were shown and used as prompts for discussion among the groups; other activities were devised and opportunities for collective reflection were provided, offering most learners an unusual opportunity to engage with the emotional content of the material. Some comments from piloters are included here:

> *[The session offered] good insight into other people's stories—made me think more.*
>
> *I feel this is an excellent way to deliver new information and extend knowledge within palliative care.*
>
> *Raises interesting moral and ethical dilemmas; made me think about difficult situations with relatives of patients.*
>
> *[The session was] 'very enlightening.'*
>
> *It gave me pause for thought.*
>
> *Personal stories were good—and thought provoking.*
>
> *I found the videos really moving.*
>
> *The session highlighted the difficulties that patients and family members face during a final illness and the ways in which a healthcare professional can impede their journey.*
>
> *[I was] thinking about what I would do in these situations and what is morally right.*
>
> *Thought-wrenching—makes you think about your own practice and how you could come across to patients.*
>
> *The importance of establishing the human connection and the impact this has.*
>
> *Reiterates importance of communication and how patients, families/carer are affected. Leaves memories that last whether good or bad.*

Despite promoting online availability of the learning resource, no one took up this option. Many piloters felt that face-to-face facilitated sessions were more appropriate for the content of the resource than isolated online learning and appreciated the opportunities for discussion, for example: *Small group discussions were helpful.*

However, a number of responses also indicated that the ability to review the materials online would also allow for a different kind of experience: 'a more personal, more private experience,' while others suggested that it would be helpful to be able to revisit the materials online and work through them in their own time.

In the light of feedback from the pilot, modules were broken down into shorter topics, with a view to making it easier for learners to plan their time (a topic could be completed in 20 minutes, whereas a module could take more than an hour). The number of modules was also reduced from 12 to 7, to eliminate repetition and provide a more logical, streamlined structure that would be easier for busy students and professionals to fit into their already-pressured lives.

Finding interprofessional groups to pilot the resource proved challenging and, in the end, only one of the groups was actually interprofessional; our experience is, perhaps, indicative of the difficulties of bringing interprofessional groups together for any kind of educational experience (Freeth et al. 2005; Howkins and Bray 2008). Other groups spanned a range of professions, including social workers, healthcare assistants, nurses, and medical students, but the discussions took place, necessarily, within these clinical groups.

Conclusion

This project provided an innovative and unusual opportunity to offer a different kind of teaching and a different kind of learning in relation to end-of-life care. The creation and use of digital stories by people spanning the interprofessional spectrum were at the very core of the programme, establishing the content, and serving as prompts for discussion and reflection with the potential to break down professional silos by promoting communication and collaboration between professional groups.

So, while the goal of developing an interprofessional educational resource was achieved, the reality of delivering the programme to interprofessional groups has, with some justification, proved to be more difficult. The experience of professionals learning and talking about end-of-life care is emotionally challenging and research evidence (Atkins 1998; Howkins and Bray 2008) demonstrates that when professionals feel threatened, they will seek the comfort and security of their own safe professional role. Interprofessional learning requires professionals to come out of their comfort zone to take time to share and listen to other voices.

In the opening quote to this chapter, Dame Cicely Saunders makes the same point when she writes *if we can gain the confidence to approach our fellows without hiding behind a professional mask instead meeting as one person to another, both aware of the depths of a pain that somehow has its healing within itself. In this discovery we may find out as much about living as about dying. People at the end of their lives will then be our teachers.*

To date, the resource has been piloted with just under 200 people, the majority of whom have praised the use of stories to prompt reflection and discussion and the opportunity to explore emotions, values, and ethical issues; people also praised the facilitative style of teaching, rather than the more traditional didactic approach.

Having tested this developmental design as an approach to creating a learning resource in end-of-life care, it is clear that the model could fruitfully be used in other clinical areas, especially those where there is a high level of interprofessional activity, such as, for example, renal care. Future developments should focus on developing similar resources across a range of clinical areas, and on working with interprofessional groups to reinforce this essential aspect of collaborative care not only at the end of life, but throughout life.

Key Points

- The creation of digital stories by professionals and family carers provided a sound, yet flexible, framework for the development of the educational resource.
- Reflective digital stories can provide the 'hook' on which to hang the curriculum for a particular topic area.
- The development of an educational resource designed to develop compassion, resilience, and EI must be approached in a very different way from the development of skills- or competency-based training.
- Implementing IPE continues to provide a challenge, despite its centrality in the design and delivery of safe, high-quality care.
- Facilitators need to be prepared with the skills to support and organise interprofessional learning.
- Exploring ways to encourage professional/personal digital story telling is worth further consideration.

References

Atkins, J. (1998). Tribalism, loss and grief: Issues for multiprofessional educa-tion. *Journal of Interprofessional Care, 12*(3), 303–307.

Ballatt, J., & Campling, P. (2011). *Intelligent kindness: Reforming the culture of healthcare*. London: RCPsych Publications.

Bayer, T. (2015). *Don't wait*. Pilgrim Projects Limited. http://www.patientvoices.org.uk/flv/0915pv384.htm. (2017 printing).

CAIPE. (2002). *Interprofessional education: A definition*. Retrieved from www.caipe.org

CAIPE. (2011). *Principles of interprofessional education*. Retrieved from www.caipe.org

Chochinov, H. M. (2007). Dignity and the essence of medicine: The A, B, C, and D of dignity conserving care. *BMJ, 335*(7612), 184–187. doi:10.1136/bmj.39244.650926.47.

CIHC. (2010). *A national interprofessional competency framework*. Vancouver: Canadian Interprofessional Health Collaborative.

DH. (2010). *Equity and excellence: Liberating the NHS*. London: DH.

DH. (2012). *Health and Social Care Act: White paper*. London: DH.

DH. (2015). *Delivering high quality, effective, compassionate care: Developing the right people with the right skills and the right values*. Leeds: DH.

Francis, R. (2013). *The Mid Staffordshire NHS Foundation Trust Public Enquiry*. Press Statement.

Freeth, D., Hammick, M., Reeves, S., Koppel, I., & Barr, H. (2005). *Effective interprofessional education*. Oxford: Blackwell Publishing.

Frenk, J., Chen, L., Bhutta, Z. A., Cohen, J., Crisp, N., Evans, T., Fineberg, H., Garcia, P., Ke, Y., & Kelley, P. (2010). Health professionals for a new century: Transforming education to strengthen health systems in an interdependent world. *The Lancet, 376*(9756), 1923–1958.

GMC. (2009). *Tomorrow's doctors: Outcomes and standards for undergraduate medical education*. Manchester: General Medical Council.

Gordon, F., & Walsh, C. (2005). A framework for interprofessional capability: Developing students of health and social care as collaborative workers. *Journal of Integrated Care, 13*(3), 26–33. doi:10.1108/14769018200500023.

Hall, P., Weaver, L., Fothergill-Bourbonnais, F., Amos, S., Whiting, N., Barnes, P., & Legauult, F. (2006). Interprofessional education in palliative care: A pilot programme using popular literature. *Journal of Interprofessional Care, 20*(1), 51–59.

Hardy, P. (2007). An investigation into the application of the Patient Voices digital stories in healthcare education: Quality of learning, policy impact and practice-based value. MSc dissertation, University of Ulster, Belfast.

Hardy, V. P. (2016). Telling tales: The development and impact of digital stories and digital storytelling in healthcare. Doctoral thesis, Manchester Metropolitan University, Manchester.

Howkins, E., & Bray, J. (2008). *Preparing for interprofessional teaching: Theory and practice*. Oxford: Radcliffe Publishing.

Kingston, E. (2015). *All hope is gone*. Pilgrim Projects. http://www.patientvoices. org.uk/flv/0918pv384.htm. (2017 printing).

NHS England. (2014). *Actions for end of life care: 2014–16*. Leeds: NHS England.

O'Connor, F. (1969). *Mystery and manners: Occasional prose*. New York: Farrar.

Saunders, C. (2007). Foreword. In M. Kearney (Ed.), *Mortally wounded*. New Orleans, Louisiana: Spring Journal Books.

Schmitt, M., Blue, A., Aschenbrener, C. A., & Viggiano, T. R. (2011). Core competencies for interprofessional collaborative practice: Reforming health care by transforming health professionals' education. *Academic Medicine, 86*(11), 1351. doi:10.1097/ACM.0b013e3182308e39.

Sumner, T. (2009). *The power of e-flection: Using digital storytelling to facilitate reflective assessment of junior doctors' experiences in training*. Paper presented at the Learning for a Complex World, University of Surrey, 31 March 2009.

Elizabeth Howkins is an educational consultant working in the field of inter-professional education and collaborative practice. She was the immediate past chair of the Centre for the Advancement of Interprofessional education. Prior to that she was Head of the Department of Health and Social Care at the University of Reading.

Pip Hardy is a co-founder of the Patient Voices Programme and a director of Pilgrim Projects Ltd, an education consultancy specialising in open learning and healthcare quality improvement. She also serves as Curriculum and Learning Lead for NHS England's School for Change Agents. Pip has an MSc in lifelong learning, and her PhD considers the potential of digital storytelling to transform healthcare.

22

The DNA of Care: Digital Storytelling with NHS Staff

Karen Deeny, Pip Hardy, and Tony Sumner

Introduction and Background

Employee engagement emerges as the best predictor of NHS trust outcomes. No combination of key scores or single scale is as effective in predicting trust performance on a range of outcomes measures as is the scale measure of employee engagement. (West et al. 2017)

This is a book about stories and, while stories are most often conveyed through words, numbers can tell stories too. So we would like to start with some statistics to help set the scene for why we felt it was so important to work with healthcare staff to create digital stories about their experiences of working in the NHS.

K. Deeny (✉)
Patient Experience Team, NHS England,
Quarry Hill, Leeds, UK

P. Hardy • T. Sumner
Patient Voices Programme, Pilgrim Projects Ltd,
Landbeach, Cambridge, UK

© The Author(s) 2018
P. Hardy, T. Sumner (eds.), *Cultivating Compassion*,
https://doi.org/10.1007/978-3-319-64146-1_22

Some Numbers to Set the Scene

The NHS in England serves a population of 54.3 million and employs around 1.3 million people. It is estimated that 1 million patients are cared for every 36 hours. Between January and March 2015 the average sickness absence rate among NHS staff was 4.44%; 33% of staff report suffering from work-related stress and 30% of NHS sick leave is due to workplace stress. Annual direct staff absence costs account for £1.7 billion of NHS resources (Boorman 2009).

So, what do we know about how NHS staff are feeling?

In total, 80% of NHS staff believe that the state of their health affects patient care. In the 2016 NHS Staff Survey, 60% of staff said that they would recommend their organisation as a place to work and 70% reported that if a friend or relative needed treatment they would be happy with the standard of care provided by their organisation.

More than 60% of NHS staff in England reported having recently attended work despite not feeling well enough to perform their duties (Boorman 2009).

Poor mental health is associated with a quarter of staff absences (Boorman 2009).

Self-reported stress affects around one-third of NHS employees (NHS Employers 2014).

Death by suicide is highest amongst the caring professions (Meltzer et al. 2008).

Since 1997, evidence has shown that NHS staff are almost 10% more likely to suffer damaging levels of stress than the general population (Wall et al. 1997).

Stress and mental health issues have overtaken musculoskeletal disorders as the main reason for sickness absence (NHS Employers 2014).

On the other hand, we know that positive staff experiences can have an important impact on outcomes for both staff and patients. Positive staff experiences are associated with an average 50% cost reduction in relation to workplace accidents. Alertness, concentration and judgement are all improved, as are staff retention rates and resilience. Patient care is safer, outcomes are better and patient experience is enhanced (West and Dawson 2012).

As long ago as 2009, the Boorman Report highlighted the pressing need to prioritise staff engagement and health and well-being. It is clear that staff well-being is a key driver, rather than a consequence, of experiences and outcomes of care for patients (Maben et al. 2012). While there has been a steady general improvement in most areas of the NHS Staff Survey since 2012, in the face of increased activity, demand and system pressures, this is arguably far from the transformational change that is needed to ensure the continued well-being of staff and the delivery of safe, high-quality care for patients.

There is much written elsewhere in this book about the importance of patients' experiences. So what do we really mean when we talk about patient experience and staff experience?

'Patient Experience' is defined by the Beryl Institute (www.theberylinstitute.org) as *the sum of all interactions, shaped by the culture of the organisation or system, that influence patient and carer perceptions across their pathways* (Wolf et al. 2014). We believe that the same definition can be applied to staff. Put simply, staff and patient experiences are two sides of the same coin. As a patient leader who is contributing to the NHS England staff experience work programme puts it: *'When my outpatient appointments go well for me, they go well for my consultant. And when they go badly for me, they go badly for him too. We are in this together – it's a shared experience'.*

Delivering consistently responsive, safe and high-quality care is possible only if staff too have the practical and emotional support they need because *'both staff and patients need care, compassion and respect'* (West 2014).

As the Point of Care Foundation urges, *'now is the time to act to improve staff experience as high-quality, patient-centred care depends on managing staff well, allowing staff to exercise control over their work, listening to what they have to say, involving them in decisions, training and developing them and paying attention to the physical and emotional consequences of caring for patients'* (Cornwell 2014).

NHS England Work Programme

The *Five Year Forward View* (NHS England 2014) recognises that closing the three widening gaps—in health and well-being, care and quality, and funding and efficiency—and delivering the necessary changes to do this will require investment in our current and future workforce. More empowered and engaged patients and communities depend on more empowered and engaged staff.

Learning from other sectors, notably the manufacturing and logistics industry, makes a strong case for more integrated staff and patient experience programmes and initiatives (Foundation Trust Network 2013). While designing for employee experience in order to deliver an intended customer experience is relatively rare in any sector, it is even less common in NHS settings.

With such a compelling evidence base about the significance of the experiences of healthcare staff for patients' outcomes and experiences of care, in late 2015 the NHS England Patient Experience team established a work programme specifically focused on driving improved outcomes and experiences for patients through improving staff experience.

Underpinning this work programme is the urgent need to focus on the relationship between staff and patient experience; this could be one of the most important moves the healthcare system makes to increase productivity and improve experiences of care for millions of people—both the 1.3 million staff and the 1 million patients experiencing care every 36 hours.

When we talk about staff, and when we talk about patients, should we think of them as separate groups of people, people delivering care and people receiving care? Perhaps a better approach would be to make clearer connections between the two sets of experiences, in order to make better sense of how they relate and what this means for our work to improve experiences of care for both staff and patients. Making better connections between staff and patient experience is a key feature of the NHS England staff experience work programme, as is the development of compassion throughout the health service; it is becoming increasingly obvious that staff need to be treated with compassion in order to deliver compassionate care.

The Role of Compassion

In a book about compassion in healthcare, it is encouraging to note that the significant role of compassion, and particularly compassionate leadership, has recently gained increasing attention (West et al. 2017; Massie and Curtis 2017). *'Developing People—Improving Care'* (NHS Improvement 2016) is an evidence-based national framework, co-developed by key national stakeholder organisations. It focuses on *'four critical capabilities'* that will help *'protect and improve services … in the short term and for the next 20 years'*. One of these four critical capabilities is the kind of compassionate leadership that ensures that staff are *'listened to, understood and supported'*. The partner organisations behind this framework have committed to implementing the framework and to making the required changes happen, pledging to *'model inclusive, compassionate leadership'* (NHS Improvement 2016). We believe that the creation and sharing of digital staff stories has a part to play in making this a reality and in promoting healthcare that is more dignified, more humane and more compassionate for everyone, whether they are delivering or receiving care.

Engaging People's Feelings

Kenneth Schwartz, a Boston healthcare lawyer, who founded the Schwartz Centre for Compassionate Healthcare (https://www.theschwartzcenter.org) a few days before his death from lung cancer, made powerful feelings-driven observations about the connections between staff and patients … between people. He said:

> *I cannot emphasise enough how meaningful it was to me when caregivers revealed something about themselves that made a personal connection to my plight. The rule books, I'm sure, frown on such intimate engagement between caregiver and patient. But maybe it's time to rewrite them.*

While many of us are becoming familiar with Schwartz Rounds, we have arguably more progress to make in the direction of the Schwartz Centre mission that makes compassion a priority for staff, patients and families alike.

One step in this direction is the partnership work between NHS England and Patient Voices. The DNA of Care staff digital stories project offered NHS staff the chance to attend Patient Voices workshops to create their own digital stories about working in healthcare. We felt that sharing stories in this way could contribute to improving experiences of care for both staff and patients and to helping experiences of care to become more dignified, more humane and more compassionate for everyone.

What We Did

Getting Organised

With a plan for five workshops comfortably in place, we set about recruiting storytellers. Word-of-mouth, twitter and email were the main vehicles for the initial programme of activity aimed at publicising the project and recruiting storytellers. However, even though the team were well connected organisationally through NHS England, had broad contacts in digital storytelling in healthcare through the Patient Voices Programme network of contacts, and reasonably large profiles on social media, it was, nevertheless, difficult to fill the workshops.

We worked to mitigate three main challenges to recruitment that are common to most Patient Voices workshops. The first of these is funding. This issue was addressed by making workshop places fully funded for staff, and supporting travel and accommodation costs where necessary. The message in our recruitment materials was clear, as can be seen in Fig. 22.1, which aimed to play on the fact that the NHS is also free at the point of need.

The second challenge was timing, and the annual pattern of pressing service demand. The demands of the Quality and Outcomes Framework

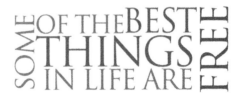

Fig. 22.1 Some of the best things in life are free

in February impact on potential release of staff from primary care settings (Hardy et al. 2012) and seasonal demands in hospital settings mean that winter is often a difficult period too. This issue was addressed by re-scheduling workshops away from these times.

Third, the organisational challenge of releasing staff for three consecutive workshop days was addressed by re-scheduling workshops to provide longer lead times for staff rostering, along with offering a variety of workshop locations and timings, some of which took place over weekends to allow for greater flexibility in time management.

A Wide Range of Staff

The workshops began to fill. Our intention, based on the learning from dropout rates from previous Patient Voices workshops, was to over-recruit: we aimed to register ten people for each workshop in the hope of having eight participants. One NHS Trust in the North-East filled an entire workshop. Several organisations actively supported staff to participate in the project. Other storytellers heard about the programme and signed up as individuals, in many cases taking annual leave in order to attend. At one point, every workshop was full and we had a waiting list. Inevitably, however, as the workshops approached, illness and pressure of work led some people to drop out. In the end there were 33 storytellers, representing a wide range of professions and geographical areas, as Table 22.1 illustrates.

The Workshops

Four out of the five workshops were held at Pilgrim Projects/Patient Voices' base near Cambridge. The venue is reasonably central for people travelling from around the country; it attracts no additional cost and it supports our commitment to hospitality, providing a comfortable, safe space in which often-painful stories can be told and shared. Nearby accommodation was secured and catering was duly arranged, taking into account the various dietary needs and preferences of a diverse group of people.

Table 22.1 DNA of Care workshop participants by profession and place

Consultant anaesthetist & clinical lead for customer experience, London	Mortuary and bereavement service manager, Teesside
Consultant in complex pain, London	Nurse lecturer, Chelmsford
Consultant in paediatric allergy, London	Organisation Development practitioner (community nursing), Teesside
Critical care nurse & Organisation Development practitioner, Teesside	Out of hours service manager, Leicester
Director, art therapy, Sheffield	Palliative care/oncology nurse and educator, Teesside
GP and medical educator (ethics), Manchester	Patient engagement lead, Kent
Haematology laboratory manager, Luton	Patient experience director, Sussex
Health Care Assistant in Emergency Assessment Unit, Teesside	Physiotherapist, Teesside
Head of staff experience, NHS England	Physiotherapist/lecturer, National Institute for Health Research Fellow, Teesside
Infection control nurse, Teesside	Lead psychologist, community services, Sheffield
Maternity support worker, Birmingham	Public health consultant, Lothian/School for Change Agents
Matron, pain management, Nottingham	Service manager lead for medicine, Harlow
Mental Health nurse, CERT Manager, Sheffield	Speech and language therapist—head and neck cancer, Cambridge
Respiratory ward manager, Nottingham	Trainee psychiatrist, Gloucester
Midwife (home births), Birmingham	Transformation officer, Teesside
Midwife, Royal College of Midwives	Urology ward sister, Nottingham

The fifth workshop was held at Crathorne Hall, a quiet, country house hotel in North Yorkshire. Having worked there before, we knew that the venue suited our requirements for comfort and hospitality and was within easy travelling distance for the storytellers based in the north east.

Storytellers were all briefed before the workshops, with extensive notes about the workshop process, the purpose of the project, the five themes and what needed to be done in preparation. They were encouraged to view some existing Patient Voices digital stories, and a short explanatory video about the Patient Voices workshop process was created (Hardy and

Sumner 2016). There were phone conversations with a number of story-tellers, many of whom were uncertain about what story to tell, whether they had any story to tell or whether it would simply be too painful to tell the story they really wanted to tell. Nevertheless, everyone to whom I spoke turned up to their workshop and made a story.

A Fine Balance: Courage and Vulnerability

Each of the five workshops followed the established Patient Voices three-day workshop model described in Chap. 4. Although the workshops were like many others we have facilitated over the years, one difference that struck us, particularly after the second workshop, was the delicate balance between, on the one hand, creating an environment that feels safe enough for people to tell the story they really need to tell and, on the other hand, ensuring that the story feels safe enough to release. While we have always been aware of this tension, wishing to respect storytellers' wishes at the same time as delivering relevant stories to the workshop sponsor, perhaps it had never seemed quite so obvious as it did when, on the last day of the second workshop, one storyteller said, almost with surprise, that she wasn't sure whether she could or would release her story as she felt so vulnerable. We were concerned, of course, as the purpose of the project had been very clear and we had, we thought, explained the need for release of the stories; concern turned to alarm when several others followed her lead and announced that they were also uncertain about releasing their stories.

We explored possibilities that might help storytellers feel safer and less vulnerable, including making the stories anonymous, using first names or initials only, and suggested that people go away to watch and reflect on their stories. We reassured them that we would respect their decisions, whatever these might be.

We brought up the issue with our clinical supervisor in our regular post-workshop supervisions, who suggested that we might consider artic-ulating the tension and explaining that it is our role to ensure a safe envi-ronment conducive to telling important stories about things that matter and also to ensure that the stories feel safe enough for storytellers to release them. This we duly did, adding that we would do our best to hold this apparent tension and ensure safety at every stage of the process.

This approach seemed to be successful as the issue was not raised at any subsequent workshops and, in the end, all the storytellers from the second workshop also released their stories.

What Storytellers Said

Without exception, storytellers claimed to have had a positive experience of the workshops. Many spoke of the value of connection and reconnection—with colleagues, with vocation, with their reasons for going into healthcare in the first place, with themselves:

> It's rare for me to feel I've made as much connection with as many people as I have this weekend.
> If we can connect with each other then there's hope for the NHS.
> For me, it's been so important to reconnect with why I came into healthcare.
> There's something very important about the **collective process** as well as the collective product. My story is the product of everyone here as well as my own.

Others spoke of the value of sharing stories in this way:

> Since sharing the story I have felt a sense of peace and contentment as it really allowed me to understand exactly why I am here in this job.
> It's taken a lot of guts to share this deeply, and not hide behind our professional selves. It's important for our colleagues and policy makers to know that it's OK to share. This should help us all communicate better in the future.

What Are We Learning?

The section above describes some of our learning about the process of running workshops for staff, and the immediate feedback from storytellers. A great deal of learning has also emerged through different ways and experiences of exploring and sharing the stories; these ranged from a large, formal launch event through to a webinar and individual storytellers sharing their stories with their organisations, colleagues and networks.

We knew from the scoping carried out within the NHS England staff experience work programme that there was a clear need to provide evidence for, and convey the compelling relationship between, staff and patient experience more effectively in a range of ways for different audiences. In particular, there was a need to highlight the significance of investing in, and paying attention to, the experiences of staff. The DNA of Care project responded to the established recognition that the relationships between providers and receivers of care are deeply interconnected.

Re-writing the Rules of Engagement

At the formal launch event for the 'DNA of Care' stories, held at the Institute for Contemporary Arts in London in late 2016, we learned a great deal from the storytellers' courage in sharing their stories with a large multi-professional and multi-agency audience.

We learned that the audience were moved not only by the digital stories, but also by the honesty and willingness of the storytellers to share so much of themselves. Our sense is that in this way, digital staff stories are one way of responding to Kenneth Schwartz's plea for caregivers to reveal something about themselves, as he had learned the importance of how that made a personal and very comforting connection to his own plight. Perhaps the making and sharing of digital staff stories is one way of re-writing the rule books about the engagement between givers and receivers of care. We recognise and understand, however, the courage, commitment and belief in the power of their stories that is needed in order for staff storytellers to share their feelings and experiences.

Changing the Conversation

As the storytellers shared their stories during this event, a strong theme began to emerge, that is, how far the stories in different ways spoke to the interface between the personal and professional selves of the storytellers and how this interface was deeply connected with their values as well as their identities. Members of the audience were invited to share their reflections and responses to each of the stories in turn, allowing plenty of time for conversation between the storytellers and those who had just watched and listened to their stories. We learned that the sharing of stories in this way seemed to give the audience a kind of permission to share their own stories and experiences. In other words, the digital stories that had been created by NHS staff seemed to have the ability to change the conversation.

We are beginning to understand more about the impact the stories have in changing conversations and driving improvement, although there is still more to discover. Having told a personal professional story *Stickers* (Gore 2016b), in her first workshop, Claudia Gore gained insight into a methodology that would enable her to tell and share, in a respectful and safe way, one of the most difficult stories faced by clinicians, that of a Serious Incident (SI). She returned to another Patient Voices workshop later in 2016 and successfully created that story, *Pieces* (Gore 2016a). That story has already prompted change in her own organisation (the provision of a bereavement service for nurses) as well as creating a space in which other clinicians can share similar stories.

Leadership, Improvement and Change

Early in 2017, we presented an 'Edge Talk' webinar '*The DNA of Care: the importance of listening to staff stories*' (Hardy and Deeny 2017). We were joined by three of the storytellers, who presented their stories. They revealed what really mattered to them along with their personal accounts of the experiences of sharing their stories and the impact this has had on them, the ways they work, their leadership and their approaches to change and improvement. We learned through the listener responses to the webinar that staff are making important connections between the stories and their potential both to inform and support quality improvement. The processes of making and sharing stories seem to have transformational effects in personal, conversational and organisational contexts.

'*Leading Change, Adding Value: a framework for nursing, midwifery and care staff*' (NHS England 2016) highlights the '*need to focus on what is important and connect with each other so we achieve more for our patients and people and also for our professions'*. Commitment 6 within this framework focuses specifically on '*what matters most*' for healthcare staff. It recognises that '*we must show the same care and consideration to ourselves and our colleagues, as we do to those we serve*' and goes on to say that one way of meeting commitment 6 is to '*embed the key question "What matters to you?" alongside the delivery of consistently compassionate leadership*'. We are learning that the creation and sharing of digital staff stories is one way of translating this important commitment into practical and meaningful action.

What Next?

Stories from Both Sides

When telling their stories, patients often refer to a staff member's role or actions and the impact of these. Similarly, we have learned that staff stories often include references to patients. Indeed, when we analysed the words in the scripts that the storytellers had used to present their stories, the most frequently used word was 'patient'. Very rarely, however, do we tell, or listen to and learn from both accounts, both sets of insights and experiences of the same circumstances, services or events. In other words, to date, we have rarely had the opportunity to listen to and learn from the inter-connectedness of the experiences of people delivering and receiving care.

One next step is to explore further the potential to develop examples of this interconnected approach, where both staff and patients together tell the intertwined story of their shared and separate experiences and perspectives of the same circumstances, service or event. One of the storytellers, a consultant in pain, was so inspired by the experience of making and sharing her own story, '*Impermanence*' (Curran 2016), that she commissioned digital storytelling workshops for her team members and patients to enable them to share their experiences of working in and with the complex pain team at University College London Hospital (Patient Voices 2017).

After making her own 'DNA of Care' story, *Stickers* (Gore 2016b), a paediatric allergy consultant developed a research proposal and a successful bid for funding to work with the Patient Voices team to run 'Terrific Teens' a pair of simultaneous, parallel Patient Voices workshops. One was for parents of young people with extremely severe allergic conditions and the other was for the young people themselves. At the end of the two workshops, the groups and their stories were brought back together to share and reflect on their joint experiences (Patient Voices 2016). The storytellers—young people and parents alike—all commented on the benefits of participating in the workshop and, in particular, of spending time with others who understand the particular problems they face on a daily basis. The stories have been used to educate and raise awareness among staff, patients and parents about the effects of severe, life-limiting allergies, while the research seeks to explore in greater depth, partly through the stories that have been created, the lived experience of young people and families affected by severe, chronic conditions. The 'Terrific Teens' stories have also prompted development of a further bid for funding to create more stories and use them more intentionally via a 'story bringer' to educate staff.

Initial scoping with NHS colleagues has revealed support for the principles of these emerging approaches, and organisations where staff and patients are potentially open to contributing stories have been identified.

Research and Evaluation of Impact

Many storytellers have shared their stories with their colleagues, organisations, professional networks, patients and public groups, and after the workshops, several formed informal professional support networks via social media. From one of those support groups sprang the inspiration for a midwife storyteller to base her master's research on investigating the impact of the process on those storytellers who had shared it with her. We are keen to learn more about how different stories, shared in different ways, have a different kind of impact; we want to understand what works well and less well in terms of using the stories as catalysts for improvement.

We have embarked on a process of tracking the ways the digital stories have been used and gathering data about what happened as a result, to help us develop greater insight into their impact.

A formal evaluation of the DNA of Care project is currently being undertaken and we hope that the results will reveal valuable insights into the benefits and uses of the stories as well as the impact of the process on the staff who created them.

Conclusion

It is no surprise that staff working in the NHS have important stories to tell; stories created by staff have been a part of the Patient Voices Programme since its inception and we know that many staff have been waiting very patiently for their stories to be heard. What has been, perhaps, less expected is the willingness to be open and vulnerable in the desire to share experiences and the hope of making things better. This has resulted in change and growth for individuals and, often, their teams and, sometimes, their organisations, particularly when staff who participated in workshops have been inspired to set up other digital storytelling projects; thus, the ripples started by the stories are really beginning to have an impact.

Key Points

- Pressure of staff time and resources mean that long lead times for initiatives are needed.
- Digital staff stories are a practical response to the pressing need to focus more effectively on the significance of the experiences of healthcare staff for patients' outcomes and experiences of care.
- Digital staff stories can have powerful transformational effects on personal decision-making, improvement conversations and at organisational levels.
- Taking part in a Patient Voices digital storytelling workshop can provide staff with a vision of how to communicate and safely share difficult experiences, such as serious incidents (SIs).

- Digital stories illuminate the importance of compassion for staff and how this might be achieved through understanding and actively responding to '*what matters most*' for them.

References

Boorman, S. (2009). *The final report of the independent NHS health and well-being review*. London: Department of Health.

Cornwell, J. (2014). *Staff care: How to engage staff in the NHS and why it matters*. London: The Point of Care Foundation.

Curran, N. (2016). *Impermanence*. Pilgrim Projects. Retrieved May 2017, from http://www.patientvoices.org.uk/flv/1028pv384.htm

Foundation Trust Network. (2013). *Realising the benefits of employee engagement*. Unipart Consulting.

Gore, C. (2016a). *Pieces*. Pilgrim Projects. Retrieved May 2017, from http://www.patientvoices.org.uk/flv/1039pv384.htm

Gore, C. (2016b). *Stickers*. Pilgrim Projects. Retrieved May 2017, from http://www.patientvoices.org.uk/flv/1003pv384.htm

Hardy, P., & Deeny, K. (2017). *The DNA of care: The importance of listening to staff stories NHS horizons*. Retrieved from http://theedge.nhsiq.nhs.uk/march-2017-dna-care-importance-listening-staff-stories/. (2017 printing).

Hardy, P., McKee, A., Sumner, T., & Teggin, M. (2012). Developing multi-professional learning organisations in primary care: Opportunities and challenges (a report for the Eastern Deanery). Pilgrim Projects, Cambridge.

Hardy, P., & Sumner, T. (2016). *NHS staff stories: Introduction to the DNA of care*. Pilgrim Projects.

Maben, J., Peccei, R., Adams, M., Robert, G., Richardson, A., Murrells, T., & Morrow, E. (2012). *Exploring the relationship between patients' experiences of care and the influence of staff motivation, affect and wellbeing*. Final Report. Southampton: NIHR Service Delivery and Organization Programme.

Massie, S., & Curtis, V. (2017). *Compassionate leadership – More important than ever in today's NHS*. London: The Kings Fund.

Meltzer, H., Griffiths, C., Brock, A., Rooney, C., & Jenkins, R. (2008). Patterns of suicide by occupation in England and Wales: 2001–2005. *The British Journal of Psychiatry, 193*(1), 73–76.

NHS Employers. (2014). *Guidance on the prevention and management of stress in the workplace*. London: NHS Employers.

NHS England. (2014). *Five year forward view.* NHS England.

NHS England. (2016). *Leading change, adding value: A framework for nursing, midwifery and care staff.* NHS England.

NHS Improvement. (2016). *Developing people – Improving care: A national framework for action on improvement and leadership development in NHS-funded services.* National Improvement and Leadership Development Board.

Patient Voices. (2016). *Terrific teens.* Pilgrim Projects. Retrieved May 2017, from http://www.patientvoices.org.uk/terrificteens.htm

Patient Voices. (2017). *Complex pain, complex teams.* Pilgrim Projects. Retrieved May 2017, from http://www.patientvoices.org.uk/complexpainteam.htm

Wall, T. D., Bolden, R., Borrill, C., Carter, A., Golya, D., Hardy, G., Haynes, C., Rick, J., Shapiro, D., & West, M. (1997). Minor psychiatric disorder in NHS trust staff: Occupational and gender differences. *The British Journal of Psychiatry, 171*(6), 519–523.

West, M. (2014). Both staff and patients need care, compassion and respect. *Nursing Times.*

West, M., & Dawson, J. (2012). Employee engagement and NHS performance. *The King's Fund,* 1–23.

West, M., Eckert, R., Collins, B., & Chowla, R. (2017). *Caring to change: How compassionate leadership can stimulate innovation in health care.* London: Kings Fund.

Wolf, J. A., Niederhauser, V., Marshburn, D., & LaVela, S. L. (2014). Defining patient experience. *Patient Experience Journal, 1*(1), 12.

Karen Deeny led the Staff Experience Programme within the NHS England Patient Experience team. With a clinical background in speech and language therapy and a passion for improvement, Karen has worked as a clinician, manager, researcher, author and coach in health, education and social care. Her PhD research focused on learning from both staff and patients' experiences to drive improvement.

Pip Hardy is a co-founder of the Patient Voices Programme and a director of Pilgrim Projects Ltd, an education consultancy specialising in open learning and healthcare quality improvement. She also serves as Curriculum and Learning Lead for NHS England's School for Change Agents. Pip has an MSc in lifelong learning, and her PhD considers the potential of digital storytelling to transform healthcare.

Tony Sumner is a co-founder of the Patient Voices Programme and a director of Pilgrim Projects. With degrees in physics and astronomy and astrophysics, and many years' experience working in the software industry, he is particularly interested in how technology and storytelling can intersect to promote deep reflection.

23

'The Stories Are All One': Care, Compassion and Transformation

Tony Sumner and Pip Hardy

The Journey to Transformation

Our vision is to move away from an outdated system towards a new model where the voice of the patient is heard through every level of the service, acting as a powerful lever for change and improvement. (DH 2001)

Storytelling is the mode of description best suited to transformation in new situations of action. (Schön 1988)

We began this book by describing the development of the Patient Voices approach to using stories and storytelling to transform healthcare and social care. Specifically, we looked at the methodology developed by the Patient Voices Programme, and then let colleagues and partners describe their own experiences working with—and learning from—Patient Voices in their own areas and on their own projects.

T. Sumner (✉) • P. Hardy
Patient Voices Programme, Pilgrim Projects Ltd,
Landbeach, Cambridge, UK

© The Author(s) 2018
P. Hardy, T. Sumner (eds.), *Cultivating Compassion*,
https://doi.org/10.1007/978-3-319-64146-1_23

When we first tried to conceptualise this approach, the model that seemed most appropriate was that of a journey to transformation, informed, illuminated and encouraged by stories that had been shared, heard and reflected upon.

The model in Fig. 23.1 was influenced by our work in developing learning programmes and materials, where the concept of a 'learning journey' had particular resonance for us—not least because, when we first formed Pilgrim Projects, that concept influenced our choice of the company's name, which we intended to reflect our approach to learning, development and education. That model was captured in the diagram from Pip's MSc dissertation (Hardy 2007).

In structuring the sections of this book, we looked at the aims, motivations and achievements of the projects described by each contributor and found that they fell into several thematic areas:

- Involvement, impact and improvement
- Transformational learning
- The healing power of the process
- Gathering the evidence of experience
- Co-production

When those thematic areas, and the projects that describe them, are overlaid on the Patient Voices journey, they demonstrate the continuity and integrity of the process that the model seeks to describe.

Learning from Patient Voices

Just as we have tried to share some of our learning journey in this and other publications, each of our contributors wanted to share some of their own learning. They show how an appropriate, safe and carefully facilitated, reflective, digital-storytelling process—and the stories created within that process—can illuminate, catalyse and pay testament to the transformation of care at individual, organisational and potentially systemic levels.

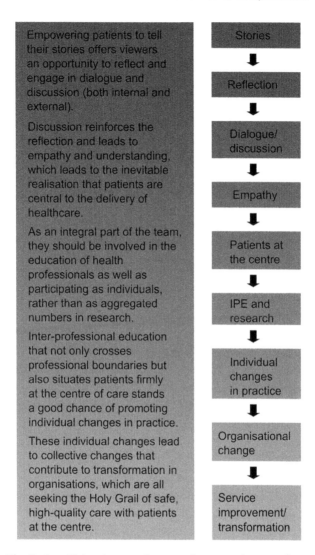

Empowering patients to tell their stories offers viewers an opportunity to reflect and engage in dialogue and discussion (both internal and external).

Discussion reinforces the reflection and leads to empathy and understanding, which leads to the inevitable realisation that patients are central to the delivery of healthcare.

As an integral part of the team, they should be involved in the education of health professionals as well as participating as individuals, rather than as aggregated numbers in research.

Inter-professional education that not only crosses professional boundaries but also situates patients firmly at the centre of care stands a good chance of promoting individual changes in practice.

These individual changes lead to collective changes that contribute to transformation in organisations, which are all seeking the Holy Grail of safe, high-quality care with patients at the centre.

Stories ⬇ Reflection ⬇ Dialogue/discussion ⬇ Empathy ⬇ Patients at the centre ⬇ IPE and research ⬇ Individual changes in practice ⬇ Organisational change ⬇ Service improvement/transformation

Fig. 23.1 The Patient Voices journey from stories to service transformation

Involvement, Impact and Improvement

As Paul Stanton describes in Chap. 5, Patient Voices reflective digital stories do not intentionally seek to provide solutions to problems within health and social care systems. However, the process does provide an empowering methodology through which storytellers may reflect on, distil, express and share the experiences that matter to them. The resulting stories can then produce in the viewer what he describes as 'the pin-drop effect', drawing the attention of viewers to the message they see and hear within the story. This appeal to the hearts, as well as the heads, of those designing and delivering healthcare can lead to greater compassion at all levels in the healthcare system, reinforcing Kotter and Cohen's finding that, when seeking change and improvement,

> *the central issue is never strategy, culture or systems. All those elements and others are important. But the core of the matter is always about changing the behaviour of people, and behaviour change happens in highly successful situations mostly by speaking to people's feelings.* (Kotter and Cohen 2002)

The experience of the Arthur and Co. project (described in Chap. 6) has shown that the stories have a timeless nature that gives them relevance and utility for many years after their creation. This reflects the statistics that we gather on the Patient Voices website: some of the older stories are more frequently viewed than newer ones, and the balance shifts continually. For the storytellers, attention to their needs, and expert facilitation that carefully manages group dynamics is key to successfully beginning a journey that extends beyond the completion of their stories.

Just as the stories will continue to involve and engage viewers for many years, the transformative aspect of the storytelling process and the relationships that build within the group can help storytellers to move on in their own journey, becoming more involved and engaged in education, research and improvement activities.

The emotional power of the stories to connect policymakers, managers and commissioners directly to the experiences of staff or service users is a foundation stone in a key programme of aviation safety as eloquently described by Cathy Jaynes in Chap. 7. Her experience with safety stories also reinforces the timelessness, flexibility and universality of the stories, enabling them to be used far beyond the original medical transport industry context for which they were intended, and contributing to the creation of a much wider culture of safety.

The stories created in a Patient Voices context, and through this process, are capable of carrying and delivering powerful experiences and key messages about the storytellers' experience in such a way that they are effective channels for involvement and impactful drivers of improvement. This, as we have seen at Manchester Mental Health and Social Care Trust (the subject of Chap. 8), can drive improvements in care and reductions in cost through changing culture, even in large healthcare organisations.

As Matthew Hodson shows us in Chap. 9, clarity of purpose on the part of the sponsors of a Patient Voices workshop helps enormously when recruiting storytellers. Getting them involved is a key part of giving them the opportunity to tell involving stories, and this is underpinned by clear briefings and targeted recruitment strategies; this is sometimes referred to as 'readiness'. Where clinicians also take part in a workshop as storytellers, they gain a greater understanding of their patients due to their deeper involvement with their stories and appreciation of their lived experiences.

Transformational Learning

Transformational learning can occur for those within the reflective digital-storytelling process as storytellers, and those outside the process observing the products of the process as story viewers. The insight and interprofessional learning that can occur within the process is powerful, highly valued and of long-lasting effect for storytellers. This was described in Chap. 10 by Liz Anderson and Dan Kinnair of the University of Leicester but, crucially, driven home by the testimonies of students who went through the programme. Steve Corry, Matthew Critchfield and Weehaan Pang reflect, in Chap. 11, on their own experience as storytellers, eloquently describing the powerful effect that the process has had on their professional development and professional identity, five years on.

Gemma Stacey reports, in Chap. 12, on her experience of working with newly qualified mental health nurses, and discovers in the digital-storytelling process the potential to heal, prepare and educate both the nursing students and the educational and professional staff who teach and support them. We hear about the benefits of using the stories as reflective prompts to provoke thoughtful discussion among final-year students, as well as the use of stories as *agent-provocateurs* of reflective and reflexive learning, demanding mindful, creative and aware deployment by educators.

How Was That for You? The Healing Power of Digital Storytelling

The reflective digital-storytelling process can be a cathartic, empowering and healing one, both intra- and interpersonally and professionally—and this, as the authors in this section showed, applies to patients, service users, carers, professionals and teams. One of the factors that contributes to this healing, we suspect, arises from one of our earliest goals on the Patient Voices Programme, that is, to move away from a patriarchal model of patient and service-user experience that used verbs like 'harvest', 'capture' or even 'take'. The role of a facilitative approach to service-user experiences, the consequent empowerment and resulting healing experienced by storytellers was powerfully captured by Julie Walters in Chap. 13, in which she explores some of the characteristics of digital storytelling and how these may contribute to the transformative nature of the process.

In Chap. 14, Mark Shea's research investigation into the digital-storytelling experience reveals that creating a digital story, although challenging, can have short- and long-term beneficial effects. His findings are borne out in the stories of those storytellers who have returned to make second, third and even fourth stories, Pep Livingstone (Livingstone 2008, 2009), Ian Porritt (Porritt 2008, 2009) and Eva Heymann (Heymann 2008, 2009a, b, 2010) among them.

A powerful and affecting experience such as this needs skilful and experienced facilitation, with due regard given to informed consent and release processes that will ensure that a powerful process is also a safe and supportive one, particularly where vulnerable people are concerned—and staff, as we have learned, can be particularly vulnerable. This issue is clearly explored in Amy Stabler's Chap. 15 on the challenges of implementing a

Patient Voices workshop to promote emotional resilience in teams that had been in difficulty.

Contributing to Evidence (the Evidence of Experience)

The place that reflective digital stories can take within a spectrum of research approaches and evidence types, and their power to enhance traditional forms of qualitative data presentation was described in Karen Taylor's account, in Chap. 16, of her use of the Patient Voices approach at the National Audit Office. She concludes that digital stories should assume their rightful place within this hierarchy of evidence, where they can provide valuable insights to those developing high-level policy in the health service.

In Chap. 17, Carol Haigh shows us, through her own experience, the inherent ability of reflective digital stories to provide policymakers and researchers with new forms of evidence. By dint of their distilled (or *'clear, pure and potent'*) nature (Stacey and Hardy 2011), they can contain, communicate and conserve the *'evidence of experience'* (Hardy 2006). They can convey key messages rapidly and powerfully; they can form valuable qualitative data and, perhaps most importantly, they can signpost the direction for further research based on what really matters to patients.

Finally, in Chap. 18, Nick Harland recognises that, although the creation of the stories requires careful integration when being incorporated within research activities, the process can provide a space where clinician storytellers' own messages can take centre stage, allowing them to engage with the research process in a deeper, more proactive and more empowered manner.

Doing It Together: A Model for Co-production

'Co-production' is a word used often and widely in discussions of the development and management of care. The projects described in Part VI serve to remind us that co-production, whether of a story, a care pathway or an educational programme, needs to diffuse through all aspects of those processes. In Chap. 19, Rosie Stenhouse and Jo Tait used a deeply reflective and creative approach to their own experiences of working with and writing about creating digital stories with people affected by dementia. They remind us that, within a digital-storytelling workshop, facilitators must be aware of their place and potential voice in the stories—especially when working on a power/voice gradient; they must be adaptive and attentive to the widely varied needs of storytellers.

True co-production does not leave the storyteller usurped or replaced by the story; rather it allows the creation of new ways of working between all stakeholders in care and education systems. This was a key message from Elspeth McLean in Chap. 20. In so doing, the stories can catalyse, enhance and enliven education programmes, allowing service users and carers to play a part in the co-production of interprofessional education.

The need for effective interprofessional collaboration is great and, arguably, nowhere greater than in end of life care, when many people from many different organisations are involved in care for patients and their families. In order to develop an educational resource that would promote this kind of collaboration, and would also focus on emotional intelligence, self-awareness, empathy and compassion, relies on involving everyone: patients, carers and clinicians across the spectrum. The design and development of such a project, with digital stories created by all these people at its core, is the subject of Elizabeth Howkins' and Pip Hardy's Chap. 21.

Although stories from staff have been a feature of Patient Voices since the earliest days, it has only recently been officially recognised that there is a deeply intertwined relationship between the experiences of staff and those of patients or—as we prefer to refer to them—people who receive care and people who give care. The stories of NHS staff, as Karen Deeny, Pip Hardy and Tony Sumner explain in Chap. 22, reveal what really matters to those clinicians and have created ripples that are still spreading outward, prompting transformation not only for the storytellers but also for their colleagues, teams and organisations.

Cultivating Compassion

The Japanese concept of the *gemba*—literally 'the actual place' (Imai 1997), is the place within a system where the real work happens, where value is created. In healthcare this is where care happens—the very heart of care. It is here, at the very centre of the care system, that we locate the stories that the Patient Voices Programme seeks to facilitate, share and use as social capital. From this place, the stories and the storytelling process can facilitate reflection, model patient involvement and engagement, generate empathic bridges between groups, prompt dialogue, allow patient involvement, enhance interprofessional working and drive change.

The Patient Voices Mandala (Hardy 2007), shown in Fig. 23.2, was an attempt to visualise this concept as a non-linear process. It followed on from the original Patient Voices Rationale (Hardy 2004) which expressed the wish that:

> ... *those who devise and implement strategy, as well as clinicians directly involved in care, may carry out their duties in a more informed and compassionate manner.*

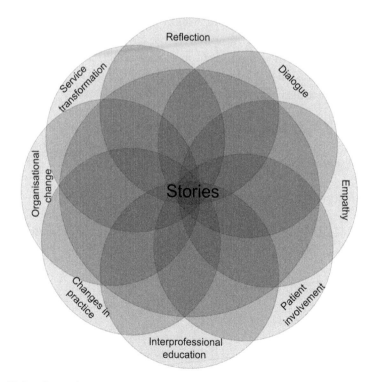

Fig. 23.2   The Patient Voices Mandala

Critical friends cautioned us against using the word 'compassion' if we wanted to be taken seriously. They also worried about words like 'healing', 'reconciliation', 'collaboration' and 'touching hearts', let alone the use of stories in an attempt to improve healthcare!

We were resolute and, through some combination of stubbornness and idealism, the 'C' word—along with those other worrying words and phrases—remained in our rationale. Like the stories we seek to facilitate, the cultivation of compassion lay, we knew, at the very heart of our work, forming the core of our intentions. It is more than gratifying to see compassion blossom in every Patient Voices workshop. The story below is just one example of this phenomenon.

A Story of Compassion

At the end of a particularly powerful and gruelling workshop, we held our usual story premiere and feedback session with storytellers. When invited to consider whether he had learned anything new about himself, one young man recovering from drug and alcohol abuse, self-harm, homelessness, attempted suicide, diagnosed with (among other things) schizophrenia and attention deficit disorder, reflected on the three days thus:

> *I found out that I'm very demanding and impatient. Even though I'm getting over mental health, I feel I'm a bit selfish, asking for help all the time, instead of being understanding that other people need help as well.*

The first response from the group was:

> *I think you were the opposite – you've been really thoughtful, checking that others are ok and making tea. I see something different from what you've described.*

Someone else in the group added:

> *And you told us good jokes!* (Hardy 2013)

And so the round of appreciative comments continued. All were thoughtful, touching, encouraging, positive, showing compassion to the young man. The session continued, with storytellers sharing their completed stories with each other. Quietly, respectfully, he watched the digital story made by a mother whose son is serving 25 years in prison for murder—a story about *her* compassion for the mother of the man her son had killed. Then he watched a story made by another mother whose son had died of pneumonia, homeless, failed by mental health and social services. Eyes bright with tears, he said:

> *I watched your two stories and see how much you are suffering. It made me think of my mum. And I thought "F**k it, I'm not going back on drugs again. I don't want my mother to have to go through what you've gone through."*
> (Hardy 2013)

Kindness and Kinship

In their book *Intelligent Kindness* (Ballatt and Campling 2011) recognise that the good of all depends on the good of each one, and that the degree to which we feel that we belong to a community, or have a sense of kinship with our families, our friends, our colleagues will, in large part, determine the way we experience the world. Having discovered some compassion for himself, the young man above was more keenly aware of the suffering of others and able to make a direct connection between that suffering and the desire to mitigate it. As Jean Vanier describes:

> *People reach greater maturity as they find the freedom to be themselves and to claim, accept and love their own personal story, with all its brokenness and its beauty.* (Vanier 2004)

Many of the Manchester storytellers have gone on to participate in the Trust's transformation activities. They and their stories are disseminating the compassion they have experienced and cultivated and the compassion carried within their stories throughout the organisation in a wide variety of ways, from education and mentoring through to recruitment and training; you will know about the impact of their stories from the discussion of the dignity and respect project in Chap. 8.

The experience in Manchester, and the success of Patient Voices stories in transforming services through changing organisational culture, highlights the centrality of compassion in healthcare, and its inherently essential nature in those who give and receive care. Care that is compassionate, dignified and respectful can change the culture of an organisation. As Manchester Mental Health and Social Care Trust continues to show compassion by listening to, believing in and acting on the stories created by service users, carers and staff, awareness continues to grow that responsibility for the design and delivery of great care must be shared between all those involved in that care.

When the Chief Executive admits to being humbled by a story (Moran 2014) and exhorts the Board to acknowledge mistakes so that they can learn from them and improve services, it is clear that transformation is occurring, even at the highest levels of healthcare organisations. When service users are involved in recruiting staff for their values, emotional intelligence and compassion, a culture of openness, transparency and kindness is likely to be strengthened (Sumner 2013).

Compassion and Suffering

Now, 14 years after we began the Patient Voices Programme, stories are everywhere and everyone is talking about compassion. The failure to learn from the Bristol Royal Infirmary Inquiry (Kennedy 2001) has resulted in a string of reports of poor care, instances of abuse and neglect, untoward numbers of deaths and unimaginable suffering for the patients, carers and staff involved. The Francis (2013) report identified a lack of compassion as contributing significantly to the failings at Mid Staffordshire Hospital. Atrocities such as those that came to light at Winterbourne View (DH 2012), where staff were found to be abusing patients with learning difficulties, force us to acknowledge that not all care staff are caring, let alone compassionate although, in our experience, the vast majority of staff really do want to provide the best possible care for their patients. Indeed, this was reinforced by the word cloud which emerged from the collected scripts from the DNA of Care project, shown in Fig. 23.3, which reveals that the word that appeared most frequently in the 34 scripts was 'patient'.

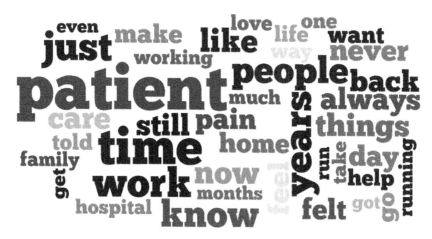

Fig. 23.3 DNA of Care word cloud

In response to these and more recent failings that have come to light, the Chief Nursing Officer has developed the 6Cs, defined as care, compassion, competence, communication, courage and commitment (Cummings 2012) so that nurses can be trained in compassion; the NHS Leadership Academy plans to train leaders in compassion; books are being written about it; attempts are being made to measure it; even doctors are talking about the importance of compassion! The term has become almost ubiquitous; indeed, an acquaintance recently commented, 'Compassion is the new mindfulness'.

Herein lies something of a paradox. The desire to improve the quality of care is laudable, and one of the fundamental drivers of the Patient Voices Programme. However, it is our view that compassion is not something that can be taught. It does not lend itself to frameworks, audits, targets, tick box exercises or assessment. Along with many other things that really matter, compassion cannot easily be measured; we know it by its absence, which contributes to and prolongs suffering.

Suffering and compassion lie close to one another. Both cover vast realms of experience. Both are difficult to quantify—is your suffering worse than mine? Is he more compassionate than she is?

If we are intent on reaching the land of compassion, we must first be willing to explore the territory of suffering.

Beyond the 6Cs

Because there is no need for compassion without suffering we cannot explore the meaning of one without the other. And the exploration of suffering is not something that most people are eager to engage with. And yet, it is one of the things that makes us human. So, at one level, compassion is a willingness to examine what it means to be human in this world and to 'simply be' with suffering—our own and that of others. This can present enormous challenges, especially when the most compassionate act may simply be to be present, to be still, to listen with our whole being, to accept without judgement another's pain. Asked to reflect on a recent clinical experience to form the basis of a digital story, a clinical psychologist realises the truth of this. Her story, *Only connect*, reveals her new insight into the need for connection and the nature of compassion (Hennessey 2013).

Compassion arises in unexpected places. We have seen the way compassion blossomed in a young man who had probably experienced very little compassion in his own life. Another recent story, *Night shift* (Vaitkunas 2013), told by a security guard, offers a moving illustration of compassion in action.

In our suffering lies our truth. Facing our dragons and, in many cases, overcoming them allows us to discover our courage, our resilience, our resourcefulness and, ultimately, to transform. That individual transformation will, inevitably, have an impact on other people.

After seeing the story *Getting to the bottom of things* (Bailey-Dering 2007), a newly qualified doctor responded by saying:

> *I had no idea of the impact of her condition on her marriage, her working life and her economic situation, her ability to socialise ... from now on, I won't make the first question I ask about the level of pain but, instead, I will ask the patient how things are for them.*

Digital storytelling offers time to look at, contemplate, examine and explore in a non-judgemental way and with curiosity, an experience of suffering; this is itself an act of compassion to the storyteller.

Watching a digital story is also an exercise in mindfulness. For two or three minutes, we direct our attention entirely to the words and images that take us into the heart of another's experience. At the end of the story, we are invited to consider how the story makes us feel and what we would do differently? If the response is a deep desire to alleviate suffering, that is the beginning of compassion.

And so we see compassion arise in storytelling workshops, in boardrooms, in lecture theatres and conference halls, wherever a few people get together to tell, share, listen to and reflect on stories. The courage of storytellers who are willing to go deeply into their own suffering results in the potential for greater understanding, not only between those in their own workshop group, but in all those who view the stories and share the storyteller's reality for just a few moments.

'In My End Is My Beginning'

We shall not cease from exploration
And the end of all our exploring
Will be to arrive where we started
And know the place for the first time. (Eliot 1959)

When we began Patient Voices, way back in 2003, there was one book about digital storytelling, that is, Joe Lambert's (2002) *Digital Storytelling: Capturing Lives, Creating Community*. There were certainly no books (or articles) about digital storytelling in healthcare. When we first met Joe Lambert in 2006, he expressed the hope that digital storytelling would become an accepted genre.

There is a growing body of evidence supporting the value of digital stories and digital storytelling and we are pleased to be part of an international community of people who are committed to the practice of 'listening deeply', as the StoryCenter strapline recommends, and to the importance of individual stories. The last few years have seen a proliferation of books, journal articles and PhDs about the application of digital storytelling across a range of contexts, including primary and secondary education, higher education, public health, community development and migration (see, e.g., Jamissen et al. 2017; Ohler 2013; Hartley and McWilliam 2009; Gubrium and Harper 2013; Pleasants and Salter 2014;

Dunford and Jenkins 2017), accompanied by scholarly work providing crucial underpinning theory for the emerging genre of digital storytelling (see, e.g., Couldry 2010; Thumim 2012; Alexandra 2008, 2013) and others now too numerous to mention. As far as we know, the first edition of this book remains the only book about the application of digital storytelling in healthcare, and so we were delighted to be interviewed by Nicole Matthews for inclusion in the recently published *Digital Storytelling in Health and Social Policy: Listening to Marginalised Voices* (Matthews and Sunderland 2017).

With the rise of social media and its growing power to influence, together with the abuse of that power by those who peddle 'fake news', the opportunity for people to tell and share the stories about what really matters to them is more important than ever. It has been our great privilege to contribute to the development of the digital-storytelling genre and it is our intention to continue to practice, study, explore and evaluate the use of digital stories and digital storytelling in healthcare.

Our Once and Future Stories

> *Each affects the other and the other affects the next, and the world is full of stories, but the stories are all one.* (Albom 2003)

Digital stories and digital storytelling, product and process, individuals and groups, people who give care and people who receive care, reflection and distillation, compassion and transformation; for well over a decade, Patient Voices reflective digital-storytelling workshops have been offering a safe space for storytellers to look at, contemplate, examine and explore, in a non-judgemental way and with curiosity, their experiences; to cultivate compassion, to celebrate our shared humanity and to inspire and initiate transformation.

We hope that initiatives such as the Patient Voices Programme can continue to highlight and offer evidence of compassion in care (or the lack of it) through stories that are '*markers and guides, comfort and warning*' (Winterson 2004); we hope this book has given you a glimpse of the potential for transformation at many different levels, and in many different contexts, offered by the telling and sharing of stories. We hope that you have been inspired by the Patient Voices projects that have been described here, and energised by the potential for compassionate care delivered with intelligent kindness.

We will leave you, as we often do in Patient Voices presentations and workshops on storytelling and transformation, with some questions on which to reflect:

What stories do you need to tell?
What stories do you need to hear?
What will you do then?

Thank you for reading—and listening to—the stories, experiences and insights we and our colleagues have shared with you in this book.

References

Albom, M. (2003). *The five people you meet in heaven* (1st ed.). New York: Hyperion.

Alexandra, D. (2008). Digital storytelling as transformative practice: Critical analysis and creative expression in the representation of migration in Ireland. *Journal of Media Practice, 9*(2). doi:10.1386/jmpr.9.2.101/1.

Alexandra, D. (2013). *Visualizing voice, embodied objects, and implicating practice: Applied visual anthropology in Ireland.* Dublin: Dublin Institute of Technology (DIT).

Bailey-Dering, J. (2007). *Getting to the bottom of things.* Pilgrim Projects. Retrieved March 2014, from http://www.patientvoices.org.uk/flv/0110pv384.htm

Ballatt, J., & Campling, P. (2011). *Intelligent kindness: Reforming the culture of healthcare.* London: RCPsych Publications.

Couldry, N. (2010). *Why voice matters: Culture and politics after neoliberalism.* Los Angeles, CA: Sage Publications.

Cummings, J. (2012). *Compassion in practice. Nursing, midwifery and care staff, our vision and strategy.* London: Department of Health.

DH. (2001). *Shifting the balance of power within the NHS: Securing delivery.* Great Britain, London: Department of Health.

DH. (2012). *Transforming care: A national response to Winterbourne View Hospital.* London: HMSO.

Dunford, M., & Jenkins, T. (2017). *Digital storytelling: Form and content.* London: Palgrave Macmillan. doi:10.1057/978-1-137-59152-4.

Eliot, T. S. (1959). *Four quartets.* London: Faber & Faber.

Francis, R. (2013). *The final report of the Mid Staffordshire NHS Foundation Trust Public Inquiry.*

Gubrium, A., & Harper, K. (2013). Participatory visual and digital methods (Developing Qualitative Inquiry Series, vol. 10). Walnut Creek, CA: Left Coast Press.

Hardy, P. (2004). *Patient Voices: The rationale.* Pilgrim Projects. http://www.patientvoices.org.uk/about.htm

Hardy, P. (2006). *Patient Voices: Hearing the stories at the heart of healthcare.* Paper presented at the Nurse Education Tomorrow, University of Durham, UK.

Hardy, P. (2007). *An investigation into the application of the Patient Voices digital stories in healthcare education: Quality of learning, policy impact and practice-based value.* MSc dissertation, University of Ulster, Belfast.

Hardy, P. (2013). *Fieldnotes: Storytellers' reflections on a digital storytelling workshop in Manchester*, November 2013.

Hartley, J., & McWilliam, K. (2009). *Story circle: Digital storytelling around the world.* New York: John Wiley & Sons.

Hennessey, S. (2013). *Only connect.* Pilgrim Projects. Retrieved June 2014, from http://www.patientvoices.org.uk/flv/0690pv384.htm

Heymann, E. (2008). *Standing on my own two feet.* Pilgrim Projects. Retrieved March 2014, form http://www.patientvoices.org.uk/flv/0249pv384.htm

Heymann, E. (2009a). *A chocolate watch.* Pilgrim Projects. Retrieved March 2014, from http://www.patientvoices.org.uk/flv/0412pv384.htm

Heymann, E. (2009b). *From darkness into light: New worlds.* Pilgrim Projects. Retrieved March 2014, from http://www.patientvoices.org.uk/flv/0345pv384.htm

Heymann, E. (2010). *The sun also rises.* Pilgrim Projects. Retrieved March 2014, from http://www.patientvoices.org.uk/flv/0517pv384.htm

Imai, M. (1997). *Genba kaizen: A commonsense low-cost approach to management.* New York: McGraw-Hill Professional.

Jamissen, G., Hardy, P., Nordkvelle, Y., & Pleasants, H. (2017). *Digital storytelling in higher education.* London: Palgrave Macmillan. doi:10.1007/978-3-319-51058-3.

Kennedy, I. (2001). *The report of the public inquiry into children's heart surgery at the Bristol Royal Infirmary 1984–1995. Learning from Bristol* (pp. 325–332). London: Stationery Office.

Kotter, J. P., & Cohen, D. S. (2002). *The heart of change: Real-life stories of how people change their organizations.* Boston, MA: Harvard Business School Press.

Lambert, J. (2002). *Digital storytelling: Capturing lives, creating community* (1st ed.). Berkeley, CA: Digital Diner Press.

Livingstone, P. (2008). *Once upon a time.* Pilgrim Projects. Retrieved May 2017, from http://www.patientvoices.org.uk/flv/0208pv384.htm

Livingstone, P. (2009). *Tell me your story.* Pilgrim Projects. Retrieved May 2017, from http://www.patientvoices.org.uk/flv/0402pv384.htm

Matthews, N., & Sunderland, N. (2017). *Digital storytelling in health and social policy: Listening to marginalised voices. Routledge advances in the medical humanities.* Oxford and New York: Routledge.

Moran, M. (2014). *CEO blog – Listen, believe, act.* Chief Executive's Blog, vol. 2014. Manchester Mental Health and Social Care Trust, Manchester.

Ohler, J. B. (2013). *Digital storytelling in the classroom: New media pathways to literacy, learning, and creativity.* Thousand Oaks, CA: Corwin Press.

Pleasants, H. M., & Salter, D. E. (2014). *Community-based multiliteracies and digital media projects: Questioning assumptions and exploring realities.* New York: Peter Lang.

Porritt, I. (2008). *A long and troubled road.* Pilgrim Projects. Retrieved May 2017, from http://www.patientvoices.org.uk/flv/0209pv384.htm

Porritt, I. (2009). *A clearer road ahead.* Pilgrim Projects. Retrieved May 2017, from http://www.patientvoices.org.uk/flv/0388pv384.htm

Schön, D. (1988). Coaching reflective teaching. In G. L. Erickson & P. P. Grimmett (Eds.), *Reflection in teacher education* (pp. 19–29). New York: Teachers College Press.

Stacey, G., & Hardy, P. (2011). Challenging the shock of reality through digital storytelling. *Nurse Education in Practice, 11*(2), 159–164. doi:10.1016/j.nepr.2010.08.003.

Sumner, T. (2013). How we can recruit for compassion. *Health Service Journal.*

Thumim, N. (2012). Introduction: Self-representation and digital culture. In N. Thumim (Ed.), *Self-representation and digital culture* (pp. 1–18). London: Palgrave Macmillan.

Vaitkunas, D. (2013). *Night shift.* Pilgrim Projects. Retrieved June 2014, from http://www.patientvoices.org.uk/flv/0685pv384.htm

Vanier, J. (2004). *Drawn into the Mystery of Jesus through the Gospel of John.* New York: Paulist Press.

Winterson, J. (2004). *Lighthousekeeping.* London: Harper Perennial. (2005 printing).

Tony Sumner is a co-founder of the Patient Voices Programme and a director of Pilgrim Projects. With degrees in physics and astronomy and astrophysics, and many years' experience working in the software industry, he is particularly interested in how technology and storytelling can intersect to promote deep reflection.

Pip Hardy is a co-founder of the Patient Voices Programme and a director of Pilgrim Projects Ltd, an education consultancy specialising in open learning and healthcare quality improvement. She also serves as Curriculum and Learning Lead for NHS England's School for Change Agents. Pip has an MSc in lifelong learning, and her PhD considers the potential of digital storytelling to transform healthcare.

Afterword

I am an avid reader and a lover of stories. I love that bittersweet moment at the end of a great book when you realise you will have to have a little break from reading, as the last story was irreplaceable.

In my work with the English National Health Service, I find myself surrounded by irreplaceable stories. Every day, they offer us important lessons if we could only slow down and take the time to hear them.

The tragic failures in health and social care in the UK and elsewhere over the past two decades have many similarities. One important similarity I have observed is that:

>...*people always knew what was taking place. WE KNEW.*

The public enquiries always reveal that, for a long time, people within the system had told stories that alerted us to impending disaster. The system chose not to listen, not to hear, not to believe, not to be curious, not to explore.

For me this is the greatest tragedy. If we had listened to the stories, we might have saved a life—many lives. Often told in anger, with frustration and sadness, the stories are telling us what people see, what they hear and what they feel.

© The Author(s) 2018
P. Hardy, T. Sumner (eds.), *Cultivating Compassion*,
https://doi.org/10.1007/978-3-319-64146-1

These are irreplaceable stories.

The collection of work within this book demonstrates the power of stories from and across many walks of life. It offers us the opportunity to view the world from numerous positions, so we can understand more and better, and cultivate our compassion. As organisational leaders, we must also cultivate the culture of storytelling.

I have learned that two simple questions can act as a catalyst to help people tell their stories:

What brought you here, now?
Why do you carry on doing what you are doing?

Try them, see what you learn ….
I am pretty sure you will hear an irreplaceable story.

Organisation Development   Maxine Craig
Hart Consultancy Services
Hartlepool, UK

Index

© The Author(s) 2018
P. Hardy, T. Sumner (eds.), *Cultivating Compassion*,
https://doi.org/10.1007/978-3-319-64146-1

Printed by Printforce, the Netherlands